Prehabilitation for Cancer Surgery

Arunangshu Chakraborty
Ashokka Balakrishnan
Editors

Prehabilitation for Cancer Surgery

Springer

Editors
Arunangshu Chakraborty
Department of Anaesthesia
Critical Care and Pain, Tata Medical Center
Newtown, Kolkata, West Bengal, India

Ashokka Balakrishnan
Department of Anaesthesia
National University Health System
Singapore, Singapore

ISBN 978-981-16-6496-0 ISBN 978-981-16-6494-6 (eBook)
https://doi.org/10.1007/978-981-16-6494-6

This Springer imprint is published by the registered company Springer Nature Singapore Pte Ltd.
The registered company address is: 152 Beach Road, #21-01/04 Gateway East, Singapore 189721, Singapore

Contents

Part I

Introduction

Prehabilitation for Cancer Surgery: Introduction to the Concept

1

Arunangshu Chakraborty and Ashokka Balakrishnan

1.1 Introduction

In the twenty-first century, with the improvement of healthcare facilities across the world, we now have an ageing population at hand with a higher life expectancy than ever before. The global average life expectancy at birth has increased from 50 to 75 in the last seven decades [1].

Life Expectancy by Country and in the World (2021) While the scourge of deadly infectious diseases have been contained to a great extent, particularly in the developed nations, cancer has come up as a leading cause of death. As per the Centers for Disease Control and Prevention (CDC) of the United States of America, cancer is a leading cause of death in the USA, taking about 600,000 lives annually, which is only second to heart diseases [2]. The World Health Organisation (WHO) estimates the global burden of cancer cases at above 18 million in 2018, amongst which 9.6 million died. Globally, death due to cancer stands at the number two spot, just after heart diseases [3]. If we look at surgical mortality in the USA, the average mortality for major cancer surgeries such as gastrectomy, pancreas surgery, etc. range from 8% to 15%, which comes to about 10,000 deaths only in the United States of America [4].

If we extrapolate these numbers across the world, considering the varying standard of medical treatment and care, the number of people dying each year from cancer surgery would be a staggering 160,000.

Solid organ malignancies make up the bulk of the global cancer burden. Nearly 70% of the global cancer burden is from solid organ tumours, lung cancer being the

A. Chakraborty (✉)
Department of Anaesthesiology, Critical Care and Pain, Tata Medical Center, Kolkata, West Bengal, India

A. Balakrishnan
Department of Anaesthesia, National University Health System, Singapore, Singapore

A. Chakraborty, A. Balakrishnan (eds.), *Prehabilitation for Cancer Surgery*,
https://doi.org/10.1007/978-981-16-6494-6_1

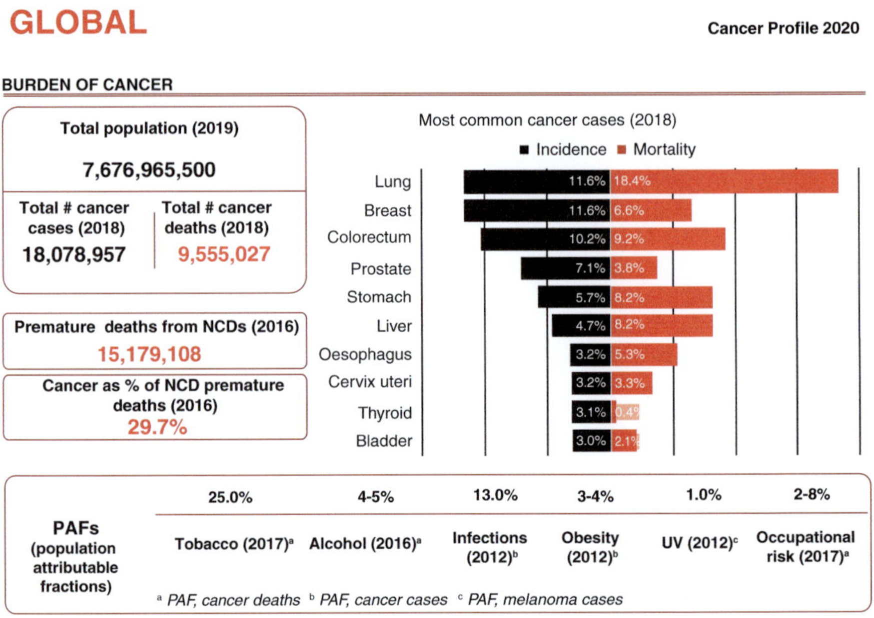

Fig. 1.1 Global cancer burden (Image source: WHO-CancerReport-2020-Global Profile, https://www.who.int/cancer/country-profiles/Global_Cancer_Profile_2020.pdf accessed on 05/02/2021)

commonest, followed by breast, colorectum, prostate, stomach, liver, oesophagus, cervix uteri, thyroid and urinary bladder cancers. As per mortality, above 65% are from solid organ tumours (Fig. 1.1).

Surgery is the mainstay of treatment in most of the solid organ malignancies. Though upfront surgery as soon as the patient presents with a tumour would be the ideal course of treatment, often there are factors which delay the surgery for a considerable period, sometimes exceeding 4 weeks from the initial reporting to the hospital. After initial reporting and a general plan of surgery, further imaging, PET CT scan, histopathological diagnosis, etc. are required for staging of the disease before the final decision for operation can be made. Once the patient is selected for an upfront surgery, they are sent for preanaesthetic evaluation for risk stratification for the kind of anaesthesia the patient would have to undergo to have the surgery. Then comes the waiting list. Apart from surface surgery such as breast and some amputations, most cancer surgeries are complicated and take a long time, limiting the number of operations that can be done in a working day, creating a waiting list for each surgical subspecialty. Some patients present with a tumour that is so large and locally invasive that they require neoadjuvant chemotherapy before the operation to shrink down the tumour as well as to restrict the spreading potential of the disease. All of these factors contribute towards a waiting period for surgery that can extend from 2 to 6 weeks.

However sophisticated the surgery may be, still it is a calculated assault on the body, causing pain, stress, inflammation and wasting of muscle mass. Many of the cancer patients would have a comorbid condition such as diabetes, heart failure, chronic obstructive pulmonary disease (COPD), etc. The perioperative stress may further complicate these comorbid conditions leading to a crisis. Regaining strength and mobility after the surgery is a serious challenge that requires a multidisciplinary approach and dedicated team work. While the postoperative challenges are known and discussed frequently, another aspect pertaining to the situation is often overlooked. The baseline condition of the patient in terms of exercise capacity, muscle mass and general fitness of the vital systems such as the cardiovascular, pulmonary, endocrine, etc. It can be easily understood and the evidence suggests that the healthier a patient is before surgery, the better is the outcome of the surgery in terms of healing and postoperative morbidity. The American Society of Anesthesiologists (ASA) had developed a physical status classification system over 60 years ago, which has enjoyed popularity and acceptance worldwide as it gave an idea of the degree of perioperative complications based on preoperative assessment of the patient. It could be easily assumed that an ASA grade IV patient would have more risks of perioperative complications compared to grade III. From this premise it can be extrapolated that if through a multidisciplinary approach a patient's severity of comorbid conditions can be eased to a less severe status, the patient would have a lesser risk of perioperative complications.

If we apply this understanding to a cancer patient who is waiting for his/her elective surgery and have a few weeks of time before he/she goes under the scalpel, it is obvious that some measures can be taken to improve the patient's physical status that would help the patient endure the surgery and help him/her recuperate from it. This effort of building up the patient's physical reserve and treating the comorbid conditions is known as prehabilitation.

The very first idea of prehabilitation in the modern times dates back to the times of the Second World War, when it was found that a 2 months programme of education, nutrition and physical training could transform almost all of the 'substandard recruits' amongst the enlisted men into 'Standard recruits'. The very first publication titled 'Prehabilitation, rehabilitation, and revocation in the army' was published in 1946 in the British Journal of Anaesthesia [5]. In one of the earliest systematic reviews consisting of 1245 patients recruited to 12 randomised controlled trials, it was found that patients undergoing cardiac and abdominal surgery experienced shorter hospital stays and reduced postoperative pulmonary complication rates if they had received preoperative exercise therapy. The authors concluded that preoperative exercise therapy should be considered as standard preoperative care in patients undergoing cardiac or abdominal surgery [6].

A more recent review by Santa Mina et al. [7] looked at 21 trials involving 1371 patients who had undergone either orthopaedic, abdominal, cardiac, or thoracic surgery. In the majority of the trials, preoperative exercise improved physical function and reduced postoperative complications, postoperative pain, and length of hospital and intensive care stay. Reduction in length of stay was found to be statistically significant on meta-analysis. The authors also reported an overall adverse event rate of just 0.5%, demonstrating that preoperative exercise is safe.

The earliest comprehensive meta-analyses were published by Wang et al. [8] and Moran et al. [9] who reviewed patients who had undergone joint replacement surgery and intra-abdominal surgery, respectively. Wang et al. found statistically significant improvements in postoperative function and pain in patients who had undergone prehabilitation but felt that the improvements were too small and too short-lived to be clinically important. The main statistically significant findings in the Moran et al. study were improved preoperative fitness and reduced postoperative complications. Neither meta-analysis could demonstrate a significant reduction in length of stay.

Cancer prehabilitation is a developing area in its own right. Patients with cancer face a unique set of circumstances not experienced by other surgical populations. Chemotherapy and chemoradiotherapy are cardiotoxic and may substantially impair cardiorespiratory fitness, cause endocrine disorders and electrolyte disturbances. In conjunction with the functional decline due to major surgery, this results in a significant 'dual hit' [10]. On the other hand, with survival adversely affected by delays in cancer treatment, the time-critical nature of the cancer pathway poses challenge to the institution of an effective prehabilitation programme in a population that could arguably benefit the most.

Loughney et al. [10] conducted the first systematic review of the effects of exercise training on patients scheduled for 'dual-hit' cancer treatment (i.e. neoadjuvant chemotherapy or chemoradiotherapy plus cancer surgery). The authors found that exercise training in the neoadjuvant setting was both safe and feasible in patients awaiting breast and rectal cancer surgery, and compliance rates were acceptable. Significant improvements in physical fitness were achieved but the effect on other outcomes, such as health-related quality of life and fatigue, was inconclusive.

1.2 The Pillars and the Foundation of Prehabilitation

Prehabilitation is a complex multidisciplinary process that aims to optimise the patient's vital systems in the given time between presentation at the prehabilitation clinic to the day of surgery. For the ease of understanding it can be compared with a building with three pillars and a foundation (Fig. 1.2). The three pillars of prehabilitation are:

1. Nutrition.
2. Physiotherapy and exercise capacity build-up.
3. Psychiatric support and help with coping.

Additionally, the management of existing comorbid conditions and addiction control measures such as smoking cessation and reduction of alcohol intake form the foundation of prehabilitation [11].

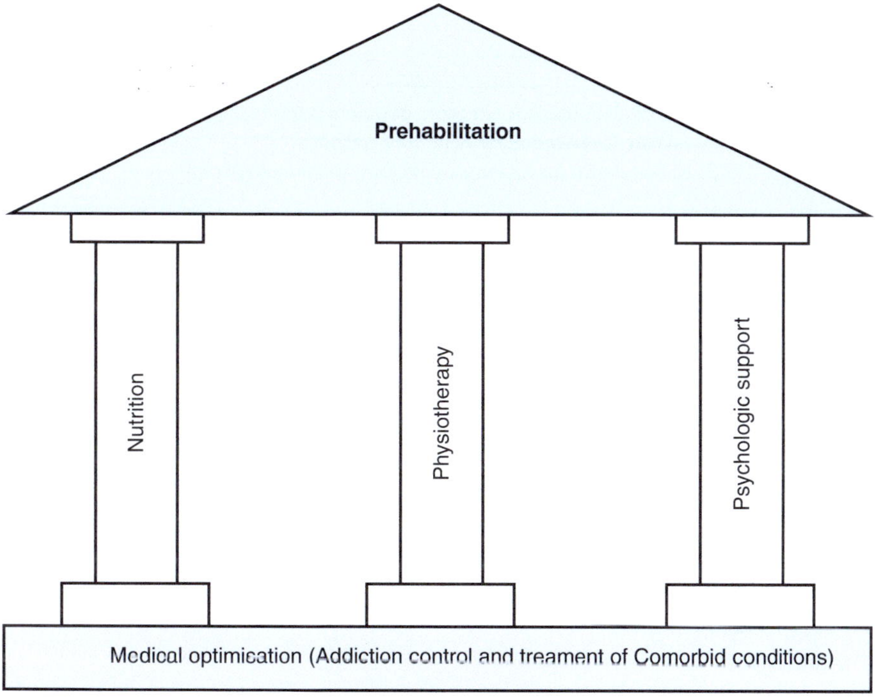

Fig. 1.2 The three pillars and foundation of prehabilitation

1.3 Setting Up a Prehabilitation Programme

1.3.1 The Prehabilitation Clinic

While setting up a prehabilitation programme, it is important to remember the time imperative. Multiple referrals must be avoided. A central facility (Prehabilitation clinic) with protocolised flowcharts covering the key elements of prehabilitation should be the first step. The clinic can be manned by a senior nurse and one physician drawn from the specialities of either internal medicine, physical medicine or anaesthesia.

Once the patient comes to the clinic, a thorough initial evaluation is done, including general survey and systemic survey. Available bloodwork and imaging must be reviewed and if needed, additional investigations ordered. After the initial assessment, the deficient areas are identified and a set of targets is to be set for each patient and it should be discussed with the patient and next of kin available at the time of consultation. The patient should be provided with a booklet of the prehabilitation programme that contains the exercises, diet and additional nutritional enhancements information. Parts relevant to the patient are highlighted and explained by the prehabilitation team. Considering the high volume of patients going to the clinic, available manpower, etc., ASA grade I and II patients can be managed by the specialised nurse, whereas grade III onwards patients should consult the team of prehabilitation physicians (Fig. 1.3).

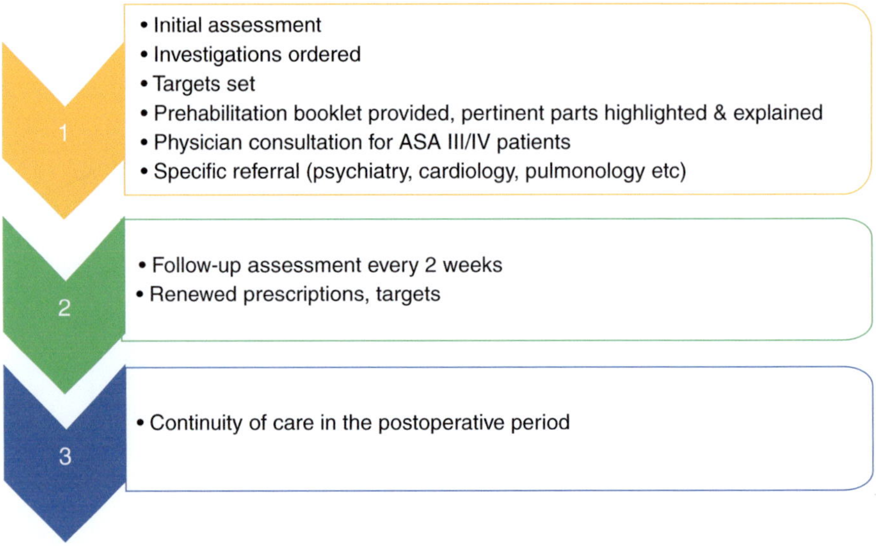

Fig. 1.3 Prehabilitation workflow

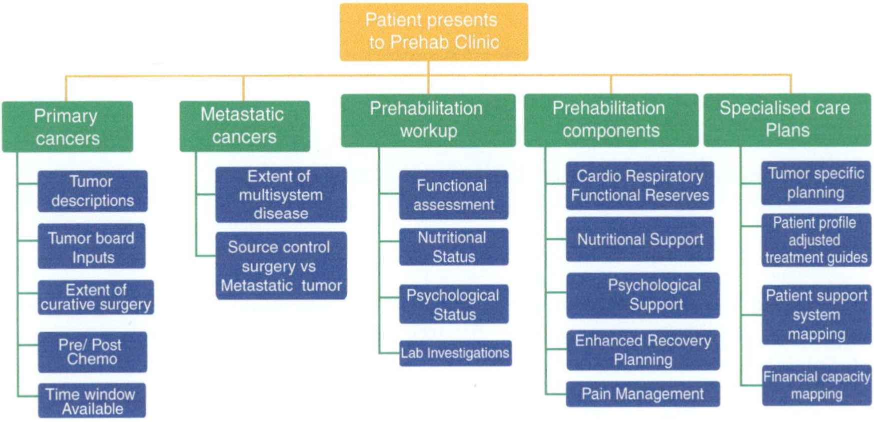

Fig. 1.4 Patient journey in prehabilitation clinics

For ASA III and IV patients, the prehabilitation would include optimisation of comorbid conditions apart from the three pillars of nutrition, exercise and psychological support.

Cancer patients planned for surgery need to be reviewed in the prehabilitation clinic that has a structured approach in organising the discussions and decisions about the tumour, assessment of present functional status of the patient, further evaluation of readiness for surgery, introduction of the various components of prehabilitation and also provision of specialised care plans for the patient (Fig. 1.4).

The initial stratification of patients into primary tumours and metastatic tumours would help in stratifying the cancer management plans. Metastatic tumour tend to have multisystem issues, more severe cachexia and poorer functional reserves with poor prognostic indicators of survival. These patients need early coordinated planning with palliative teams for managing pain, nutrition, psychological support, etc. When surgery is indicated in metastatic tumours, it needs additional measures when compared to primary tumours.

Assessment in prehabilitation includes the evaluation of functional reserves, nutritional status, psychological milieu, and investigations to stratify the level of optimisation. The majority of components would include methods and measures for improvement in cardiorespiratory functional reserves, nutritional and psychological support and plans for multimodal pain management.

Specialised care planning includes approaches that suit the biopsychosocial and socioeconomic perspectives of the patient. These include adjustments in care plans based on the patient's struggles and unique experiences with the tumour, chemotherapy and the coping mechanisms. These include the social and family support for care at home, while accompanying for visits to healthcare facilities and options for daily and emergent support when frailty is a concern. Financial paradigms need to be explored and documented early in the consultations to ensure smooth planning and avoidance of acute distress that arises from inability to afford options that could be equivocal in clinical benefits but can add significant stress to the therapeutic alliance.

1.3.2 Referrals

Many patients would need a referral to the allied specialties such as psychiatry, internal medicine, cardiology, pulmonology, etc. These referrals need to be completed with a priority in a time bound manner. Necessary framework must be created to reduce turnaround time. These are facilitated by presence of multidisciplinary consensus about thresholds for correction of abnormal parameters and criteria for clearance in fitness for surgery and perioperative chemotherapy.

1.3.3 Follow-Up

Regular follow-up of the patient, at least in a two weekly interval should be done to monitor the progress, review or renew prescriptions and boost psychological well-being in general. While patients are prepared for surgery, deployment of prehabilitation care coordinators facilitates the initiation, follow-up and continuity of care until definitive surgery and management thereof. Pain relief and opioid use can be a specialised area of expertise and effectiveness of addiction control is enhanced through follow-up discussions and troubleshooting.

1.3.4 Care Continuum

It is important to enter each patient in a database for continuity of care after the operation. A surveillance programme should be set to find out the effectiveness of the programme. Periodic reviews should include cancer-specific measures and other methods for global wellness of the patients. Prehabilitation coordinators and cancer-specific coordinators need to maintain a database of event, care and treatment logs and requires transparent sharing of proposed plans for ensuring the continuity of management.

1.4 Conclusion

The 65th World Health Assembly took the resolution of reducing the non-communicable disease burden by at least 25% by 2025 [12].

While reducing the disease burden requires a multidisciplinary approach from an entirely different angle, adopting the practices of prehabilitation, we can achieve up to 30% reduction in postoperative complications in major cancer surgery, which itself is no mean feat. Prehabilitation is a promising paradigm. Conceptually intuitive, and based on sound theoretical principles, the emerging evidence is encouraging. In this book we try to provide a roadmap about how best to utilise this tool, with detailed insights into each of the pillars of prehabilitation. In the near future, as interest grows and knowledge accumulates, prehabilitation may play as significant a role in the management of the high-risk surgical patient as rehabilitation and enhanced recovery protocols, bringing benefits to patients and the overburdened public health system through shorter hospital stays, reduced readmission rates, reduced dependence on social care, and earlier functional recovery.

References

1. https://www.worldometers.info/demographics/life-expectancy/
2. Kochanek KD, Xu JQ, Arias E, Mortality in the United States. NCHS Data Brief, no 395. Hyattsville, MD: National Center for Health Statistics; 2019. p. 2020.
3. https://www.who.int/news-room/fact-sheets/detail/cancer
4. Finlayson EV, Goodney PP, Birkmeyer JD. Hospital volume and operative mortality in cancer surgery: a national study. Arch Surg. 2003;138(7):721–5; discussion 726. https://doi.org/10.1001/archsurg.138.7.721.
5. Anon. PREHABILITATION, rehabilitation, and revocation in the Army. Br Med J. 1946;1:192–7.
6. Valkenet K, van de Port IG, Dronkers JJ, de Vries WR, Lindeman E, Backx FJ. The effects of preoperative exercise therapy on postoperative outcome: a systematic review. Clin Rehabil. 2011;25:99–111.
7. Santa Mina D, Clarke H, Ritvo P, et al. Effect of total body prehabilitation on postoperative outcomes: a systematic review and meta-analysis. Physiotherapy. 2014;100:196–207.
8. Wang L, Lee M, Zhang Z, Moodie J, Cheng D, Martin J. Does preoperative rehabilitation for patients planning to undergo joint replacement surgery improve outcomes? A systematic review and meta-analysis of randomised controlled trials. BMJ Open. 2016;6:e009857.

9. Moran J, Guinan E, McCormick P, et al. The ability of prehabilitation to influence postoperative outcome after intra-abdominal operation: a systematic review and meta-analysis. Surgery. 2016;160:1189–201.
10. Loughney L, West MA, Kemp GJ, Grocott MP, Jack S. Exercise intervention in people with cancer undergoing neoadjuvant cancer treatment and surgery: a systematic review. Eur J Surg Oncol. 2016;42:28–38.
11. Banugo P, Amoako D. Prehabilitation. BJA Educ. 2017;17(12):401–5. https://doi.org/10.1093/bjaed/mkx032.
12. World Health Organization. Sixty-fifth world health assembly resolutions, decisions, annexes. 2012 May 21–26; Available from: http://www.who.int/mediacentre/events/2012/wha65/en/. WHA65/2012/REC/1.

Functional Assessment

2

Rakhi Khemka, Sumantra Sarathi Banerjee, and Arunangshu Chakraborty

Abbreviations

6MWT	6 minute walk test
ACC	American College of Cardiology
ACCP	American College of Chest Physicians
AHA	American Heart Association
ANP	Atrial natriuretic peptide
ASA-PS	American Society of Anesthesiologist physical status
AT	Anaerobic threshold
ATS	American Thoracic society
BNP	Brain natriuretic peptide
BP	Blood pressure
CCI	Charlson comorbidity index
CO_2	Carbon dioxide
COPD	Chronic obstructive pulmonary disease
CPET	Cardiopulmonary exercise testing
DASI	Duke Activity Status Index
DLCO	Diffusion capacity of lung for carbon monoxide
ECG	Electrocardiogram
ECOG-PS	Eastern Cooperative Oncology Group Performance Score
ERS	European Respiratory Society

R. Khemka (✉) · S. S. Banerjee · A. Chakraborty
Department of Anaesthesiology, Critical Care and Pain, Tata Medical Center, Kolkata, West Bengal, India

A. Chakraborty, A. Balakrishnan (eds.), *Prehabilitation for Cancer Surgery*,
https://doi.org/10.1007/978-981-16-6494-6_2

ESTS	European Society of Thoracic Surgery
FEV1	Forced expiratory volume in first second
FVC	Forced vital capacity
LT	Lactate threshold
MACE	Major Adverse Cardiac Events
MET	Metabolic equivalent of task
MI	Myocardial infarction
OR	Odds ratio
PFT	Pulmonary function test
PPC	Postoperative pulmonary complications
PPO	Predicted postoperative
RCRI	Revised cardiac risk index
$V'O_2$	Peak oxygen consumption
V_E/VCO_2	Ventilatory equivalent for CO_2

2.1 Introduction

Worldwide every year around 300 million people undergo major surgery, many of them are at risk for post-operative cardiovascular and pulmonary complications [1, 2]. As per the recommendations of the clinical practice guidelines, preoperative risk stratification is an important part of any planning aimed to prevent these complications [3]. Risk-stratification algorithms proposed by international guidelines lay lot of importance on the assessment of preoperative fitness or functional capacity [3, 4]. American College of Cardiology and American Heart Association (ACC & AHA) guidelines recommend that the patients can be allowed to proceed directly to elective major non-cardiac surgery if they are found to be capable of performing more than four metabolic equivalents of activity without symptoms. Preoperative assessment of functional capacity is a versatile measure of perioperative risk since it may stratify risk for non-cardiovascular complications such as pneumonia, respiratory failure and infection [5–9].

The preoperative evaluation of the patient undergoing non-cardiac surgery can be performed for reasons such as: assessment of perioperative risk (which can be used to inform the decision to proceed or the choice of surgery), determining the need for changes in management, and identification of cardiovascular conditions or risk factors requiring longer-term management. This can lead to change in the management plan, the decision to perform further cardiovascular interventions, or recommendations about post-operative monitoring. This may also guide the perioperative team about the optimal location and timing of surgery and intensity of post-operative monitoring [3].

The goal of preoperative evaluation in patients coming to hospitals for oncosurgeries is to involve the patient and their caregivers into shared decision making by providing them with clear, understandable information about perioperative cardiovascular risk in the perioperative period and long-term disability.

As assessment of functional capacity is a complex concept, so no single test could serve the purpose adequately. The commonest way for a clinician to assess the functional capacity is by asking the patient its capacity to walk or climb stairs or perform certain activities. Therefore, most of the scores used as tools to assess functional capacity are based on clinicians own assessment such as metabolic equivalent score (METs) [10], Eastern Cooperative Oncology Group Performance Score (ECOG-PS) [11] or Duke Activity Status Index (DASI) [12] which is a 12-point based standard questionnaire. Other non-invasive tests such as 6 minute walk test (6MWT) [10, 13] and spirometry can also be used for assessing the functional capacity of the patient in the preoperative period. Cardiopulmonary exercise testing (CPET) is considered the gold standard assessment of physiological performance. It provides objective information on the integrated cardiopulmonary and musculoskeletal function [14]. Serum concentration of N-terminal pro-B-type natriuretic peptide (NT-pro BNP), which is biomarker for heart failure or cardiac ischaemia is also used [15].

2.2 Metabolic Equivalent Score (MET)

Metabolic Equivalent of Task, or popularly known as MET is a frequently used and widely popular tool for assessment of functional capacity. MET is frequently quantified by anaesthesiologists during the preoperative visit by asking questions about general activity level and from that information formulating a subjective assessment of the patient's functional capacity. Its popularity stands on the simplicity of its application and interpretation and all these can be done in a single visit just by asking simple questions about daily functional activity. One MET approximately represents the rate of oxygen consumption while sitting at rest which is 3.5 ml/min/kg of body weight.

MET has its own limitations. Being a subjective tool is not accurate in assessing functional capacity as recollection of functional status is associated with either increased or decreased reporting. In one multicentric trial for non-cardiac surgery, anaesthesiologists assessment of functional status on the basis of subjective analysis attained only 19% sensitivity and 95% specificity [16]. Subjective assessment is also poorly correlated with well-validated questionnaire based functional assessment tool [17, 18]. Furthermore, subjective assessment is associated with poor prediction of post-operative morbidity and mortality. Few multicentre and single centre studies had shown poor predictability of subjective tools in assessing post-operative outcome [16, 19]. So, assessment of functional capacity in the preoperative period can be improved by using structured questionnaire based assessment (like Duke Activity Status Index or DASI) which is better validated with gold standard of functional assessment [12].

Despite its subjective nature and limitations, MET is still used widely due to its simplicity and familiarity of anaesthesiologists with it. Although studies have shown poor predictability of MET for post-operative outcome, there are studies that states exercise tolerance is a major determinant of predicting perioperative risk [20]. Inability to achieve 4 METs which is equivalent to inability to climb a flight of stairs is highly predictive of (89%) post-operative cardiopulmonary complication [21]. Preoperative lower MET score was found to be associated with significantly prolonged hospital stay after radical cystectomy and urinary diversion in a multinational study [22].

Results from 2014 ACC/AHA guideline for non-cardiac surgery with cardiac comorbidities incorporated MET in their algorithm. It is to be considered when the patient's estimated perioperative risk of Major Adverse Cardiac Events (MACE) becomes elevated based on clinical and surgical risk factors [3]. MET is also considered as a baseline preoperative functional assessment tool in case of pulmonary resection surgery, where MET value of less than 2 calls for deferring surgery and medical optimisation [23, 24]. Prospective assessment has shown that higher levels of MET-hour/week were associated with lower risk of developing digestive system cancer [25]. Many studies have shown that certain MET-hour/week increment in exercise capacity independently improved cancer specific and cardiovascular mortality in colon, breast and adult survivors of childhood cancer subsets [26–28]. So, improvement in MET score in serial follow-up can be a predictor of mortality in malignancy.

2.3 Eastern Cooperative Oncology Group Performance Score (ECOG-PS)

The scale was developed by the Eastern Cooperative Oncology Group (ECOG), now part of the ECOG-ACRIN Cancer Research Group, and published in 1982. Cooperative Oncology Group Performance Status Scale (ECOG-PS) is a simple physician rated score which is widely used for preoperative assessment of the functional status of patients suffering from cancer. It is calculated subjectively by the attending physician by asking questions to the patient about his capacity to perform activities. The score describes a patient's level of functioning in terms of their ability to take care of themselves, daily activity, and physical ability [11].

Refer to Table 2.1 for finding out the criteria for scoring the patients which depends on their level of functional status is.

The score is commonly used by clinicians to assess the functional status of the patients suffering from cancer and planned for surgical treatment to predict complications, morbidity and mortality in the post-operative period. Studies have found that functional performance using ECOG-PS score was independently associated with mortality after high-risk emergency laparotomy or laparoscopy, the higher the ECOG performance score, the greater was the risk of 30-day post-operative mortality [29].

A study from 2015 suggested that inclusion of ASA-PS and ECOG performance score alone or in combination, improved risk adjustment models after cancer surgery [30].

Table 2.1 Grades of ECOG performance status (Developed by the Eastern Cooperative Oncology Group [11][a]

Grade.	ECOG performance status
0	Fully active able to carry on all pre disease performance without restriction
1	Restricted in physical sirens activity but ambulatory and able to carry out work of a light or sedentary nature, e.g. light house work, office work, etc.
2	Ambulatory and capable of self-care, but unable to carry out any work activities, up and about for more than 50% of waking hours
3	Capable of only limited self-care, confines to bed or chair more than 50% of waking hours
4	Completely disabled, cannot carry on any self-care, totally confined to bed or chair
5	Dead

[a]Oken M, Creech R, Tormey D, et al. Toxicity and response criteria of the Eastern Cooperative Oncology Group. *Am J Clin Oncol.* 1982;5:649–655

Chou et al. found that ECOG-PS scale was found to be one of the most influencing factor in predicting 3-month post-operative mortality in elderly patients undergoing radical surgeries for solid tumour resection. Patients with a good ECOG scale (0–1) and fewer comorbidities with low Charlson comorbidity index (CCI 0–2) had the lowest probability of 3-month post-operative mortality after cancer surgery. The highest probability of 3-month post-operative mortality (55.2% and 47.8%) after cancer surgery was observed among patients with a poor ECOG scale [3–4] and multiple comorbidities (CCI >2) [3]. Charlson comorbidity index is a tool used to predict 10-year survival in patients with multiple comorbidities [31].

2.4 Duke Activity Status Index (DASI)

The Duke Activity Status Index (DASI) is a questionnaire, originally published in 1989 [12] to assess the functional capacity. Since then, DASI has been used mainly to evaluate patients with cardiovascular diseases [32, 33].

It is a 12-item self-reported questionnaire that assesses daily activities such as personal care, ambulation, household tasks, sexual function, and recreation with respective metabolic costs. Each item has a specific weight based on the metabolic cost (MET). The participants are asked to identify each activity they are able to do. The final score ranges between zero and 58.2 points. The higher the score, the better the functional capacity [12]. Refer to Table 2.2 to know the questions asked for scoring.

In 2018, a multicentric trial was published using the DASI questionnaire as one of the tools for preoperative assessment of functional capacity for patients scheduled for major non-cardiac surgery. The study found that the DASI questionnaire improved prediction of post-operative 30day myocardial infarction or death. The authors suggested using objective scales such as DASI to assess functional capacity as it can be easily implemented into most perioperative practice settings [16].

Table 2.2 Duke Activity Status Index [12]

Can you	Weight
1. Take care of yourself, that is eating, dressing, bathing or using the toilet?	2.75
2. Walk indoors, such as around your house?	1.75
3. Walk a block or two on level ground?	2.75
4. Climb a flight of stairs or walk up a hill?	5.50
5. Run a short distance?	8.00
6. Do light work around the house like dusting or washing dishes?	2.70
7. Do moderate work around the house like vacuuming, sweeping floors or carrying groceries?	3.50
8. Do heavy work around the house like scrubbing floors or lifting or moving heavy furniture?	8.00
9. Do yard work like raking leaves, weeding or pushing a power mower?	4.50
10. Have sexual relations?	5.25
11. Participate in moderate recreational activities like golf, bowling, dancing, double tennis, or throwing a baseball football?	6.00
12. Participate in strenuous sports like swimming, single tennis, football, basketball or skiing?	7.50
Total score ______________	

DASI scoring: positive responses are summed up to get a total score, which ranges from 0 to 58.2. Higher scores, higher functional capacity

Very recently, Measurement of Exercise Tolerance before Surgery (METS) study was published to characterise the association of preoperative DASI scores with post-operative death or complications. The study recruited more than 1500 participants (>40 yr. of age) at an elevated cardiac risk who had inpatient non-cardiac surgery. It was found that self-reported functional capacity better than a DASI score of 34 was associated with reduced odds of 30-day death or myocardial injury (odds ratio: 0.97 per 1 point increase above 34; 95% confidence interval [CI]: 0.96–0.99) and 1 yr. death or new disability (odds ratio: 0.96 per 1 point increase above 34; 95% CI: 0.92–0.99). Self-reported functional capacity worse than a DASI score of 34 was associated with increased odds of 30-day death or myocardial infarction (odds ratio: 1.05 per 1 point decrease below 34; 95% CI: 1.00–1.09), and moderate-to-severe complications (odds ratio: 1.03 per 1 point decrease below 34; 95% CI: 1.01–1.05). Therefore, it was concluded that DASI questionnaire should help the preoperative identification of patients at an elevated risk of post-operative morbidity [34].

Although DASI scores are easy to implement, it is suggested that further studies are needed to define optimal riskspecific thresholds in DASI scores, and develop reliable nonEnglish versions of the questionnaire [16].

2.5 Minute Walk Test (6MWT)

6 Minute Walk Test (6MWT) is an objective test which is simpler to perform and interpret but provides very basic information about exercise capacity and all the systems that jointly contribute to alter exercise capacity. Balke developed this

simple technique of measuring functional capacity through walking within a specified time period in the early 1960s [10]. Initially the time period for walking was 12 min [35]. But, as it was found to be too laborious for most respiratory disease patients, and a 6 minute walk was also better tolerated, so the latter was adopted and continued in current practice [13].

6 MWT better represents the functional capacity of daily physical activities as it requires sub maximal level of exercise capacity mimicking daily activities. 6MWT represents the integrated global performance of all the systems involved in exercise. It neither presents the individual status of the different organ systems nor the basis of exercise limitation [36]. The patient is required to walk on a flat, hard surface and the results of 6MWT simply represent the distance covered by the patient.

6MWT is most commonly used to measure the response to medical intervention in case of moderate-to-severe heart and lung disease and to evaluate functional capacity and predict mortality and morbidity [37]. Although, the 6MWT does not determine peak oxygen uptake, it has shown very good correlation with peak oxygen uptake ($r = 0.73$) in patients with end stage lung disease [9]. 6MWT is indicated for pretreatment and post-treatment comparisons of functional capacity in case of lung resection surgeries [38].

Unstable angina, and acute myocardial infarction in the last 1 month are absolute contraindications for performing 6MWT. A resting heart rate of more than 120/min, systolic blood pressure of more than 180 mmHg and diastolic blood pressure of more than 100 mmHg are relative contraindications for the test [37]. All patients should have a resting electrocardiogram within 6 months and it should be evaluated beforehand. Patients with stable angina can go through the test after taking their antianginal medication and nitrates should be kept ready nearby [8]. Before undergoing the test, the patients should have rated their baseline dyspnoea and overall fatigue by using the Borg scale.

An optimal cut-off value of 6MWT distance in case of single test is not yet available and standardised. Factors like age, height, weight and sex independently affect the distance travelled and they should be considered during interpretation of results [8]. A mean value of 6MWT was found 630 m in one study with healthy adults [39], while another study found median distance of 580 m for healthy men and 500 m for healthy women [40]. The result of 6MWT performed before and after an intervention should be interpreted as absolute difference between the two readings. Similarly, different studies have found different cut-off values for patients to be interpreted as significant. In one study, if the preoperative 6MWT distance was less than 500 m before lobectomy, there was an increased propensity for post-operative complications and prolonged hospital stay [41]. Another study showed patients who underwent single lobectomy for lung cancer, a 6MWT distance travelled 400 m or more had less post-operative cardiopulmonary complications than patients with shorter 6MWT distance [42].

ACCP and European societies have not recommended 6MWT for lung resection as there are studies with conflicting results [23], whereas American Thoracic society (ATS) has recommended that 6MWT should be used as a supplement but not as a substitute to CPET [37]. Although validity of 6MWT is tested in the scenario of lung resection surgery mostly, patients with non-lung cancers, posted for oncosurgeries also had 6MWT as the preoperative workup as part of the functional capacity assessment. The 6MWT was found to predict postoperative pulmonary complications (PPC) in patients undergoing both thoracic and non-thoracic surgeries.

Patients with lower 6MWT distance in perioperative setting had significantly higher PPC in the post-operative period [43]. Particularly 6MWT of 325 m or less can predict postoperative pulmonary complications (PPC) with 77% sensitivity and 100% specificity and comparable to that of FEV1% [44]. In thoracic and abdominal oncosurgeries, 6 minute walk distance of less than 390 m correlates with longer duration of ICU and hospital stay [45]. The CATCH-LUNG study predicted that patients of non-small cell lung cancer with moderate risk and short distance (that is, less than 400 m) covered in 6MWT were having increased chances of developing postoperative pulmonary complications [46]. A systematic review with meta-analysis that includes studies from 2007 to 2020, claims that 6MWT is quite a relevant assessment tool for monitoring and analysis of cardiorespiratory function in medical and exercise interventions of breast cancer survivors [47]. 6MWT can be a useful tool for functional assessment in patients with malignant pleural mesothelioma, as the distance covered was significantly correlated with inspiratory capacity and minimum recorded SpO_2 during the test correlates well with vital capacity and post-operative days of extubation [48].

2.6 Spirometry

Spirometry is a simple and frequently used objective tool for assessment of functional status of the patient in the preoperative period. It can also be repeated in the post-operative period or after other forms of therapy to evaluate the treatment response.

Spirometry is used not only for preoperative assessment and optimisation of respiratory conditions or for surgery related to the respiratory system but also for prediction of postoperative pulmonary complications (PPC) after other surgeries. Studies have shown that spirometry can be an independent predictor of postoperative pulmonary complications (PPC) in resection of malignant tumours of gastrointestinal tract [49].

Predictive value of spirometry for PPC has conflicting results among clinical studies. A study based on a large cohort of patients posted for colorectal surgery found preoperative spirometry useful. They found low percentage of preoperative vital capacity tends to be an independent risk factor (OR = 0.97, 95% CI = 0.94–0.99; $p = 0.049$) for developing post-operative pneumonia [50].

In another large cohort of gastrectomy patients revealed that preoperative abnormal spirometry values are independently associated with local wound and other surgical complications [51]. On the contrary, few others have questioned routine use of spirometry as a predictive tool for pulmonary complications, specifically, when used as a sole predictive tool in non-thoracic cases [9, 52–54]. Preoperative spirometry should be reserved for selective patients with a history of prior asthma or chronic obstructive pulmonary disease (COPD) [9].

Preoperative spirometry is useful in predicting PPC in thoracic surgeries, such as lung resections or in patients with lung cancer intended for radical treatment. Most guidelines consider Forced Expiratory Volume at 1 second (FEV1), predicted post-operative (PPO) FEV1, diffusion capacity of lung for carbon monoxide (DLCO) and predicted postoperative (PPO) DLCO as the best parameters for predicting post-operative complications and lung function after lung resection surgery.

$$\text{PPO}\,\text{FEV}_1 = \text{preoperative}\,\text{FEV}_1 \times (1 - y/z)$$

The preoperative FEV_1 is taken as the best measured post bronchodilator value. The number of functional or unobstructed lung segments to be removed is y and the total number of functional segments is z [55]. Same equation is applicable for PPO DLCO. Multiple studies have shown the role of FEV1 as an independent predictor of post-operative complications and DLCO as an independent predictor of delayed mortality and long-term survival [38, 56–63]. The European Respiratory Society (ERS) and European Society of Thoracic Surgeons (ESTS) recommends that for lung cancer surgery ppoFEV1 and ppoDLCO should be combined with other clinical parameters and their values of less than 30% of predicted is predictive of high-risk outcome [64]. Also, FEV1 and DLCO values of less than 80% of normal, warrant use of exercise tests in the preoperative period [64]. As per recommendations of American College of Physicians (ACP) ppoFEV1 and ppoDLCO values of more than 60% of predicted negate requirement of further testing in lung resections, whereas exercise test and formal cardiopulmonary exercise test (CPET) is recommended by them for ppoFEV1 and ppoDLCO values of 30–60% and less than 30%, respectively [23].

2.7 Cardiopulmonary Exercise Testing (CPET)

Cardiopulmonary exercise testing (CPET) is a relatively non-invasive and dynamic assessment which is considered the gold standard for assessment of functional capacity. It provides an overall assessment of the integrative exercise responses involving the pulmonary, cardiovascular, haematopoietic, neuropsychological, and skeletal muscle systems. CPET permits the evaluation of both submaximal and peak exercise responses, providing the physician with relevant information for clinical decision making [65].

Main indications for cardiopulmonary exercise testing are [65]:

1. Evaluation of exercise tolerance.
2. Evaluation of undiagnosed exercise intolerance.
3. Evaluation of patients with cardiovascular diseases.
4. Evaluation of patients with respiratory diseases/symptoms.
5. Preoperative evaluation.
6. Exercise evaluation and prescription for pulmonary rehabilitation.
7. Evaluation of impairment/disability.
8. Evaluation for lung, heart, and heart–lung transplantation.

In clinical scenarios, CPET should be considered when the attending physician is unable to find answers of the specific questions even after evaluating basic clinical data including history, physical examination, chest radiographs, resting pulmonary function tests, and resting electrocardiogram (ECG) [65].

Treadmill and cycle ergometer are the two common modes of exercise used commonly. Cycle ergometry is the preferable mode of exercise in most of the clinical settings, but treadmill is also an acceptable alternative [65].

Most commonly used technique is incremental physical workload on a computer-controlled, electromagnetically braked cycle ergometer, under physician supervision and in accordance with published guidelines [65]. The incremental workload exercise test usually takes 8–12 min to complete. In the beginning the participant sits on the cycle ergometer and the baseline cardiovascular and respiratory measurements are taken, and 3 min of unloaded cycling (0 W) that serves a warm-up. Pedalling resistance is then increased progressively every minute using a ramped protocol during which participants pedal at 60 revolutions per minute. Typically, work rates are increased by 10 W per minute in untrained individuals, and by up to 20–30 W per minute in well-trained participants or those that participate regularly in physical activity. After the exercise test is stopped, participants continue to pedal for a 5-min recovery period, during which the work intensity is reduced to 20 W [14].

While the participant is working on the cycle ergometer or treadmill, the physiological reserve of the heart, lungs and skeletal muscles can be quantified by monitoring ECG changes, heart rate and blood pressure responses, respiratory volumes, oxygen consumption and carbon dioxide production, as well as by grading dyspnoea and subjective feelings. Evaluation of CPET result is useful to know whether it is the cardiac or pulmonary or skeletal muscle dysfunction which is responsible for the abnormal results [65, 66].

3b. The absolute and relative contraindications for CPET are described in Table 2.3 [67, 68].

The indications for termination of exercises while performing CPET are ischaemic chest pain or ECG changes, complex ectopy, second or third degree heart block, hypotension (>20 mmHg drop from highest value during the test), hypertension (>250 mmHg systolic, >120 mmHg diastolic), sudden pallor, loss of coordination, mental confusion, dizziness, sign of respiratory failure, desaturation ($SpO_2 < 80\%$) [68–70].

CPET is gaining popularity as a tool for preoperative functional assessment as resting pulmonary and cardiac function testing cannot reliably predict exercise performance and oxygen consumption at the peak of exercise functional (VO_2 peak) in the patients with cardiopulmonary disease [36, 71–82]. Furthermore, exertional symptoms correlate poorly with resting cardiopulmonary measurements [79, 80, 83]. Although exertional dyspnoea is common in patients with respiratory disease, symptoms that limit exertions are leg discomfort, chest pain, or fatigue as well [71, 83]. The practical relevance of CPET is further highlighted by the finding that the subjective measures of a patient's quality of life reveal a stronger correlation with exercise tolerance than with either spirometry or oxygenation, hence CPET becomes

Table 2.3 Absolute and relative contraindications for CPET

Absolute	Relative
Acute MI (3–5 days)	Left main coronary stenosis
Unstable angina	Moderate stenotic valvular heart disease
Uncontrolled arrhythmia causing symptoms or hemodynamic compromise	Severe untreated arterial hypertension at rest Systolic >200 mmHg, diastolic >120 mmHg
Syncope	Tachy/bradyarrhythmias
Acute endocarditis	High degree atrioventricular block
Acute myocarditis or pericarditis	Hypertrophic cardiomyopathy
Uncontrolled heart failure	Significant pulmonary hypertension
Acute pulmonary embolism or pulmonary infarction	Advanced or complicated pregnancy
Thrombosis of lower extremity	Electrolyte abnormalities
Suspected dissecting aneurysm	Orthopaedic impairment that may compromise ability to perform exercise
Uncontrolled asthma	
Respiratory failure/room air $SpO_2 < 85\%$	
Pulmonary oedema	
Acute non-cardiopulmonary disorder that may affect exercise capacity (infection, renal failure)	
Mental impairment leading to inability to cooperate	

more relevant [84]. The 6 minute walk test (6MWT) has gained popularity. Currently, both the 6MWT and CPET are used for functional assessment. Their use depends on the need of the patient and available resources.

Several prospective studies have demonstrated strong correlation between predictive perioperative morbidity and mortality and limitation of exercise capacity as expressed by peak oxygen uptake (peak $V'O_2$) or maximal oxygen uptake [23, 64, 85–88]. Based on these data, CPET has been endorsed by the European Respiratory Society (ERS) and the European Society of Thoracic Surgery (ESTS) and incorporated in a functional algorithm for the evaluation of candidates for lung resection [64, 88]. These guidelines recommend that CPET should be performed in all patients posted for surgical intervention with forced expiratory volume in 1 s (FEV1) or with diffusing capacity of the lung for carbon monoxide (DLCO).

There are many variables (both non-invasive and invasive) that are being measured during the test, which include external work, metabolic gas exchange, cardiovascular parameters (heart rate, ECG, BP, SpO_2), ventilatory parameters, pulmonary gas exchange, arterial blood gas and symptoms (dyspnoea, chest pain, fatigue) [89]. Out of all these, the variables that are used commonly in clinical practice are clinically in perioperative practice are: anaerobic threshold (AT), peak oxygen consumption ($V'O_2$ peak) and ventilatory equivalents for CO_2 (V_E/VCO_2) [90] (see Table 2.4 for definitions of these variables).

The suggested criteria for normality of the variables measured during CPET are as follows: [36]

Table 2.4 Cardiopulmonary exercise test variables with important predictive utility in published perioperative case cohorts [90]

Variable	Definition	Interpretation
Anaerobic or lactate threshold (AT/LT)	The oxygen uptake above which lactate begins to increase and a metabolic acidosis occurs. This is identified by the associated changes in gas exchange [91]	An index of submaximal or sustainable exercise capacity. Associated with post-operative morbidity and mortality in the majority of published case series
$V'O_2$ peak	Highest oxygen uptake value achieved during an exercise test [91]	An index of maximal aerobic exercise capacity. Associated with post-operative morbidity and mortality in most published case series
V_E/VCO_2	Ventilatory equivalent for CO_2 is the ratio of minute ventilation to pulmonary CO_2 production	An index of the efficiency of gas exchange reflecting ventilation–perfusion matching. If elevated, gas exchange efficiency is reduced reflecting increased dead space [92]. It is associated with post-operative morbidity and mortality in some but not all published case series

1. Peak oxygen consumption ($V'O_2$ peak), >84% of the predicted.
2. Anaerobic threshold (AT) >40% $V'O_2$ max predicted, wide range of normal (40–80%).
3. Ventilatory equivalents for CO_2 (V_E/VCO_2) <0.28 and < 0.3 for age more than 40 years.

In 1993, Older et al. reported an association between preoperative AT and post-operative morbidity in elderly patients undergoing elective major surgery [91]. Patients with an AT of <11 ml kg^{-1} min^{-1} had a higher 'non-surgical' mortality rate than patients with an AT value >11 ml kg^{-1} min^{-1}, particularly if a low AT was coupled with ECG evidence of ischaemia early in exercise. Similar association between low preoperative exercise capacity and poor post-operative outcomes has been reported by other observational studies [92, 93]. Preoperative cardiorespiratory fitness has been associated with increased length of stay in critical care unit [94], short-term morbidity [95, 96], short-term survival (30-day mortality) [97, 98], intermediate survival (90-day mortality) [97, 98], and long-term survival (>90 day mortality) [97, 99–101]. The first multicentre study, conducted by Perioperative Exercise Testing and Training Society (POETTS) in 703 patients across six centres in UK, reported that variables derived from preoperative CPET can be used to assess risk before major elective colorectal surgery. They reported increase in morbidity associated with lower levels of oxygen uptake variables with an area under the receiver operating curve (ROC) is 0.79 for AT (cut-off 11.1 ml kg^{-1} min^{-1}) and 0.83 for $V'O_2$ peak 18.2 ml kg^{-1} min^{-1} [97].

In an observational study, in 2011, Licker et al. found that in patients posted for lung cancer resection, the incidence of cardiovascular and pulmonary complications increased in parallel with the reduction in peak $V'O_2$ during exercise testing.

Compared with patients with peak $V'O_2$ 17 ml kg^{-1} min^{-1}, those with a peak $V'O_2$ of 10 ml kg^{-1} min^{-1} had a four-fold higher incidence of cardiac and pulmonary morbidity [102].

Other studies also reported that patients with $V'O_2$ at AT <11 ml min^{-1} kg^{-1} or $V'O_2$ at peak <19 ml min^{-1} kg^{-1} were at significant risk of post-operative cardiovascular death and surgical complications following major abdominal surgery [103], and in surgery for oesophagogastric cancer [104].

To summarise, preoperative CPET can be used to assess functional capacity and evaluate physical fitness objectively. This information can be used by the treating team for individual risk stratification, collaborative decision making, to obtain inform consent and triaging the patient to ensure optimum perioperative care.

2.8 Brain Natriuretic Peptide (BNP) and N-Terminal Pro-B-Type Natriuretic Peptide (NT-Pro BNP)

Cardiac natriuretic hormones like atrial natriuretic peptide (ANP) and brain natriuretic peptide (BNP) are mainly produced by cardiomyocytes. These hormones are synthesised by cardiomyocytes as prohormones (i.e. pro ANP and pro BNP), which are then split into two fragments at the time of secretion: the longer fragment includes the inactive NT peptide (i.e. NT pro ANP and NT-pro BNP), whereas the shorter one (i.e. COOH-terminus fragment) represents the active hormone (i.e. ANP and BNP) [105]. ANP is predominantly produced in the atria, whereas BNP is mainly produced in the ventricles [106]. Unlike atria the ventricular cardiomyocytes do not usually display secretory granules at electron microscopy in the normal heart [107, 108], but such secretary granules have been observed in samples of ventricular myocardium collected during surgery or endocardial biopsies in patients with cardiac disease [105]. Therefore, under physiological conditions, ventricular myocardium produces very little BNP, but several pathophysiological mechanisms, such as ventricular hypertrophy, inflammation, and fibrosis, stimulate BNP production and release from ventricular cardiomyocytes [109–112]. Furthermore, myocardial ischemia and hypoxia can induce the synthesis and secretion of BNP and its related peptides by ventricular cells [15, 113–116].

Studies have demonstrated that elevated preoperative BNP concentrations are strong independent predictors of perioperative cardiovascular complications, such as mortality, myocardial infarction [MI], and heart failure [117, 118]. In vascular surgical cases, preoperative BNP risk stratification is found to be a better predictor than traditional subjective risk stratification [119]. European Society of Cardiology and European Society of Anaesthesiology guidelines for preoperative cardiac risk assessment have recommended preoperative measurement of natriuretic peptides in high-risk non-cardiac surgeries [120]. However, recent studies have reported that elevated post-operative NP concentrations are independently associated with post-operative cardiovascular complications [121, 122].

In 2014, a meta-analysis was published, which included 18 studies and 2179 patients. The purpose of the meta-analysis was to evaluate the prognostic value of preoperative and post-operative values of natriuretic peptide (NT) and N-Terminal fragment of pro BNP (NT-pro BNP). The study showed that a preoperative NT-pro BNP/BNP measurement was independently associated with the primary outcome (i.e. death or nonfatal myocardial infarction) at 30 days after non-cardiac surgery (OR, 3.40; 95% CI, 2.57–4.47; $p < 0.001$) [123]. Importantly, a preoperative NT-pro BNP/BNP measurement before non-cardiac surgery improved risk prediction among patients who did and did not suffer the primary outcome. Values >300 ng/L for NT-pro BNP and > 92 mg/L for BNP were identified as significant thresholds associated with an increased risk of the primary outcome. According to these thresholds, 7.6% of patients had an elevated NT-pro BNP/BNP measurement before non-cardiac surgery. Death or nonfatal myocardial infarction within 30 days after surgery occurred in 4.9% of patients with preoperative NT-pro BNP/BNP values below these thresholds compared with 21.8% of patients with NT-pro BNP/BNP values at or above these thresholds. These findings were consistent with results from previous meta- analyses [118, 123–126].

In 2017, Canadian Cardiovascular Society Guidelines on Perioperative Cardiac Risk Assessment and Management recommended measuring NT-pro BNP or BNP before non-cardiac surgery to enhance perioperative cardiac risk estimation in patients who are 65 years of age or older, are 45–64 years of age with significant cardiovascular disease, or have an revised cardiac risk index (RCRI) score ≥ 1 [127].

In 2018, a multicentric trial was published which evaluated >1400 patients posted for major non-cardiac surgery. Preoperative functional assessment was done using subjective assessment, DASI questionnaire, CPET and cardiac biomarkers. Results showed peak oxygen consumption was positively correlated with DASI scores (Spearman ρ 0.43, $p < 0.0001$), and negatively correlated with NT-pro BNP concentrations (Spearman ρ –0.21, $p < 0.0001$). There was also a negative correlation between DASI scores and NT-pro BNP concentrations [16].

Cost and accessibility are important considerations while testing for the biomarkers in the preoperative period. But compared with cardiac imaging and non-invasive cardiac stress testing, NT-pro BNP/BNP biomarkers are inexpensive and avoid the need for return visits. There are other preoperative biomarkers (e.g. high sensitivity troponin) [128] might be helpful in clinical situations where use of NT-pro BNP as a prognostic biomarker is limited such as in the presence of obesity [129], chronic renal kidney [130] or heart failure with preserved ejection fraction [131].

2.9 Conclusion

Assessment of preoperative functional capacity is a very important tool in the armamentarium of clinicians as it gives an insight about the risk of post-operative morbidity and mortality. Therefore, it helps in identifying the subset of patients who can benefit from preoperative optimisation, interventions, haemodynamic management, helps in collaborative decision making, obtaining informed consent, and triaging the patients, closer post-operative surveillance or complete avoidance of surgery.

There are various ways of assessing functional capacity, out of which the subjective assessments are easy to implement but do not accurately identify patients with poor fitness or those at increased risk for morbidity and mortality after major elective non-cardiac surgery. Clinicians could instead consider more objective measures, such as DASI questionnaires, CPET and NT-pro BNP testing for assessing perioperative cardiac risk and to predict complications after major elective non-cardiac surgery.

Cost and accessibility are very important considerations especially, for the assessments which require special set-up, skilled technicians and expensive laboratory testing. More high quality multicentric research is required to characterise the most effective means of improving patient fitness before surgery and to evaluate the impact of such improvements on surgical and disease-specific (e.g. cancer) outcomes.

References

1. Botto F, Alonso-Coello P, Chan MTV, Villar JC, Xavier D, Srinathan S, et al. Myocardial injury after noncardiac surgery: a large, international, prospective cohort study establishing diagnostic criteria, characteristics, predictors, and 30-day outcomes. Anesthesiology. 2014;120(3):564–78.
2. Weiser TG, Haynes AB, Molina G, Lipsitz SR, Esquivel MM, Uribe-Leitz T, et al. Estimate of the global volume of surgery in 2012: an assessment supporting improved health outcomes. Lancet Lond Engl. 2015;385(Suppl. 2):S11.
3. Fleisher LA, Fleischmann KE, Auerbach AD, Barnason SA, Beckman JA, Bozkurt B, et al. 2014 ACC/AHA Guideline on perioperative cardiovascular evaluation and management of patients undergoing noncardiac surgery. Circulation. 2014;130(24):e278–333.
4. Kristensen SD, Knuuti J, Saraste A, Anker S, Bøtker HE, Hert SD, et al. 2014 ESC/ESA Guidelines on non-cardiac surgery: cardiovascular assessment and management: The Joint Task Force on non-cardiac surgery: cardiovascular assessment and management of the European Society of Cardiology (ESC) and the European Society of Anaesthesiology (ESA). Eur Heart J. 2014;35(35):2383–431.
5. Anderson DJ, Chen LF, Schmader KE, Sexton DJ, Choi Y, Link K, et al. Poor functional status as a risk factor for surgical site infection due to methicillin-resistant *Staphylococcus aureus*. Infect Control Hosp Epidemiol. 2008;29(9):832–9.
6. Arozullah AM, Daley J, Henderson WG, Khuri SF. Multifactorial risk index for predicting postoperative respiratory failure in men after major noncardiac surgery. The National Veterans Administration Surgical Quality Improvement Program. Ann Surg. 2000;232(2):242–53.
7. Arozullah AM, Khuri SF, Henderson WG, Daley J, Participants in the National Veterans Affairs Surgical Quality Improvement Program. Development and validation of a multifactorial risk index for predicting postoperative pneumonia after major noncardiac surgery. Ann Intern Med. 2001;135(10):847–57
8. Chen T-Y, Anderson DJ, Chopra T, Choi Y, Schmader KE, Kaye KS. Poor functional status is an independent predictor of surgical site infections due to methicillin resistant *Staphylococcus aureus* in older adults. J Am Geriatr Soc. 2010;58(3):527–32
9. Qaseem A, Snow V, Fitterman N, Hornbake ER, Lawrence VA, Smetana GW, et al. Risk assessment for and strategies to reduce perioperative pulmonary complications for patients undergoing noncardiothoracic surgery: a guideline from the American College of Physicians. Ann Intern Med. 2006;144(8):575–80.
10. Balke B. A simple field test for the assessment of physical fitness. REP 63-6. Rep Civ Aeromed Res Inst US. 1963:1–8.

11. Oken M, Creech R, Tormey D, Horton J, Davis T, McFadden E, et al. Toxicity and response criteria of the Eastern Cooperative Oncology Group. Am J Clin Oncol. 1982;5(6):649–56.
12. Hlatky MA, Boineau RE, Higginbotham MB, Lee KL, Mark DB, Califf RM, et al. A brief self-administered questionnaire to determine functional capacity (the Duke Activity Status Index). Am J Cardiol. 1989;64(10):651–4.
13. Butland RJ, Pang J, Gross ER, Woodcock AA, Geddes DM. Two-, six-, and 12-minute walking tests in respiratory disease. Br Med J Clin Res Ed. 1982;284(6329):1607–8.
14. Wijeysundera DN, Pearse RM, Shulman MA, Abbott TEF, Torres E, Croal BL, et al. Measurement of Exercise Tolerance before Surgery (METS) study: a protocol for an international multicentre prospective cohort study of cardiopulmonary exercise testing prior to major non-cardiac surgery. BMJ Open. 2016;6(3):e010359.
15. Goetze JP. Biochemistry of pro-B-type natriuretic peptide-derived peptides: the endocrine heart revisited. Clin Chem. 2004;50(9):1503–10.
16. Wijeysundera DN, Pearse RM, Shulman MA, Abbott TEF, Torres E, Ambosta A, et al. Assessment of functional capacity before major non-cardiac surgery: an international, prospective cohort study. Lancet Lond Engl. 2018;391(10140):2631–40.
17. Melon CC, Eshtiaghi P, Luksun WJ, Wijeysundera DN. Validated questionnaire vs physicians' judgment to estimate preoperative exercise capacity. JAMA Intern Med. 2014;174(9):1507.
18. Stokes JW, Wanderer JP, McEvoy MD. Significant discrepancies exist between clinician assessment and patient self-assessment of functional capacity by validated scoring tools during preoperative evaluation. Perioper Med Lond Engl. 2016;5:18.
19. Wiklund RA, Stein HD, Rosenbaum SH. Activities of daily living and cardiovascular complications following elective, noncardiac surgery. Yale J Biol Med. 2001;74(2):75–87.
20. Chassot PG, Delabays A, Spahn DR. Preoperative evaluation of patients with, or at risk of, coronary artery disease undergoing non-cardiac surgery. BJA Br J Anaesth. 2002;89(5):747–59.
21. Girish M, Trayner E, Dammann O, Pinto-Plata V, Celli B. Symptom-limited stair climbing as a predictor of postoperative cardiopulmonary complications after high-risk surgery. Chest. 2001;120(4):1147–51.
22. Shea C, Khawaja AR, Sofi K, Nabi G. Association of metabolic equivalent of task (MET) score in length of stay in hospital following radical cystectomy with urinary diversion: a multi-institutional study. Int Urol Nephrol. 2021;53(7):1305–10. 6 [cited 2021 May 25]. https://doi.org/10.1007/s11255-021-02813-x.
23. Brunelli A, Kim AW, Berger KI, Addrizzo-Harris DJ. Physiologic evaluation of the patient with lung cancer being considered for resectional surgery: diagnosis and management of lung cancer, 3rd ed: American College of Chest Physicians evidence-based clinical practice guidelines. Chest. 2013;143(Suppl. 5):e166S–90S.
24. Licker M, Triponez F, Diaper J, Karenovics W, Bridevaux P-O. Preoperative evaluation of lung cancer patients. Curr Anesthesiol Rep. 2014;4(2):124–34.
25. Keum N, Bao Y, Smith-Warner SA, Orav J, Wu K, Fuchs CS, et al. Association of physical activity by type and intensity with digestive system cancer risk. JAMA Oncol. 2016;2(9):1146–53.
26. Meyerhardt JA, Giovannucci EL, Ogino S, Kirkner GJ, Chan AT, Willett W, et al. Physical activity and male colorectal cancer survival. Arch Intern Med. 2009;169(22):2102–8.
27. Schmid D, Leitzmann MF. Association between physical activity and mortality among breast cancer and colorectal cancer survivors: a systematic review and meta-analysis. Ann Oncol Off J Eur Soc Med Oncol. 2014;25(7):1293–311.
28. Jones LW, Habel LA, Weltzien E, Castillo A, Gupta D, Kroenke CH, et al. Exercise and risk of cardiovascular events in women with nonmetastatic breast cancer. J Clin Oncol Off J Am Soc Clin Oncol. 2016;34(23):2743–9.
29. Cihoric M, Tengberg LT, Foss NB, Gögenur I, Tolstrup M-B, Bay-Nielsen M. Functional performance and 30-day postoperative mortality after emergency laparotomy—a retrospective, multicenter, observational cohort study of 1084 patients. Perioper Med. 2020;9(1):13.

30. Young J, Badgery-Parker T, Dobbins T, Jorgensen M, Gibbs P, Faragher I, et al. Comparison of ECOG/WHO performance status and ASA score as a measure of functional status. J Pain Symptom Manag. 2015;49(2):258–64.
31. Chou W-C, Liu K-H, Lu C-H, Hung Y-S, Chen M-F, Cheng Y-F, et al. To operate or not: prediction of 3-month postoperative mortality in geriatric cancer patients. J Cancer. 2016;7(1):14–21.
32. Shaw LJ, Olson MB, Kip K, Kelsey SF, Johnson BD, Mark DB, et al. The value of estimated functional capacity in estimating outcome: results from the NHBLI-Sponsored Women's Ischemia Syndrome Evaluation (WISE) Study. J Am Coll Cardiol. 2006;47(Suppl. 3):S36–43.
33. Chung S-C, Hlatky MA, Stone RA, Rana JS, Escobedo J, Rogers WJ, et al. Body mass index and health status in the Bypass Angioplasty Revascularization Investigation 2 Diabetes Trial (BARI 2D). Am Heart J. 2011;162(1):184–92. e3
34. Wijeysundera DN, Beattie WS, Hillis GS, Abbott TEF, Shulman MA, Ackland GL, et al. Integration of the Duke Activity Status Index into preoperative risk evaluation: a multicentre prospective cohort study. Br J Anaesth. 2020;124(3):261–70.
35. Cooper KH. A means of assessing maximal oxygen intake. Correlation between field and treadmill testing. JAMA. 1968;203(3):201–4.
36. Weisman IM, Zeballos RJ. An integrated approach to the interpretation of cardiopulmonary exercise testing. Clin Chest Med. 1994;15(2):421–45.
37. ATS Committee on Proficiency Standards for Clinical Pulmonary Function Laboratories. ATS statement: guidelines for the six-minute walk test. Am J Respir Crit Care Med. 2002;166(1):111–7.
38. Holden DA, Rice TW, Stelmach K, Meeker DP. Exercise testing, 6-min walk, and stair climb in the evaluation of patients at high risk for pulmonary resection. Chest. 1992;102(6):1774–9.
39. Troosters T, Gosselink R, Decramer M. Six minute walking distance in healthy elderly subjects. Eur Respir J. 1999;14(2):270–4.
40. Enright PL, Sherrill DL. Reference equations for the six-minute walk in healthy adults. Am J Respir Crit Care Med. 1998;158(5 Pt 1):1384–7.
41. Marjanski T, Wnuk D, Dziedzic R, Ostrowski M, Sawicka W, Rzyman W. 500 Meters is a result of 6-Minute Walk Test which differentiates patients with high and low risk of postoperative complications after lobectomy—a validation study. J Clin Med. 2021;10(8):1686. 14 [cited 2021 May 25]. Available from: https://www.ncbi.nlm.nih.gov/pmc/articles/PMC8070994/
42. Wesolowski S, Orlowski TM, Kram M. The 6-min walk test in the functional evaluation of patients with lung cancer qualified for lobectomy. Interact Cardiovasc Thorac Surg. 2020;30(4):559–64.
43. Hattori K, Matsuda T, Takagi Y, Nagaya M, Inoue T, Nishida Y, et al. Preoperative six-minute walk distance is associated with pneumonia after lung resection. Interact Cardiovasc Thorac Surg. 2018;26(2):277–83.
44. Keeratichananont W, Thanadetsuntorn C, Keeratichananont S. Value of preoperative 6-minute walk test for predicting postoperative pulmonary complications. Ther Adv Respir Dis. 2016;10(1):18–25.
45. Sathyaprasad SL, Thomas M, Philip FA, Krishna KMJ. Performance in 6-min walk test in prediction of post-operative pulmonary complication in major oncosurgeries: a prospective observational study. Indian J Anaesth. 2020;64(1):55.
46. Lee H, Kim HK, Kang D, Kong S, Lee JK, Lee G, et al. Prognostic value of 6-min walk test to predict postoperative cardiopulmonary complications in patients with non-small cell lung cancer. Chest. 2020;157(6):1665–73.
47. But-Hadzic J, Dervisevic M, Karpljuk D, Videmsek M, Dervisevic E, Paravlic A, et al. Six-minute walk distance in breast cancer survivors—a systematic review with meta-analysis. Int J Environ Res Public Health. 2021;18(5):2591. 5 [cited 2021 May 25] Available from: https://www.ncbi.nlm.nih.gov/pmc/articles/PMC7967367/

48. Nagaya M, Ito S, Fukui T, Inoue T, Kawaguchi K, Nakamura S, et al. Preoperative evaluation of six-minute walk test in patients with malignant pleural mesothelioma. MacFarlane N, editor. Cogent Med. 2017;4(1):1421007.
49. Fuso L, Cisternino L, Di Napoli A, Di Cosmo V, Tramaglino LM, Basso S, et al. Role of spirometric and arterial gas data in predicting pulmonary complications after abdominal surgery. Respir Med. 2000;94(12):1171–6.
50. Tajima Y, Tsuruta M, Yahagi M, Hasegawa H, Okabayashi K, Shigeta K, et al. Is preoperative spirometry a predictive marker for postoperative complications after colorectal cancer surgery? Jpn J Clin Oncol. 2017;47(9):815–9.
51. Jeong O, Ryu SY, Park YK. The value of preoperative lung spirometry test for predicting the operative risk in patients undergoing gastric cancer surgery. J Korean Surg Soc. 2013;84(1):18–26.
52. Kocabas A, Kara K, Ozgur G, Sonmez H, Burgut R. Value of preoperative spirometry to predict postoperative pulmonary complications. Respir Med. 1996;90(1):25–33.
53. Smetana GW, Lawrence VA, Cornell JE, American College of Physicians. Preoperative pulmonary risk stratification for noncardiothoracic surgery: systematic review for the American College of Physicians. Ann Intern Med. 2006;144(8):581–95.
54. Ferguson MK. Preoperative assessment of pulmonary risk. Chest. 1999;115(Suppl. 5):58S–63S.
55. Bolliger CT, Gückel C, Engel H, Stöhr S, Wyser CP, Schoetzau A, et al. Prediction of functional reserves after lung resection: comparison between quantitative computed tomography, scintigraphy, and anatomy. Respir Int Rev Thorac Dis. 2002;69(6):482–9.
56. Markos J, Mullan BP, Hillman DR, Musk AW, Antico VF, Lovegrove FT, et al. Preoperative assessment as a predictor of mortality and morbidity after lung resection. Am Rev Respir Dis. 1989;139(4):902–10.
57. Pierce RJ, Copland JM, Sharpe K, Barter CE. Preoperative risk evaluation for lung cancer resection: predicted postoperative product as a predictor of surgical mortality. Am J Respir Crit Care Med. 1994;150(4):947–55.
58. Nakahara K, Monden Y, Ohno K, Miyoshi S, Maeda H, Kawashima Y. A method for predicting postoperative lung function and its relation to postoperative complications in patients with lung cancer. Ann Thorac Surg. 1985;39(3):260–5.
59. Ferguson MK, Siddique J, Karrison T. Modeling major lung resection outcomes using classification trees and multiple imputation techniques. Eur J Cardiothorac Surg. 2008;34(5):1085–9.
60. Ferguson MK, Little L, Rizzo L, Popovich KJ, Glonek GF, Leff A, et al. Diffusing capacity predicts morbidity and mortality after pulmonary resection. J Thorac Cardiovasc Surg. 1988;96(6):894–900.
61. Berry MF, Villamizar-Ortiz NR, Tong BC, Burfeind WR, Harpole DH, D'Amico TA, et al. Pulmonary function tests do not predict pulmonary complications after thoracoscopic lobectomy. Ann Thorac Surg. 2010;89(4):1044–51. discussion 1051-1052
62. Cerfolio RJ, Bryant AS. Different diffusing capacity of the lung for carbon monoxide as predictors of respiratory morbidity. Ann Thorac Surg. 2009;88(2):405–10. discussion 410-411
63. Ferguson MK, Dignam JJ, Siddique J, Vigneswaran WT, Celauro AD. Diffusing capacity predicts long-term survival after lung resection for cancer. Eur J Cardio-Thorac Surg Off J Eur Assoc Cardio-Thorac Surg. 2012;41(5):e81–6.
64. Brunelli A, Charloux A, Bolliger CT, Rocco G, Sculier J-P, Varela G, et al. ERS/ESTS clinical guidelines on fitness for radical therapy in lung cancer patients (surgery and chemo-radiotherapy). Eur Respir J. 2009;34(1):17–41.
65. American Thoracic Society, American College of Chest Physicians. ATS/ACCP Statement on cardiopulmonary exercise testing. Am J Respir Crit Care Med. 2003;167(2):211–77.
66. Palange P, Ward SA, Carlsen K-H, Casaburi R, Gallagher CG, Gosselink R, et al. Recommendations on the use of exercise testing in clinical practice. Eur Respir J. 2007;29(1):185–209.
67. Fletcher GF, Balady G, Froelicher VF, Hartley LH, Haskell WL, Pollock ML. Exercise Standards. Circulation. 1995;91(2):580–615.

68. ACSMs Guidelines for Exercise Testing and Prescription [Internet]. [cited 2021 May 26]. Available from: https://www.acsm.org/read-research/books/acsms-guidelines-for-exercise-testing-and-prescription
69. Löllgen H, Ulmer HV, Crean P. Recommendations and standard guidelines for exercise testing. Report of the Task Force Conference on Ergometry, Titisee 1987. Eur Heart J. 1988;9(Suppl. K):3–37.
70. Gibbons RJ, Balady GJ, Beasley JW, Bricker JT, Duvernoy WF, Froelicher VF, et al. ACC/AHA Guidelines for Exercise Testing. A report of the American College of Cardiology/American Heart Association Task Force on Practice Guidelines (Committee on Exercise Testing). J Am Coll Cardiol. 1997;30(1):260–311.
71. Hamilton AL, Killian KJ, Summers E, Jones NL. Muscle strength, symptom intensity, and exercise capacity in patients with cardiorespiratory disorders. Am J Respir Crit Care Med. 1995;152(6 Pt 1):2021–31.
72. Weisman IM, Zeballos RJ. Clinical exercise testing. Clin Chest Med. 2001;22(4):679–701. viii
73. Bye PT, Anderson SD, Woolcock AJ, Young IH, Alison JA. Bicycle endurance performance of patients with interstitial lung disease breathing air and oxygen. Am Rev Respir Dis. 1982;126(6):1005–12.
74. Carlson DJ, Ries AL, Kaplan RM. Prediction of maximum exercise tolerance in patients with COPD. Chest. 1991;100(2):307–11.
75. Keogh BA, Lakatos E, Price D, Crystal RG. Importance of the lower respiratory tract in oxygen transfer. Exercise testing in patients with interstitial and destructive lung disease. Am Rev Respir Dis. 1984;129(2 Pt 2):S76–80.
76. Sue DY, Oren A, Hansen JE, Wasserman K. Diffusing capacity for carbon monoxide as a predictor of gas exchange during exercise. N Engl J Med. 1987;316(21):1301–6.
77. Ries AL, Farrow JT, Clausen JL. Pulmonary function tests cannot predict exercise-induced hypoxemia in chronic obstructive pulmonary disease. Chest. 1988;93(3):454–9.
78. Cotes JE, Zejda J, King B. Lung function impairment as a guide to exercise limitation in work-related lung disorders. Am Rev Respir Dis. 1988;137(5):1089–93.
79. Franciosa JA, Park M, Levine TB. Lack of correlation between exercise capacity and indexes of resting left ventricular performance in heart failure. Am J Cardiol. 1981;47(1):33–9.
80. Szlachcic J, Massie BM, Kramer BL, Topic N, Tubau J. Correlates and prognostic implication of exercise capacity in chronic congestive heart failure. Am J Cardiol. 1985;55(8):1037–42.
81. Punzal PA, Ries AL, Kaplan RM, Prewitt LM. Maximum intensity exercise training in patients with chronic obstructive pulmonary disease. Chest. 1991;100(3):618–23.
82. Dillard TA, Hnatiuk OW, McCumber TR. Maximum voluntary ventilation. Spirometric determinants in chronic obstructive pulmonary disease patients and normal subjects. Am Rev Respir Dis. 1993;147(4):870–5.
83. Killian KJ, Leblanc P, Martin DH, Summers E, Jones NL, Campbell EJ. Exercise capacity and ventilatory, circulatory, and symptom limitation in patients with chronic airflow limitation. Am Rev Respir Dis. 1992;146(4):935–40.
84. Curtis JR, Deyo RA, Hudson LD. Pulmonary rehabilitation in chronic respiratory insufficiency. 7. Health-related quality of life among patients with chronic obstructive pulmonary disease. Thorax. 1994;49(2):162–70.
85. Brunelli A, Pompili C, Salati M. Low-technology exercise test in the preoperative evaluation of lung resection candidates. Monaldi Arch Chest Dis Arch Monaldi Mal Torace. 2010;73(2):72–8.
86. Benzo R, Kelley GA, Recchi L, Hofman A, Sciurba F. Complications of lung resection and exercise capacity: a meta-analysis. Respir Med. 2007;101(8):1790–7.
87. Win T, Jackson A, Sharples L, Groves AM, Wells FC, Ritchie AJ, et al. Cardiopulmonary exercise tests and lung cancer surgical outcome. Chest. 2005;127(4):1159–65.
88. Brunelli A, Charloux A, Bolliger CT, Rocco G, Sculier J P, Varela G, et al. The European Respiratory Society and European Society of Thoracic Surgeons clinical guidelines for evaluating fitness for radical treatment (surgery and chemoradiotherapy) in patients with lung cancer. Eur J Cardio-Thorac Surg Off J Eur Assoc Cardio-Thorac Surg. 2009;36(1):181–4.

89. Demark-Wahnefried W, Clipp EC, Lipkus IM, Lobach D, Snyder DC, Sloane R, et al. Main outcomes of the FRESH START trial: a sequentially tailored, diet and exercise mailed print intervention among breast and prostate cancer survivors. J Clin Oncol Off J Am Soc Clin Oncol. 2007;25(19):2709–18.
90. Richardson K, Levett DZH, Jack S, Grocott MPW. Fit for surgery? Perspectives on preoperative exercise testing and training. Br J Anaesth. 2017;119(Suppl. 1):i34–43.
91. Older P, Smith R, Courtney P, Hone R. Preoperative evaluation of cardiac failure and ischemia in elderly patients by cardiopulmonary exercise testing. Chest. 1993;104(3):701–4.
92. Smith TB, Stonell C, Purkayastha S, Paraskevas P. Cardiopulmonary exercise testing as a risk assessment method in non cardio-pulmonary surgery: a systematic review. Anaesthesia. 2009;64(8):883–93.
93. Hennis PJ, Meale PM, Grocott MPW. Cardiopulmonary exercise testing for the evaluation of perioperative risk in non-cardiopulmonary surgery. Postgrad Med J. 2011;87(1030):550–7.
94. Prentis JM, Manas DMD, Trenell MI, Hudson M, Jones DJ, Snowden CP. Submaximal cardiopulmonary exercise testing predicts 90-day survival after liver transplantation. Liver Transplant Off Publ Am Assoc Study Liver Dis Int Liver Transplant Soc. 2012;18(2):152–9.
95. West MA, Asher R, Browning M, Minto G, Swart M, Richardson K, et al. Validation of preoperative cardiopulmonary exercise testing-derived variables to predict in-hospital morbidity after major colorectal surgery. Br J Surg. 2016;103(6):744–52.
96. Barakat HM, Shahin Y, McCollum PT, Chetter IC. Prediction of organ-specific complications following abdominal aortic aneurysm repair using cardiopulmonary exercise testing. Anaesthesia. 2015;70(6):679–85.
97. Lai CW, Minto G, Challand CP, Hosie KB, Sneyd JR, Creanor S, et al. Patients' inability to perform a preoperative cardiopulmonary exercise test or demonstrate an anaerobic threshold is associated with inferior outcomes after major colorectal surgery. Br J Anaesth. 2013;111(4):607–11.
98. Hartley RA, Pichel AC, Grant SW, Hickey GL, Lancaster PS, Wisely NA, et al. Preoperative cardiopulmonary exercise testing and risk of early mortality following abdominal aortic aneurysm repair. Br J Surg. 2012;99(11):1539–46.
99. Kaibori M, Ishizaki M, Matsui K, Nakatake R, Sakaguchi T, Habu D, et al. Assessment of preoperative exercise capacity in hepatocellular carcinoma patients with chronic liver injury undergoing hepatectomy. BMC Gastroenterol. 2013;13:119.
100. Carlisle J, Swart M. Mid-term survival after abdominal aortic aneurysm surgery predicted by cardiopulmonary exercise testing. Br J Surg. 2007;94(8):966–9.
101. Thompson AR, Peters N, Lovegrove RE, Ledwidge S, Kitching A, Magee TR, et al. Cardiopulmonary exercise testing provides a predictive tool for early and late outcomes in abdominal aortic aneurysm patients. Ann R Coll Surg Engl. 2011;93(6):474–81.
102. Licker M, Schnyder J-M, Frey J-G, Diaper J, Cartier V, Inan C, et al. Impact of aerobic exercise capacity and procedure-related factors in lung cancer surgery. Eur Respir J. 2011;37(5):1189–98.
103. Older P, Hall A, Hader R. Cardiopulmonary exercise testing as a screening test for perioperative management of major surgery in the elderly. Chest. 1999;116(2):355–62.
104. Moyes LH, McCaffer CJ, Carter RC, Fullarton GM, Mackay CK, Forshaw MJ. Cardiopulmonary exercise testing as a predictor of complications in oesophagogastric cancer surgery. Ann R Coll Surg Engl. 2013;95(2):125–30.
105. Goetze JP. Biosynthesis of cardiac natriuretic peptides. Results Probl Cell Differ. 2010;50:97–120.
106. Clerico A, Recchia FA, Passino C, Emdin M. Cardiac endocrine function is an essential component of the homeostatic regulation network: physiological and clinical implications. Am J Physiol Heart Circ Physiol. 2006;290(1):H17–29.
107. Jamieson JD, Palade GE. Specific granules in atrial muscle cells. J Cell Biol. 1964;23:151–72.
108. Kisch B. Electron microscopy of the atrium of the heart. I Guinea Pig Exp Med Surg. 1956;14(2–3):99–112.

109. Vesely DL, de Bold AJ. Cardiac natriuretic peptides gene expression and secretion in inflammation. J Investig Med Off Publ Am Fed Clin Res. 2009;57(1):29–32.
110. Ma KK, Ogawa T, de Bold AJ. Selective upregulation of cardiac brain natriuretic peptide at the transcriptional and translational levels by pro-inflammatory cytokines and by conditioned medium derived from mixed lymphocyte reactions via p38 MAP kinase. J Mol Cell Cardiol. 2004;36(4):505–13.
111. Nishikimi T, Kuwahara K, Nakao K. Current biochemistry, molecular biology, and clinical relevance of natriuretic peptides. J Cardiol. 2011;57(2):131–40.
112. Walther T, Klostermann K, Heringer-Walther S, Schultheiss H-P, Tschöpe C, Stepan H. Fibrosis rather than blood pressure determines cardiac BNP expression in mice. Regul Pept. 2003;116(1–3):95–100.
113. Casals G, Ros J, Sionis A, Davidson MM, Morales-Ruiz M, Jiménez W. Hypoxia induces B-type natriuretic peptide release in cell lines derived from human cardiomyocytes. Am J Physiol Heart Circ Physiol. 2009;297(2):H550–5.
114. Chiu C-Z, Wang B-W, Chung T-H, Shyu K-G. Angiotensin II and the ERK pathway mediate the induction of myocardin by hypoxia in cultured rat neonatal cardiomyocytes. Clin Sci Lond Engl 1979. 2010;119(Pt 7):273–82.
115. Tóth M, Vuorinen KH, Vuolteenaho O, Hassinen IE, Uusimaa PA, Leppäluoto J, et al. Hypoxia stimulates release of ANP and BNP from perfused rat ventricular myocardium. Am J Phys. 1994;266(4 Pt 2):H1572–80.
116. Tan T, Scholz PM, Weiss HR. Hypoxia inducible factor-1 improves the negative functional effects of natriuretic peptide and nitric oxide signaling in hypertrophic cardiac myocytes. Life Sci. 2010;87(1–2):9–16.
117. Rodseth RN, Lurati Buse GA, Bolliger D, Burkhart CS, Cuthbertson BH, Gibson SC, et al. The predictive ability of pre-operative B-type natriuretic peptide in vascular patients for major adverse cardiac events: an individual patient data meta-analysis. J Am Coll Cardiol. 2011;58(5):522–9.
118. Karthikeyan G, Moncur RA, Levine O, Heels-Ansdell D, Chan MTV, Alonso-Coello P, et al. Is a pre-operative brain natriuretic peptide or N-terminal pro-B-type natriuretic peptide measurement an independent predictor of adverse cardiovascular outcomes within 30 days of noncardiac surgery? A systematic review and meta-analysis of observational studies. J Am Coll Cardiol. 2009;54(17):1599–606.
119. Biccard BM, Buse GAL, Burkhart C, Cuthbertson BH, Filipovic M, Gibson SC, et al. The influence of clinical risk factors on pre-operative B-type natriuretic peptide risk stratification of vascular surgical patients. Anaesthesia. 2012;67(1):55–9.
120. Poldermans D, Bax JJ, Boersma E, De Hert S, Eeckhout E, Fowkes G, et al. Guidelines for pre-operative cardiac risk assessment and perioperative cardiac management in non-cardiac surgery: the Task Force for Preoperative Cardiac Risk Assessment and Perioperative Cardiac Management in Non-cardiac Surgery of the European Society of Cardiology (ESC) and endorsed by the European Society of Anaesthesiology (ESA). Eur J Anaesthesiol. 2010;27(2):92–137.
121. Mahla E, Baumann A, Rehak P, Watzinger N, Vicenzi MN, Maier R, et al. N-terminal pro-brain natriuretic peptide identifies patients at high risk for adverse cardiac outcome after vascular surgery. Anesthesiology. 2007;106(6):1088–95.
122. Rodseth RN, Biccard BM, Chu R, Lurati Buse GA, Thabane L, Bakhai A, et al. Postoperative B-type natriuretic peptide for prediction of major cardiac events in patients undergoing non-cardiac surgery: systematic review and individual patient meta-analysis. Anesthesiology. 2013;119(2):270–83.
123. Rodseth RN, Biccard BM, Le Manach Y, Sessler DI, Lurati Buse GA, Thabane L, et al. The prognostic value of pre-operative and post-operative B-type natriuretic peptides in patients undergoing noncardiac surgery: B-type natriuretic peptide and N-terminal fragment of pro-B-type natriuretic peptide: a systematic review and individual patient data meta-analysis. J Am Coll Cardiol. 2014;63(2):170–80.

124. Ryding ADS, Kumar S, Worthington AM, Burgess D. Prognostic value of brain natriuretic peptide in noncardiac surgery: a meta-analysis. Anesthesiology. 2009;111(2):311–9.
125. Rodseth RN, Padayachee L, Biccard BM. A meta-analysis of the utility of pre-operative brain natriuretic peptide in predicting early and intermediate-term mortality and major adverse cardiac events in vascular surgical patients. Anaesthesia. 2008;63(11):1226–33.
126. Young Y-R, Sheu B-F, Li W-C, Hsieh T-M, Hung C-W, Chang S-S, et al. Predictive value of plasma brain natriuretic peptide for postoperative cardiac complications—a systemic review and meta-analysis. J Crit Care. 2014;29(4):696.e1–10.
127. Duceppe E, Parlow J, MacDonald P, Lyons K, McMullen M, Srinathan S, et al. Canadian cardiovascular society guidelines on perioperative cardiac risk assessment and management for patients who undergo noncardiac surgery. Can J Cardiol. 2017;33(1):17–32.
128. Kopec M, Duma A, Helwani MA, Brown J, Brown F, Gage BF, et al. Improving prediction of postoperative myocardial infarction with high-sensitivity cardiac troponin T and NT-proBNP. Anesth Analg. 2017;124(2):398–405.
129. Ndumele CE, Matsushita K, Sang Y, Lazo M, Agarwal SK, Nambi V, et al. N-Terminal pro-brain natriuretic peptide and heart failure risk among individuals with and without obesity: the Atherosclerosis Risk in Communities (ARIC) Study. Circulation. 2016;133(7):631–8.
130. Gregg LP, Adams-Huet B, Li X, Colbert G, Jain N, de Lemos JA, et al. Effect modification of chronic kidney disease on the association of circulating and imaging cardiac biomarkers with outcomes. J Am Heart Assoc. 2017;6(7):e005235.
131. Tromp J, Khan MAF, IJT K, Meyer S, de Boer RA, Jaarsma T, et al. Biomarker profiles in heart failure patients with preserved and reduced ejection fraction. J Am Heart Assoc. 2017;6(4):e003989.

Part II

Components of Prehabilitation

3 Cardiovascular Prehabilitation for Cancer Surgery

Priya Chockalingam

Abbreviations

ACEi	Angiotensin converting enzyme inhibitors
ARBs	Angiotensin receptor blockers
BP	Blood pressure
CABG	Coronary artery bypass graft
CAD	Coronary artery disease
CRS	Cardiotoxicity risk score
cTn	Cardiac troponin
CTRCD	Cancer therapy-related cardiac dysfunction
CVD	Cardiovascular disease
ECG	Electrocardiogram
HF	Heart failure
HFrEF	Heart failure with reduced ejection fraction
HRpEF	Heart failure with preserved ejection fraction
LV	Left ventricle
LVEF	Left ventricular ejection fraction
NT-pro BNP	N-terminal pro-B-type natriuretic peptide
PAD	Peripheral artery disease
PAH	Pulmonary arterial hypertension
PCI	Percutaneous coronary intervention
Top2β	Topoisomerase 2-beta
VEGF	Vascular endothelial growth factor
VHD	Valvular heart disease
VTE	Venous thromboembolism

P. Chockalingam (✉)
Preventive Cardiologist, Cardiac Wellness Institute, Chennai, Tamil Nadu, India
e-mail: priyachockalingam@cardiacwellnessinstitute.com

A. Chakraborty, A. Balakrishnan (eds.), *Prehabilitation for Cancer Surgery*,
https://doi.org/10.1007/978-981-16-6494-6_3

3.1 Introduction

Cardiovascular disease (CVD) remains a leading cause of death in cancer survivors (second only to cancer recurrence), largely attributable to exposure to chemotherapeutic agents, radiotherapy and immunomodulatory therapies used to treat patients with cancer, along with the emergence of new cardiovascular risk factors later in life. While metabolic derangements and deterioration in cardiovascular health can occur due to cancer therapies, the presence of cancer itself can cause cardiometabolic derangements and systemic inflammation, which in turn can lead to CVD [1].

The first example of cardiac cancer treatment toxicity was described in relation to anthracyclines more than 50 years ago [2]. The concept that chemotherapy and radiotherapy may induce potentially deadly cardiovascular side effects developed progressively and cardiologists were charged with the management of patients with these complications. The terms Cardio-Oncology and Onco-Cardiology have both been used to describe this field, encompassing a continuum of cardiovascular risk stratification, prevention and treatment that spans the timeline from cancer diagnosis into survivorship, and depends on close collaboration across cardiology and oncology specialties. This type of integrated care as provided by multidisciplinary cardio-oncology teams is now recognized as the state-of-the-art practice for prevention, diagnosis and treatment of CVD associated with cancer therapy [3, 4]. While the field of cardio-oncology has developed to evaluate and treat heart diseases in people before, during and after cancer therapy, the field of preventive cardio-oncology or cardiovascular prehabilitation is shifting from a reactive to a proactive model that focuses on:

- Early diagnosis of CVD and its risk factors in cancer patients.
- CVD risk mitigation planning prior to initiating cancer therapies.
- Multi-modal approach to optimize cardiorespiratory function from the time of cancer detection.

3.2 Shared Risk Factors

The knowledge of shared risk factors between various cancers and CVD has paved the way for cardiovascular risk assessment in tandem with screening for or managing these cancers [5].

For instance, unhealthy diet and obesity are implicated in the causation of breast cancer, smoking leads to lung cancer, and a diet rich in red meat and deficient in fibre contributes to colorectal cancers, and each of these lifestyle risk factors are closely associated with CVD. Metabolic syndrome, which refers to the clustering of various cardiometabolic risk factors such as obesity, hypertension, dyslipidaemia and insulin resistance, has been found to be associated both causally and prognostically with several cancers [6]. And our understanding of the role of psychosocial factors such as health behaviour, socioeconomic status, stress, depression, personality traits and life events in the development and progression of cancer is currently evolving [7]. In other words, each of the nine potentially modifiable risk factors

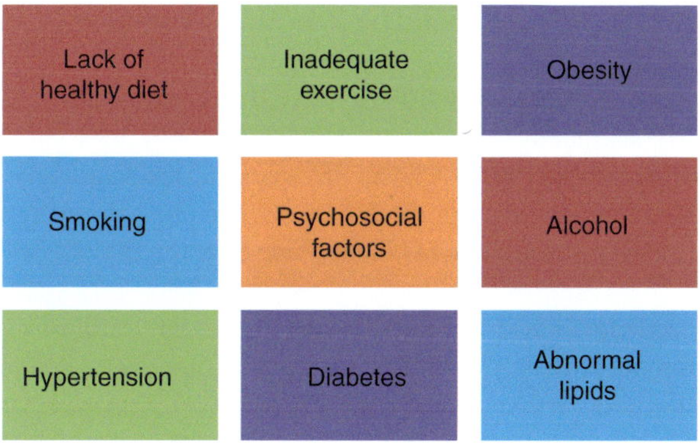

Fig. 3.1 Potentially modifiable risk factors common to CVD and cancer

implicated in myocardial infarction is also known to be associated with cancer (Fig. 3.1) [8].

Interestingly, primordial prevention of CVD and several cancers involves education, awareness and behaviour modification pertaining to diet, exercise, substance abuse, body weight management and psychosocial factors. The cardiovascular impact of therapies for cancer (and potentially the presence of cancer itself) can superimpose on pre-existing CVD risk factors to worsen cardiovascular outcomes, which is described as the 'multiple hit' hypothesis.

While there is clear evidence on the higher rate of CVD in cancer patients, the higher incidence of cancer in the heart failure population has led to the question 'can heart failure cause cancer?' And there is evidence mounting to prove that beyond shared root causes and molecular pathways, heart failure may actually promote cancerous growth [9, 10].

3.3 CVD Risk Mitigation

Surgical treatment for cancer is often preceded by chemotherapy and/or radiotherapy and both are known to have acute as well as chronic toxicity on the cardiovascular system [2].

Possible cardiovascular complications of chemotherapy and/or radiotherapy are [11]:

- Myocardial dysfunction and heart failure (HF).
- Coronary artery disease (CAD).
- Valvular heart disease (VHD).
- Arrhythmias—acquired long QT syndrome, atrial fibrillation and atrioventricular blocks.
- Arterial hypertension.
- Thromboembolic disease.
- Peripheral vascular disease and stroke.
- Pulmonary hypertension.
- Pericarditis.

3.3.1 Myocardial Dysfunction and Heart Failure (HF)

3.3.1.1 Pathophysiology, Incidence and Clinical Presentation

Myocardial dysfunction and HF are the commonest cardiovascular causes of mortality and morbidity due to cancer therapies and are frequently described as 'cardiotoxicity'. The time point when cardiotoxicity becomes clinically manifest varies substantially. Some cancer treatments induce side effects early after exposure while others generate cardiac injuries resulting in clinical problems only years later. In addition, some cancer drugs like anthracyclines can induce late cardiomyopathy by progressive cardiac remodelling as a late consequence of earlier myocyte damage, while others may cause transient cardiac dysfunction without long-term consequences. The fact that patients often receive multiple cancer drugs and radiation with the potential for cardiotoxic effects from interactions of the various therapeutic modalities makes the prediction of long-term cardiovascular prognosis challenging [11]. The incidence of left ventricular (LV) dysfunction with some of the more toxic chemotherapeutic agents is as below:

Anthracyclines (dose dependent)

- Doxorubicin (Adriamycin).
  400 mg/m^2—3 to 5%
  550 mg/m^2—7 to 26%
  700 mg/m^2—18 to 48%
- Idarubicin (>90 mg/m^2) —5 to 18%.
- Epirubicin (>900 mg/m^2)—0.9 to 11.4%.

Alkylating agents

- Cyclophosphamide 7–28%.
- Ifosfamide.
  <10 g/m^2—0.5%
  12.5 to 16 g/m^2—17%.

Antimetabolites

- Clofarabine—27%.

Monoclonal antibodies

- Trastuzumab—1.7 to 20.1%.

Small molecule tyrosine kinase inhibitors

- Sunitinib—2.7 to 19%.
- Pazopanib—7 to 11%.
- Sorafenib—4 to 8%.

Proteasome inhibitors

- Carfilzomib—11 to 25%.
- Bortezomib—2 to 5%.

The primary cause of chemotherapy-induced cardiotoxicity is anthracycline compounds, which are used extensively to treat lymphoma, sarcoma, breast cancer and paediatric leukaemia. Anthracycline-induced cardiomyopathy has been classified as early or late onset using a cut-off of 1 year after anthracycline treatment. While the cumulative incidences of cardiac events peak at 1 year after anthracycline treatment, late effects may manifest after several years (median of 7 years after treatment). Anthracycline-induced cardiac injury became a prototype of what later was named Type-I cancer therapy-related cardiac dysfunction (CTRCD), characterized by ultrastructural evidence of necrosis, dose-dependence and largely irreversible effects on cardiac muscle. In contrast, Type II CTRCD is associated with the use of molecularly targeted cancer therapeutics whose effects are not dose related, do not have molecular evidence of necrosis, and are often reversible [12].

The most commonly accepted pathophysiological mechanism of anthracycline-induced cardiotoxicity is the oxidative stress hypothesis, which suggests that the generation of reactive oxygen species and lipid peroxidation of the cell membrane damage cardiomyocytes. Topoisomerase 2-beta (Top2β), an enzyme that in humans is encoded by the *TOP2B* gene, was recently revealed as another key mediator of anthracycline-induced cardiotoxicity. Top2β deletion from the heart protects mice from anthracycline-induced cardiomyopathy, which strongly favours this hypothesis. Doxorubicin disrupts the normal catalytic cycle of topoisomerase Top 2β, causing deoxyribonucleic acid double-stranded breaks. It further changes the transcriptome, leading to defective mitochondrial biogenesis and increase in reactive oxygen species. As a result, cardiomyocytes show myofibrillar disarray and vacuolization. Dexrazoxane was shown to bind to Top2β to prevent anthracycline binding. Other mechanisms, for example, iron accumulation in haemochromatosis amplifies the reactive oxygen species response during anthracycline treatment [13].

Risk factors for anthracycline-related cardiotoxicity include lifetime cumulative dose, infusion regimen and any condition that increases cardiac susceptibility, including pre-existing cardiac disease, hypertension, concomitant use of other chemotherapies or mediastinal radiation therapy, older age (>65 years) and paediatric population (<18 years).

Other conventional chemotherapies that can induce myocardial dysfunction and HF are cyclophosphamide, cisplatin, ifosfamide and taxanes (paclitaxel and docetaxel). Cyclophosphamide cardiotoxicity is relatively rare and is primarily seen in patients receiving high doses (>140 mg/kg) before bone marrow transplantation.

Radiotherapy is known to cause radiation-induced cardiotoxicity in which marked interstitial myocardial fibrosis is common and the relative risk of fatal cardiovascular events is high. In patients with breast cancer treated in the 1980s and 1990s, the risk of cardiotoxicity was highest in patients treated with both left breast radiotherapy and cardiotoxic chemotherapy, suggesting a synergistic effect on cardiac risk. Systolic dysfunction is generally observed when radiotherapy is combined with anthracyclines. HF may also be aggravated by concomitant radiation-induced VHD and CAD, and can evolve over years.

3.3.1.2 Screening, Prevention and Management

The first step to identify patients at increased risk for cardiotoxicity is a careful baseline assessment of cardiovascular risk factors including a thorough search for heart failure, asymptomatic LV dysfunction, evidence of CAD, VHD, hypertensive heart disease, cardiomyopathy (dilated, hypertrophic, restricted), cardiac sarcoidosis and any significant arrhythmias. Risk assessment should include clinical history (prior anthracycline use and/or radiotherapy to chest and mediastinum), examination and baseline measurement of cardiac function.

Cardiac biomarkers (natriuretic peptides or troponins) may be considered in addition, preferably using the same assay that will be used during follow-up measurements, to increase comparability. It is critical to detect subclinical cardiac abnormalities, which may influence clinical decisions regarding the choice of chemotherapy, indication for cardioprotection or increased surveillance frequency (e.g. asymptomatic LV dysfunction). Finally, baseline assessment of cardiovascular risk factors allows appropriate interpretation of subsequent results/changes during regular monitoring.

Strategies for screening and detection of cardiotoxicity include cardiac imaging (echocardiography, nuclear imaging, cardiac magnetic resonance) and biomarkers (troponin, natriuretic peptides). The choice of modalities depends upon local expertise and availability. Patients at high risk for developing cardiotoxicity should be examined by a cardiologist with expertise in this field or, if necessary, by a cardio-oncology specialist team.

The Cardiotoxicity Risk Score (CRS) proposed by Mayo Clinic takes both patient and treatment risk factors into account (Table 3.1). This model addresses the a priori risk of developing CTRCD. Patients with a CRS score of ≥4 could benefit from cardiological consultation during and after chemotherapeutic treatment, and those with high-risk scores should be closely monitored during and after treatment [14]. However, this risk model has not been validated in a prospective setting and its real clinical value remains to be determined.

Due to the minimal invasiveness, limited costs, and low inter-observer variability, biomarkers constitute an appealing approach to aid in the early detection of subclinical cardiotoxicity (Fig. 3.2). Most studies have assessed the potential of

Table 3.1 Cardiotoxicity Risk Score (CRS) [14]

Medication-related risk[a]	Examples
High (risk score 4)	Anthracyclines; trastuzumab; cyclophosphamide; 5-fluorouracil
Intermediate (risk score 2)	Pertuzumab; vinblastine; capecitabine; ponatinib
Low (risk score 1)	Bevacizumab; imatinib
Rare (risk score 0)	Carboplatin; fludarabine; paclitaxel; rituximab
Patient-related risk factors (1 point per item)	
• Cardiomyopathy or heart failure • Coronary artery disease or equivalent (including peripheral artery disease) • Hypertension • Diabetes mellitus • Prior or concurrent anthracyclines • Prior or concurrent chest irradiation • Age < 15 years or > 65 years • Female gender	
Overall risk by CRS and intensity of monitoring	
>6	Very high
5–6	High
3–4	Intermediate
1–2	Low
0	Very Low

[a]The highest medication-related risk score (e.g. 4, 2, 1 or 0) is used for calculation of the CRS

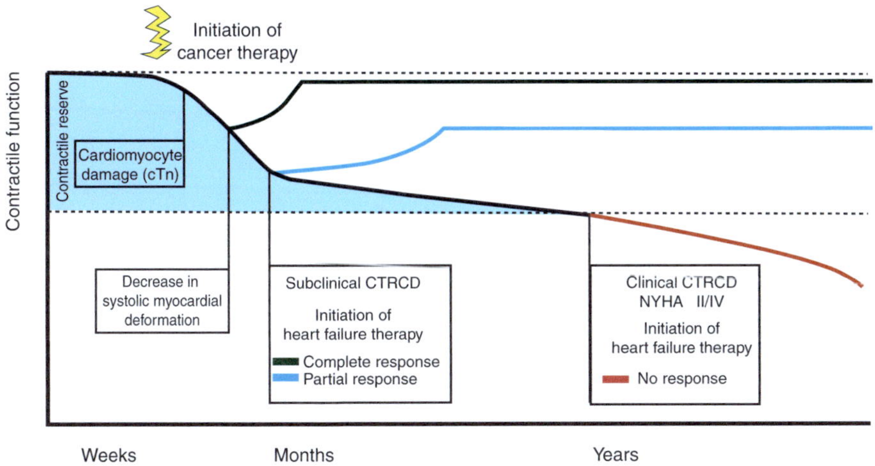

Fig. 3.2 Time frame of detection and treatment of cardiotoxicity
Early initiation of heart failure treatment (green, blue line) leads to better outcomes regarding recovery of contractile function. Initiation of heart failure treatment at time when symptoms are present (red line) results in poor outcomes regarding recovery of cardiac function. Reproduced with permission from Teske et al. [11]
cTn Cardiac troponin, *CTRCD* chemotherapy related cardiac dysfunction, *NYHA* New York Heart Association classification

classical cardiac biomarkers like cardiac troponin (cTn) and N-terminal pro-B-type natriuretic peptide (NT-pro BNP). Troponins seem to be the most promising candidates, both in patients treated with anthracyclines and various agents used for targeted therapy (e.g. trastuzumab). Nevertheless, repeated sampling is currently necessary to detect cTn elevations, as the optimal timing to reach maximal sensitivity has not yet been established [15]. Other biomarkers including microRNA, myeloperoxidase and markers of extracellular matrix turnover are more specific for detecting both acute and chronic effects of anthracyclines and other chemotherapy regimens. In other targeted cancer therapies including trastuzumab, vascular endothelial growth factor inhibitors (e.g. pazopanib, sorafenib, sunitinib) and proteasome inhibitors (e.g. bortezomib, carfilzomib and ixazomib) treatment surveillance using natriuretic peptides has more evidence for detecting subclinical LV dysfunction, predating the development of symptoms and signs consistent with HF [16].

Management of Cardiotoxicity Before Cardiotoxic Cancer Treatment
If baseline cardiotoxicity risk is high due to pre-existing CVD, previous anthracycline-containing chemotherapy or poorly controlled cardiovascular risk factors, then a very stringent optimization of risk factor control has to be obtained and a prophylactic cardioprotective medication regimen should be considered (Fig. 3.3). Cancer patients with low baseline risk but planned for high total cumulative anthracycline doses (>250–300 mg/m^2 doxorubicin or equivalent) may also be considered for prophylactic cardioprotective medication.

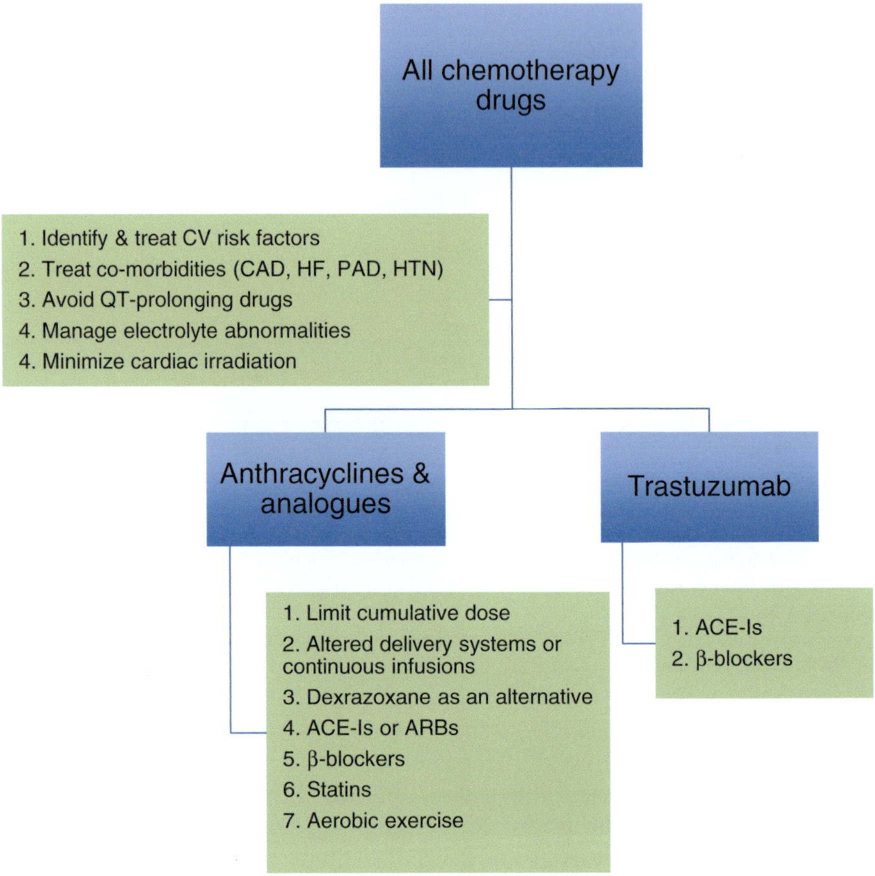

Fig. 3.3 Strategies to reduce chemotherapy-induced cardiotoxicity before initiating cancer treatment

One study randomized adults with haematological malignancies scheduled for high-dose anthracycline chemotherapy to enalapril and carvedilol at HF therapy doses versus normal care, starting cardiac drugs before the first cycle of chemotherapy. At the 6-month follow-up, there was a decrease in LV ejection fraction (LVEF) observed in the control arm which was not observed in patients receiving both cardioprotective drugs [17]. Whether patients with a low baseline risk treated with anthracyclines also profit from preventive treatment with angiotensin converting enzyme inhibitors (ACEi), angiotensin receptor blockers (ARBs) or beta-blocker therapy remains controversial, and no recommendation is available at this time. In a recent prospective, placebo-controlled trial in patients with early breast cancer treated with anthracyclines, the ARB candesartan protected against early decline in LVEF, which was not seen in the placebo or beta-blocker therapy groups [18].

Cancer patients with pre-existing clinical HF or significant LV dysfunction at baseline should be managed, if possible, by a specialist cardio-oncology team, and the risk versus benefit regarding selection of chemotherapy options should be discussed with the oncology team. Options include selection of an alternative non-cardiotoxic chemotherapy, anthracycline preparations with lower cardiotoxicity (e.g. liposomal doxorubicin), reduced-dose schedules and/or additional cardioprotective drugs (e.g. ACEi, beta-blockers, aldosterone antagonists or dexrazoxane). Dexrazoxane, an intracellular iron-chelating agent, prevents the reduction in LV function caused by doxorubicin. Currently the European license for dexrazoxane use is only for adults with advanced or metastatic breast cancer who have received a cumulative dose of >300 mg/m^2 doxorubicin or >540 mg/m^2 epirubicin and would benefit from continued anthracycline-based therapy.

Management of Cardiotoxicity During and Following Cancer Treatment
Cancer patients presenting with clinical HF, either reduced ejection fraction (HFrEF) or preserved ejection fraction (HFpEF), during or following cancer treatment should be treated according to current ESC guidelines for HF [19]. Interruption of cancer treatment may be warranted and decision on further management should be based on severity of LV dysfunction, clinical HF status, cancer prognosis and efficacy of the cancer therapy. If rechallenge with a previously cardiotoxic drug is planned, continuation with cardioprotective drug therapy such as ACEi and beta blockers is strongly recommended. Other potential options include the selection of preparations with a potentially less cardiotoxic profile (e.g. liposomal doxorubicin) or possibly other less cardiotoxic drugs (e.g. dexrazoxane) when indicated.

Treatment response in patients with a decline of LVEF to ≤45% has shown to be highly dependent on the timing of treatment initiation. The response rate is as high as 64% among patients with CTRCD that received heart failure treatment <2 months after detection of LV impairment and decreased to only 7% after 4–6 months. Remarkably, no response was observed in patients with CTRCD that received treatment ≥6 months after the last chemotherapeutic cycle (Fig. 3.4a). Detecting the development of CTRCD as soon as possible guides the optimal timing of treatment initiation, since this seems to be particularly crucial for treatment response. However, in a follow-up study by the same group, a large proportion of patients did not show recovery of cardiac function despite early initiation of conventional heart failure treatment. Only 11% showed full recovery to a mean LVEF of 61%. Cardiac function was partially restored in 71% of the patients, to a mean LVEF of 54%. Notably, 18% of patients did not respond to treatment, with a mean LVEF at the end of the study of 38% (Fig. 3.4b). Cardiac outcome for partial and non-responders is significantly worse, including heart failure requiring hospitalization and cardiac related death (Fig. 3.4c).

Sacubitril/valsartan (LCZ-696) is a combined neprilysin inhibitor and angiotensin AT1 receptor blocker approved in recent years for the treatment of chronic heart failure with reduced ejection fraction. In patients with refractory CTRCD and in experimental studies, treatment with sacubitril/valsartan has been shown to be well tolerated and to improve echocardiographic functional and structural parameters, NT-pro BNP levels and symptomatic status [20–22].

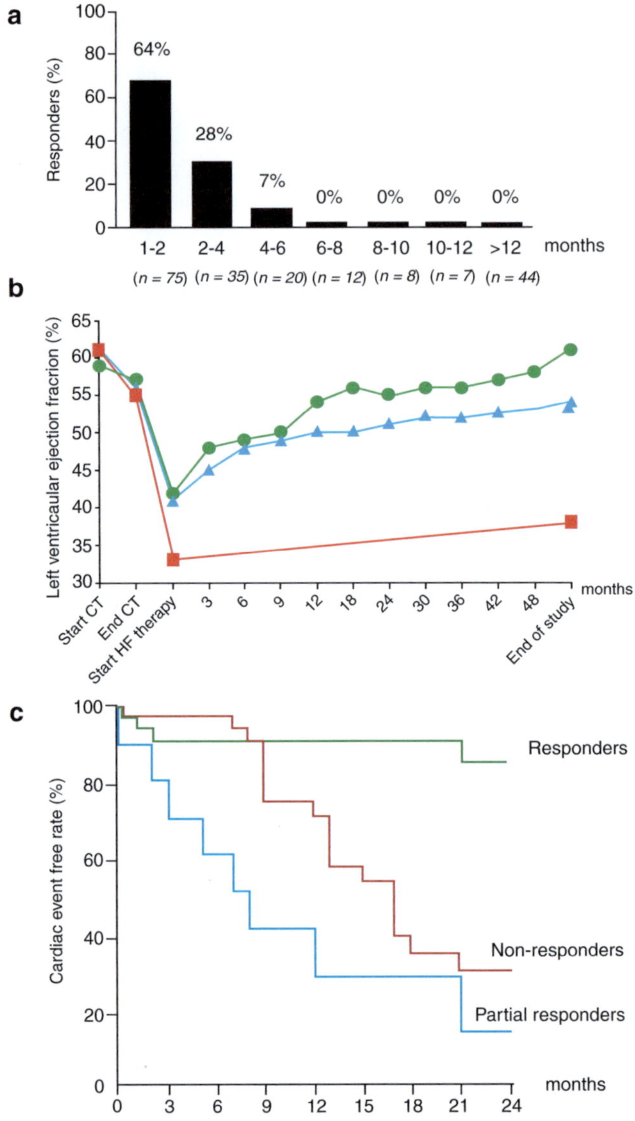

Fig. 3.4 Response and outcome to heart failure (HF) treatment in patients with chemotherapy-related cardiac dysfunction. (**a**) Percentage of (partial) responders according to the time elapsed from diagnosing left ventricular dysfunction and start of HF therapy. (**b**) Left ventricular ejection fraction in patients with cardiotoxicity and with no (*square/red*), partial (*triangle/blue*) or full (*dot/green*) recovery following heart failure therapy. (**c**) Cumulative cardiac event rate during follow-up. Reproduced with permission from Teske et al. [11]. *CT* Chemotherapy

Figure 3.5 outlines the roadmap of a working cardio-oncology unit in The Netherlands. The aim of this unit is to improve cardiac outcome in oncology patients by

- Identifying patients at high risk of developing CTRCD before chemotherapeutic treatment is initiated.

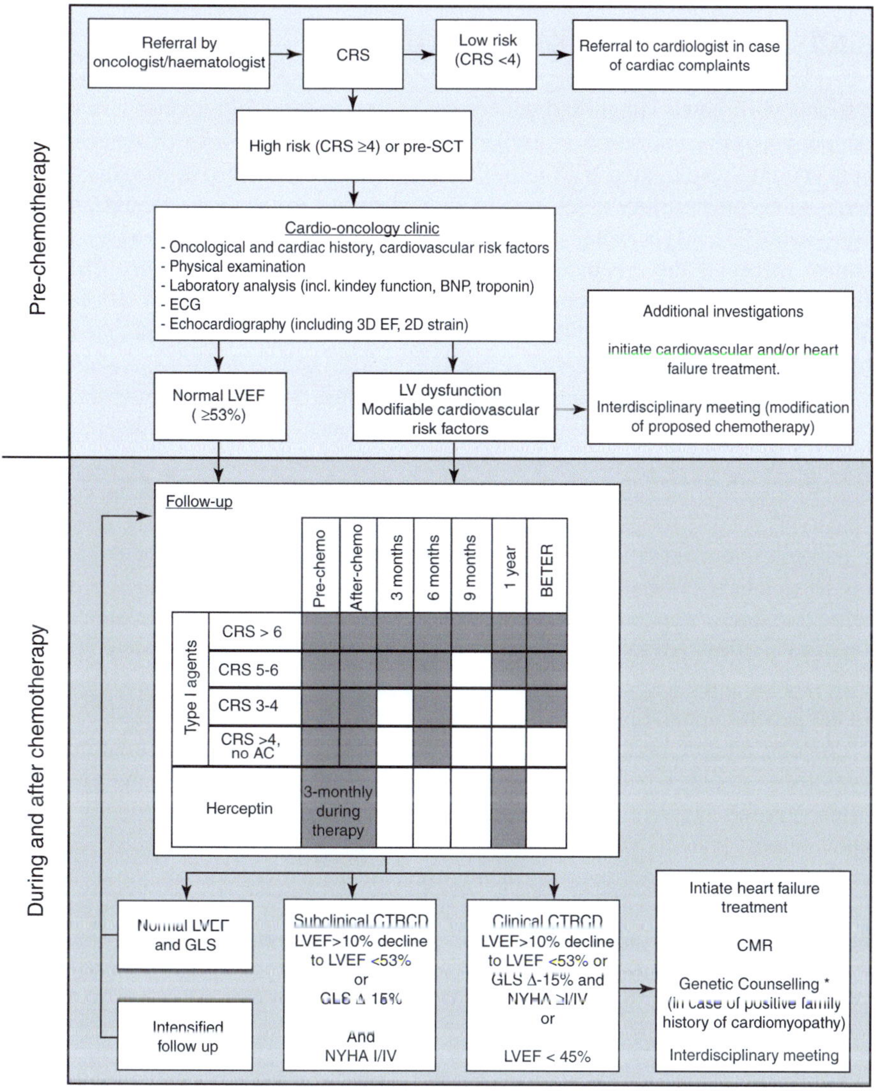

Fig. 3.5 Cardio-oncology care at the University Medical Centre Utrecht, The Netherlands. *AC* Anthracyclines, *BNP* brain natriuretic peptide, *CMR* cardiac magnetic resonance, *CRS* Cardiotoxicity Risk Score, *CTRCD* chemotherapy-related cardiac dysfunction, *GLS* global longitudinal strain, *LVEF* left ventricular ejection fraction, *SCT* stem-cell transplantation. *To be considered, depending on local policy Reproduced with permission from Teske et al. [11]

- Screening and monitoring high-risk patients to enable early detection of (sub-clinical) cardiac dysfunction.
- Initiating early treatment in order to improve overall cardiovascular outcome.

Patients are monitored up to 1 year after the end of chemotherapy, as a majority of the patients described in the literature develop CTRCD within this time frame.

3.3.2 Coronary Artery Disease (CAD)

Patients with newly diagnosed cancer are at two to threefold greater risk of incident myocardial infarction or ischaemic stroke compared with patients without cancer, and those treated with radiotherapy have an absolute risk increase of 76.4 cases of coronary artery disease and 125.5 cases of cardiac death per 100,000 person-years [23]. Myocardial ischaemia and infarction may be caused by several cancer therapies the mechanism of which includes endothelial injury (fluoropyrimidines), vasospasm, procoagulant status (Vascular endothelial growth factor—VEGF—inhibitors), arterial thrombosis (platinum compounds) and plaque rupture (radiotherapy) [11].

Supradiaphragmal and, in certain patient groups, even infradiaphragmal radiotherapy may be associated with a higher incidence of ischaemic heart disease through the development of severe atherosclerotic and non-atherosclerotic disease, complicated by plaque rupture and thrombosis, and potentially with coronary spasm. The most exposed coronaries are the left anterior descending during left breast irradiation and the left main stem, circumflex and right coronary arteries during treatment for Hodgkin lymphoma. Radiation-related cardiac disease in patients with lymphoma typically manifests 15–20 years after the initial treatment, and younger patients are more susceptible than older patients. The risk of myocardial infarction in patients treated for Hodgkin lymphoma is two to sevenfold higher than in the general population, with a cumulative incidence of 10% at 30 years.

A long latency period with asymptomatic CAD after radiation treatment and symptoms arising several years after the initial cancer therapy is common. CAD often presents atypically and the prevalence of silent ischaemia is higher than in conventional patients with CAD possibly because of concomitant neurotoxicity of radiotherapy, or chemotherapy affecting the patient's perception of angina. Sudden cardiac death in irradiated patients has been reported and linked to diffuse intimal hyperplasia of all coronary arteries or to significant left main stenosis.

The choice of optimal revascularization strategy by either a cardiac surgical procedure or percutaneous coronary intervention (PCI) in cancer patients is often complex and will depend on type and severity of CAD, age, comorbidities, bleeding risk and overall cancer prognosis. Around 1 in 10 patients undergoing PCI in the United States has current or previous cancer, with worse short-term clinical outcomes compared with patients without cancer. The prognostic impact of cancer is specific both for the type of cancer and the presence of metastases and whether the diagnosis is historical or current [24]. In fact, a concomitant cancer diagnosis is associated with a conservative medical management strategy for acute myocardial infarction, and worse clinical outcomes, compared to patients without cancer [25]. Among those undergoing coronary artery bypass graft (CABG) surgery, the prevalence of comorbid cancer has steadily increased. Outside of major bleeding, these patients appear to share similar outcomes to those without cancer indicating that CABG utilization should not be declined in cancer patients when otherwise indicated [26].

3.3.3 Valvular Heart Disease (VHD)

VHD in cancer patients is usually not a direct effect of chemotherapy but rather may be due to pre-existing valve lesions, radiotherapy, infective endocarditis and secondary to LV dysfunction. Around 10% of patients receiving radiotherapy are reportedly affected by radiation-induced VHD, which includes fibrosis and calcification of the aortic root, aortic valve cusps, mitral valve annulus and the base and mid portions of the mitral valve leaflets, sparing the mitral valve tips and commissures [11].

Echocardiography is the modality of choice for assessment, and 3D echocardiography may be useful, particularly for the evaluation of mitral valve commissures. Baseline and repeated echocardiography after radiation therapy involving the heart are recommended for the diagnosis and follow-up of VHD. Cardiac surgery is also frequently challenging in such patients because of mediastinal fibrosis, impaired wound healing and associated coronary artery, myocardial and pericardial disease. Transcatheter valve implantation (e.g. transcatheter aortic valve implantation) may be a suitable option in patients in need of valve replacements.

3.3.4 Arrhythmias

Patients with cancer may experience a wide spectrum of cardiac arrhythmias, including sinus tachycardia, bradyarrhythmias or tachyarrhythmias, and conduction defects. Arrhythmias can be present at baseline in 16–36% of cancer patients [11].

QT prolongation can be caused by cancer therapies, electrolyte disturbances, predisposing factors and concomitant medications (e.g. anti-emetics, cardiac medications, antibiotics, psychotropes) and can lead to life-threatening arrhythmias such as torsade de pointes. Arsenic trioxide, which is used to treat some leukaemias and myelomas, prolongs the QT interval in 26–93% of patients, and life-threatening ventricular tachyarrhythmias is not uncommon.

Arrhythmias in patients with cancer can occur before, during and shortly after treatment. Management should be individualized and decisions on the use of anti-arrhythmic drugs or device therapy (implantable or external wearable cardioverter defibrillators) should consider the competing risks of cardiac- and cancer-related life expectancy, quality of life and complication risks. Electrocardiogram (ECG) and electrolyte monitoring during treatment should be considered at baseline, 7–15 days after initiation or changes in dose, monthly during the first 3 months and then periodically during treatment depending on the chemotherapy drug and patient status. Patients experiencing diarrhoea should be monitored more frequently, and those receiving treatment with arsenic trioxide should be monitored weekly with ECG. Treatment discontinuation or alternative regimens should be considered if the QTc is >500 ms, QTc prolongation is >60 ms or dysrhythmias are encountered.

3.3.5 Arterial Hypertension

Hypertension is a frequent, and arguably the most common, comorbidity in patients with cancer and can also be a causative factor, such as in renal cancer. VEGF inhibitors have a high risk (11–45%) of inducing new hypertension or destabilizing previously controlled hypertension, including severe hypertension in 2–20% of cases. VEGF inhibition may also cause renal thrombotic microangiopathy [11].

All patients should undergo a formal evaluation and documentation of pretreatment risk for CVD. Blood pressure (BP) values and proteinuria should be assessed before initiation of treatment, and if hypertension is present (BP ≥ 140/90) antihypertensive treatment should be started first. The purpose of this assessment is to identify patients at high risk for chemotherapy-induced hypertension, especially if VEGF inhibitors are being considered. There is evidence that pre-existing hypertension in cancer patients confers worse prognosis with increasing mortality. The main goal of treatment is to reduce BP to <140/90. In high-risk patients, particularly those with diabetes or chronic kidney disease, stricter targets should be utilized aiming for <130/80. In patients already taking antihypertensive medication, adherence to treatment should be initially verified and compliance ensured. In patients adherent to medication where the BP is still above their target range, a second agent should be introduced. Hypertension should not preclude initiation of chemotherapy unless the treating physician deems the risk of hypertension too high [27].

Aggressive pharmacological management of hypertension is recommended with ACEi or ARBs, beta-blockers and non-dihydropyridine calcium channel blockers (amlodipine, felodipine) as first-line therapies. ACEi and beta-blockers are the preferred antihypertensive drugs in patients with HF or at risk of HF or LV dysfunction. Because decreased nitric oxide signalling plays a key role in the pathogenesis of hypertension, drugs that increase nitric oxide signalling, such as the beta1-blocker nebivolol, may represent a valuable option in this population. Other beta-blockers with vasodilatory effects, such as carvedilol, can be considered. Diltiazem and verapamil inhibit cytochrome P450 3A4, and because many VEGF inhibitors are a substrate of this isoenzyme, this combination results in increased drug plasma levels and should therefore be avoided. Inhibitors of phosphodiesterase-5, such as sildenafil and tadalafil, may also offer an antihypertensive therapy option, although available data are limited in patients with arterial hypertension. Diuretics should not be used as first-line therapy due to their risk of electrolyte depletion and consequent QT prolongation.

3.3.6 Thromboembolic Disease

Tumour cells can trigger coagulation through different pathways, including procoagulant, antifibrinolytic and pro-aggregating activities; release of pro-inflammatory and pro-angiogenic cytokines and interaction with vascular and blood cells through adhesion molecules. Intra-arterial thrombotic events are rare in patients with cancer, occurring mostly in metastatic pancreatic, breast, colorectal and lung cancers, under anthracyclines and taxane- and platinum-based chemotherapies, and affected patients have a poor prognosis. Venous thrombosis and venous thromboembolism (VTE) occur frequently in patients with cancer, may affect up to 20% of hospitalized patients and are frequently under-recognized. They can be related to chemotherapy, including its administration route (use of indwelling venous catheters), and also to the cancer itself and the patient's previous risk of venous thrombosis. As VTE is the most common cause of death after surgery for cancer, antithrombotic prophylaxis should be given for a minimum of 4 weeks after surgery [11].

The decision to administer anticoagulation for VTE prevention in patients with cancer should always take into consideration the patient's bleeding risk and life expectancy, both of which may change over time warranting periodic reassessment. Treatment of a confirmed episode of acute VTE in haemodynamically stable patients consists of low-molecular-weight heparin given over a period of 3–6 months. As cancer is a strong risk factor for VTE recurrence, chronic anticoagulation after the acute phase of treatment, and until the cancer is considered cured, should be considered. The choice of anticoagulation discontinuation or maintenance under low-molecular-weight heparin or switching to Vitamin K antagonists should be discussed on an individual basis after considering the cancer therapy success, the risk of VTE recurrence and bleeding, as well as the patient's preference. A vena cava filter, either definitive or retractable, may be implanted when anticoagulation is contraindicated or failing. However, the risk of filter thrombosis and occlusion leading to distal propagation of thrombosis with post-thrombotic syndrome should be considered.

3.3.7 Peripheral Vascular Disease and Stroke

Severe atherosclerotic and non-atherosclerotic peripheral artery disease (PAD) in the lower extremities can occur (in up to 30%) in patients treated with nilotinib, ponatinib or tyrosine kinase inhibitor used for chronic myeloid leukaemia, even in the absence of CVD risk factors, although the latter increases the likelihood of PAD. PAD can occur as early as in the first months of therapy or as a late effect several years after treatment. Other cancer therapy-related peripheral arterial toxicity includes Raynaud's phenomenon and ischaemic stroke (i.e. with L-asparaginase, cisplatin, methotrexate, 5-FU and paclitaxel) [11].

The risk of stroke more than doubles after mediastinal, cervical or cranial radiotherapy. Endothelial damage and thrombus formation may occur after irradiation of cerebral small vessels. In medium or large vessels, three mechanisms are described: vasa vasorum occlusions with medial necrosis and fibrosis; adventitial fibrosis and accelerated atherosclerosis, leading to increased carotid stiffness and intima-media thickness and advanced atherosclerosis (occurring >10 years after radiotherapy). Similar consequences are reported for the aorta and other peripheral arteries, including the subclavian and iliofemoral, with ischaemic limb symptoms.

The recommended assessment of PAD risk at baseline includes risk factor assessment, clinical examination and ankle–brachial index measurement.

Antiplatelet drugs should be considered mostly in symptomatic PAD. In case of severe PAD at baseline or during cancer therapy, revascularization should be individualized and discussed in a multidisciplinary meeting with experts in haematology, vascular surgery and cardio-oncology. Patients irradiated for head and neck cancer or lymphoma should undergo cerebrovascular ultrasound screening, especially beyond 5 years after irradiation. Duplex imaging may be considered at least every 5 years, or earlier and/or more frequently if the results of the first examination are abnormal.

3.3.8 Pulmonary Hypertension

Pulmonary hypertension is a rare but serious complication of some cancer agents and stem cell bone marrow transplantation. Imatinib, a tyrosine kinase inhibitor improves haemodynamics in patients with advanced pulmonary arterial hypertension (PAH). However, a drug of the same tyrosine kinase inhibitor family, dasatinib, used as second-line treatment for chronic myelogenous leukaemia, can induce severe precapillary pulmonary hypertension. This condition appears 8–40 months after exposure to dasatinib, with clinical and haemodynamic presentation suggestive of PAH. Unlike other forms of PAH, this is often reversible after drug discontinuation or replacement with another tyrosine kinase inhibitor, such as nilotinib [11].

3.3.9 Pericarditis

Acute pericarditis may occur with the use of several chemotherapeutic drugs (predominantly anthracyclines, but also cyclophosphamide, cytarabine and bleomycin). Pericarditis has become uncommon during radiotherapy and is usually associated with pericardiac mediastinal tumours. Acute pericarditis with typical chest pain, fever, ST-T changes and large effusions, even leading to tamponade, may develop 2–145 months after thoracic radiotherapy, with an absolute cumulative incidence of 2–5%. Transthoracic echocardiography is the method of choice for the evaluation of patients with suspected pericardial disease due to chemotherapy, but computerized tomography can be of help, particularly to identify calcification. Treatment of pericardial effusion consists primarily of non-steroidal anti-inflammatory drugs and colchicine. Pericardiocentesis may be required for large effusions and those causing haemodynamic compromise, eventually followed by surgical pericardial windowing [11].

3.3.10 Preoperative Cardiovascular Evaluation for Cancer Patients

Because cancer itself as well as the chemotherapy received prior to elective or emergency surgery puts the cancer patient at a higher cardiovascular risk category, a careful preoperative assessment is mandatory especially for detecting patients with subclinical heart failure. While heart failure and left ventricular dysfunction are the main findings of chemotherapy-related cardiotoxicity, QT prolongation, arrhythmias, myocardial ischaemia, pericarditis and/or myocarditis-like syndromes, and changes in blood pressure are other significant side effects. These overt or subclinical changes require a careful pre-, intra- and post-operative anaesthetic management in patients with history of anticancer therapy [28].

Similarly, an active pursuit for risk factors and evidence of stroke in preoperative cancer patients is imperative. Cancer patients are at a high risk of embolic stroke due to severe carotid artery stenosis. Head and neck cancer patients require special considerations due to higher incidence of carotid artery disease, particularly following the radiation treatment. Carotid duplex ultrasonography is the screening modality of choice for the detection of cervical carotid artery disease. Surgical carotid endarterectomy remains the gold-standard therapy for all symptomatic patients with severe carotid artery stenosis. Carotid stenting is a minimally invasive alternative treatment for symptomatic patients deemed high risk for carotid endarterectomy either due to medical or anatomical reasons [29]. When it comes to asymptomatic carotid artery stenosis, presence of any cancer, chronic obstructive pulmonary disease, congestive heart failure and chronic kidney disease (the 4C model) renders patients a higher risk of 5-year mortality and therefore a lower priority for aggressive management such as carotid endarterectomy [30].

3.4 Neoplastic and Paraneoplastic CVD

In the course of their evolution, cancers are known to directly or indirectly act on the endocardium, myocardium and pericardium as well as on the venous and arterial vascular trees [31]. Having elaborated on the cancer treatment induced CVD in the previous section, this section focuses on the rare but recognized effects of the malignancies themselves on the heart and blood vessels.

3.4.1 Cardiomyopathy Syndromes

Takotsubo cardiomyopathy, a clinical syndrome that generally presents as acute coronary syndrome or as an acute heart failure characterized by severe left ventricular systolic dysfunction in response to stress, is known to occur in association with several malignancies. The potential triggers for Takotsubo cardiomyopathy in cancer patients include emotional turmoil of the diagnosis, the inflammatory state of cancer, and the physical stress of various cancer treatments, including chemotherapy. In addition, it has been hypothesized that the circulating paraneoplastic mediators may modify the adrenoreceptors in cardiac tissue, leading to contractile dysfunction [32]. In a retrospective cohort study of 50 patients with Takotsubo cardiomyopathy, 18% had a previous history of malignancy, with another 14% developing malignancies over a follow-up of 3 years, supporting the hypothesis that this might be a paraneoplastic phenomenon [33].

Several anti-neoplastic agents, particularly 5-fluorouracil, capecitabine, combretastatin, rituximab, vascular endothelial growth factors inhibitors, other angiogenesis inhibitors and taxols have been implicated to be associated with this condition but it is currently an under-recognized and thus under-diagnosed disease entity among cancer patients receiving chemotherapy. Data suggests that coexisting malignancy has a significantly higher mortality, length of hospital stay and healthcare costs than Takotsubo cardiomyopathy without malignancy. The management of haemodynamically stable patients involves the initiation of standard guideline-directed medical therapy for heart failure with reduced ejection fraction, which includes beta-blocker therapy and an ACEi or ARB and diuretics as necessary to treat volume overload. In patients who require further cancer treatment, re-challenging with the culprit anti-neoplastic therapy poses a major clinical dilemma and should be escalated to the expertise of a cardio-oncology team [32].

While dermatomyositis, an idiopathic inflammatory myopathy has been established as one of the many paraneoplastic phenomena, there is anecdotal evidence to show that cardiac involvement can also occur with dermatomyositis. Persistently elevated cardiac troponin I despite the absence of cardiac symptoms and a subsequent negative ischaemic workup and normalization of cardiac enzymes after administration of intravenous steroids and treatment of the underlying renal cell carcinoma, suggest a paraneoplastic aetiology of cardiac manifestations [34].

3.4.2 Paraneoplastic Vasculitis, Vasculopathy and Hypercoagulability

The vasculitides comprise a group of heterogeneous autoimmune disorders characterized by inflammation of the blood vessels resulting in tissue ischaemia with end-organ damage. Paraneoplastic vasculitides are estimated to represent 2–5% of all vasculitides. The spectrum of clinical manifestations in vasculitis can range from localized single-organ involvement to life-threatening disease, with multiple major organs affected. The mechanistic associations between malignancy and vasculitis include a dysfunctional immune system associated with autoimmunity, cytotoxic drug therapies used for the management of vasculitis such as cyclophosphamide, and paraneoplastic phenomenon as in the case of polyarteritis nodosa with hairy cell leukaemia [35]. Although rare, vasculitis and cancer may occur concurrently. While the mechanisms by which cancer could result in manifestations of vasculitis are not clearly understood, numerous hypotheses have been suggested. These include impaired clearance of immune complexes, immunogenicity related to cancer antigens which may share homology to vascular antigens, or an immunologic response to either deposition of neoantigens or alteration of self-antigens in vessel walls.

Resolution of vasculitis following effective treatment of the putatively linked malignancy and recurrence of vasculitis concurrently with progression of cancer provides strong additional support for vasculitis being a true paraneoplastic syndrome [36]. It is important to note that:

- Malignancy may present initially with an acute vasculitis.
- 2.5–5% of patients with vasculitis have a related malignancy that may not be obvious at presentation.
- Chronic or persistent vasculitis with poor response to usually effective therapy, especially in elderly patients, should be evaluated bearing in mind the possibility of them being paraneoplastic.
- Recurrence of a tumour might be suspected when vasculitis appears or relapses in patients diagnosed as having malignancy.

Vasculopathies are rarer than vasculitides, but are associated with specific malignancies. Malignancy is an important risk factor for venous thromboembolism and about 5% of patients with an unprovoked venous thrombus are found to have an occult malignancy. Hypercoagulability is a well-documented neoplastic phenomenon with an increased risk of thrombosis in the setting of positive anti-phospholipids. Disseminated intravascular coagulation has been reported to occur in 6.8% of patients with solid organ tumours, most frequently in association with adenocarcinomas.

Most neoplastic and paraneoplastic vascular syndromes require no specific treatment outside of treatment of the underlying malignancy. The two key exceptions are primary angiitis of the central nervous system, because of its poor prognosis, and erythromelalgia, in which aspirin is an effective agent [37].

3.4.3 Metastatic Involvement of the Heart

Secondary tumours of the heart are rare but are anticipated to increase with extended survival of oncologic patients thanks to improved diagnostic and therapeutic modalities. The leading causes for cardiac metastasis are melanoma, carcinoma (lung, breast, oesophagus and rarely colorectal) and haematologic malignancies (leukaemia and lymphoma). Over 90% of secondary tumours of the heart are clinically silent, and are often diagnosed only postmortem. Therefore, early detection of these tumours is extremely challenging. Thus, if an oncologic patient presents with a new onset of cardiac symptoms, clinicians should be aware of the possibility of cardiac metastases and perform further investigations. Metastatic cardiac tumours may present as right-sided heart failure, arrhythmias, ischaemia and cardiac tamponade [38].

Diagnostic modalities include imaging (echocardiography, cardiac magnetic resonance, computerized tomography), tissue histology (malignant cells in pericardial effusions) and endomyocardial biopsy. Cardiac metastases are most often found in patients with multiple metastases and a profound burden of disseminated disease. Therefore, the most important goals of intervention are palliation of symptoms and prevention or delay of symptom recurrence [39].

3.5 Special Populations

Some special considerations are warranted in the paediatric, geriatric and pregnant population receiving cancer treatment [2].

3.5.1 Paediatric Cancer Population

The lifelong risk of childhood cancer survivors having cardiovascular toxicity from cancer therapies is eightfold higher than in the normal population. This population is continuously increasing due to the greatly enhanced survival rates. Anthracyclines and/or RT are the most used cardiotoxic agents for cancer in paediatric patients; therefore, lifelong follow-up of these patients is recommended.

3.5.2 Elderly Cancer Population

The elderly population is the other group most affected by the cardiotoxicity of cancer therapy, due largely to the prevalence of classic CVD risk factors and cardiovascular comorbidities or diabetes. Also, general illnesses such as kidney or liver dysfunction lead to pharmacokinetic or pharmacodynamic impairment with altered drug elimination. All of these conditions make the elderly patient more vulnerable to the additional burden of chemotherapy or radiotherapy.

3.5.3 Pregnant Women

Very little is known about the maternal risk of chemotherapy induced cardiotoxicity. Pharmacokinetic and pharmacodynamic changes and the circulatory overload occurring during pregnancy may lead to toxic effects. Close monitoring, including clinical cardiac assessment and echocardiographic evaluation before chemotherapy and re-evaluation before every dose, should be considered in the pregnant condition.

A long-term observational case report seemed to demonstrate no significant long-term cardiotoxic effects in children born from mothers treated with chemotherapy during pregnancy [40].

3.6 Multi-Modal Approach to Cardiovascular Prehabilitation

Over the past decade, it has become increasingly evident that successful surgery is not dependent solely on the operation alone but rather, on the patient's ability to return to a physically and psychologically healthy state. As low cardiorespiratory fitness limits access to curative therapies, a higher proportion of elderly patients with a cancer diagnosis are deemed ineligible for surgery. A multi-modal approach during the preoperative period should include medical and pharmacological optimization, correction of anaemia, alcohol and smoking cessation, as well as exercise and physical activity, nutritional optimization and anti-anxiety strategies [41].

With the role of multidisciplinary teams in the prevention and rehabilitation of CVD being established firmly in developing countries like India [42], the multi-modal approach to cardiovascular prehabilitation (and other systemic prehabilitation) is likely to be the next big game-changer in the care of cancer patients globally.

3.7 Future Directions and Conclusion

Recent advances in cardiac biomarkers, human induced pluripotent stem cell technology, molecular imaging, pharmacogenomics and personalized medicine are expected to advance our understanding of the disease phenotype in cancer patients exposed to potential cardiotoxins as well as to guide us in the appropriate pre-surgical workup of cancer patients [15, 43–45]. Larger scale studies are however needed to further identify susceptibility markers and to develop superior risk-profiling tools to improve quality of life and life expectancy in cancer survivors.

In conclusion, cardiovascular prehabilitation is a growing field and one that holds tremendous promise in improving the outlook of cancer patients. When a stable or a critically ill CVD patient gets diagnosed with cancer or a newly diagnosed cancer patient is unearthed with an underlying CVD, it is imperative to treat the CVD adequately, risk stratify the patient prior to initiating cancer therapy, apply the cumulative knowledge to provide the most effective and safe cancer treatment and finally follow up the patient rigorously after treatment, ensuring personalized care all along (Fig. 3.6). Though several questions remain unanswered in the etiopathogenesis and outcomes of cancer, it is crystal clear that a multidisciplinary team approach is the cornerstone in cancer management and cardiovascular prehabilitation truly epitomizes this integrated approach.

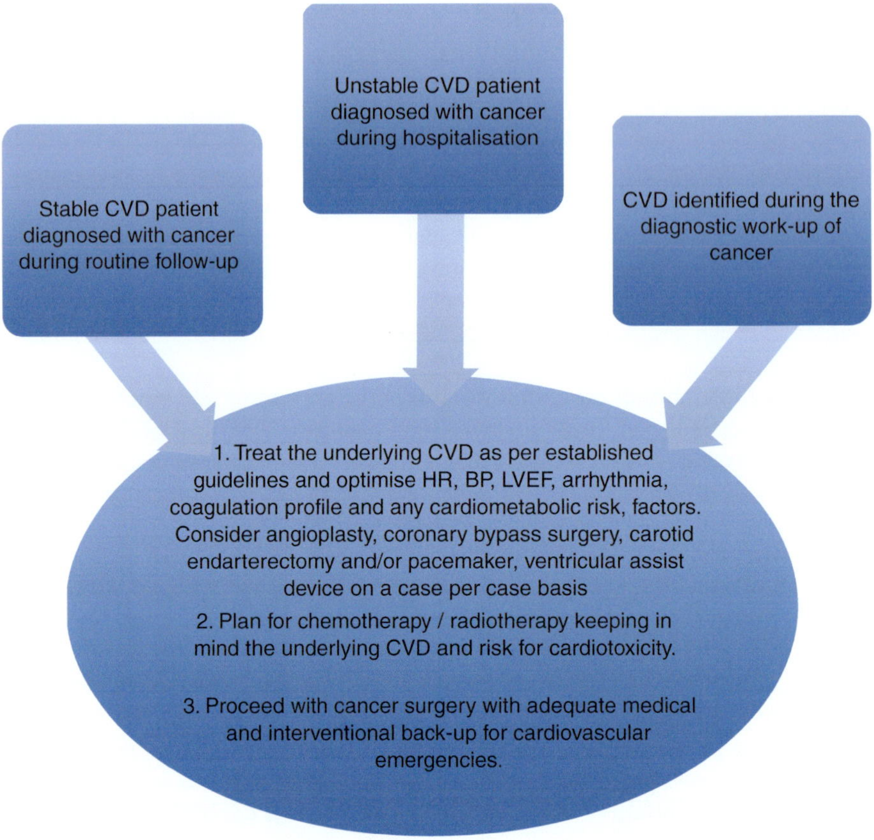

Fig. 3.6 Summary of cardiovascular prehabilitation for cancer surgery

References

1. Brown SA. preventive cardio-oncology: the time has come. Front Cardiovasc Med. 2020;6:187.
2. https://www.escardio.org/Journals/E-Journal-of-Cardiology-Practice/Volume-16/Cardio-oncology-principles-and-organisational-issues.
3. Totzeck M, Schuler M, Stuschke M, Heusch G, Rassaf T. Cardio-oncology—strategies for management of cancer-therapy related cardiovascular disease. Int J Cardiol. 2019;280:163–75.
4. Lancellotti P, Suter TM, López-Fernández T, Galderisi M, Lyon AR, Van der Meer P, et al. Cardio-oncology services: rationale, organization, and implementation. Eur Heart J. 2019;40:1756–63.
5. Handy CE, Quispe R, Pinto X, Blaha MJ, Blumenthal RS, Michos ED, et al. Synergistic opportunities in the interplay between cancer screening and cardiovascular disease risk assessment: together we are stronger. Circulation. 2018;138:727–34.
6. Esposito K, Chiodini P, Colao A, Lenzi A, Giugliano D. Metabolic syndrome and risk of cancer: a systematic review and meta-analysis. Diabetes Care. 2012;35:2402–11.
7. Lang-Rollin I, Berberich G. Psycho-oncology. Dialogues Clin Neurosci. 2018;20:13–22.

8. Yusuf S, Hawken S, Ounpuu S, Dans T, Avezum A, Lanas F, INTERHEART Study Investigators, et al. Effect of potentially modifiable risk factors associated with myocardial infarction in 52 countries (the INTERHEART study): case-control study. Lancet. 2004;364:937–52.
9. Richards AM. Can heart failure cause cancer? Nat Rev Cardiol. 2019;16:7–8.
10. Kitsis RN, Riquelme JA, Lavandero S. Heart disease and cancer: are the two killers colluding? Circulation. 2018;138:692–5.
11. Zamorano JL, Lancellotti P, Rodriguez Muñoz D, Aboyans V, Asteggiano R, Galderisi M, ESC Scientific Document Group, et al. ESC Position Paper on cancer treatments and cardiovascular toxicity developed under the auspices of the ESC Committee for Practice Guidelines: The Task Force for cancer treatments and cardiovascular toxicity of the European Society of Cardiology (ESC). Eur Heart J. 2016;37:2768–801.
12. Barac A, Murtagh G, Carver JR, Chen MH, Freeman AM, Herrmann J, et al. Cardiovascular health of patients with cancer and cancer survivors: a roadmap to the next level. J Am Coll Cardiol. 2015;65:2739–46.
13. Vejpongsa P, Yeh ET. Prevention of anthracycline-induced cardiotoxicity: challenges and opportunities. J Am Coll Cardiol. 2014;64:938–45.
14. Teske AJ, Linschoten M, Kamphuis JAM, et al. Cardio-oncology: an overview on outpatient management and future developments. Neth Heart J. 2018;26:521–32.
15. Ananthan K, Lyon AR. The role of biomarkers in cardio-oncology. J Cardiovasc Transl Res. 2020;13:431–50.
16. Tan LL, Lyon AR. Role of biomarkers in prediction of cardiotoxicity during cancer treatment. Curr Treat Options Cardiovasc Med. 2018;20:55.
17. Bosch X, Rovira M, Sitges M, Domenech A, Ortiz-Perez JT, de Caralt TM, et al. Enalapril and carvedilol for preventing chemotherapy-induced left ventricular systolic dysfunction in patients with malignant hemopathies: the OVERCOME trial (preventiOn of left Ventricular dysfunction with Enalapril and caRvedilol in patients submitted to intensive ChemOtherapy for the treatment of Malignant hEmopathies). J Am Coll Cardiol. 2013;61:2355–62.
18. Gulati G, Heck SL, Ree AH, Hoffmann P, Schulz-Menger J, Fagerland MW, et al. Prevention of cardiac dysfunction during adjuvant breast cancer therapy (PRADA): a 2 Å~ 2 factorial, randomized, placebo-controlled, double-blind clinical trial of candesartan and metoprolol. Eur Heart J. 2016;37:1671–80.
19. Ponikowski P, Voors AA, Anker SD, Bueno H, Cleland JGF, Coats AJS, ESC Scientific Document Group, et al. 2016 ESC Guidelines for the diagnosis and treatment of acute and chronic heart failure: The Task Force for the diagnosis and treatment of acute and chronic heart failure of the European Society of Cardiology (ESC) Developed with the special contribution of the Heart Failure Association (HFA) of the ESC. Eur Heart J. 2016;37:2129–200.
20. Martín-Garcia A, López-Fernández T, Mitroi C, Chaparro-Muñoz M, Moliner P, Martin-Garcia AC, et al. Effectiveness of sacubitril–valsartan in cancer patients with heart failure. ESC Heart Failure. 2020;7:763–7.
21. Gregorietti V, Fernandez TL, Costa D, Ortega Chahla E, Daniele AJ. Use of Sacubitril/valsartan in patients with cardio toxicity and heart failure due to chemotherapy. Cardio-Oncology. 2020;6:24.
22. Boutagy NE, Feher A, Pfau D, Liu Z, Guerrera NM, Freeburg LA, et al. Dual angiotensin receptor-neprilysin inhibition with sacubitril/valsartan attenuates systolic dysfunction in experimental doxorubicin-induced cardiotoxicity. JACC CardioOncol. 2020;2:774–87.
23. Mamas MA, Brown SA, Sun LY. Coronary artery disease in patients with cancer: it's always the small pieces that make the bigger picture. Mayo Clin Proc. 2020;95:1819–21.
24. Potts JE, Iliescu CA, Lopez Mattei JC, Martinez SC, Holmvang L, Ludman P, et al. Percutaneous coronary intervention in cancer patients: a report of the prevalence and outcomes in the United States. Eur Heart J. 2019;40:1790–800.
25. Bharadwaj A, Potts J, Mohamed MO, Parwani P, Swamy P, Lopez-Mattei JC, et al. Acute myocardial infarction treatments and outcomes in 6.5 million patients with a current or historical diagnosis of cancer in the USA. Eur Heart J. 2020;41:2183–93.

26. Guha A, Dey AK, Kalra A, Gumina R, Lustberg M, Lavie CJ, et al. Coronary artery bypass grafting in cancer patients: prevalence and outcomes in the United States. Mayo Clin Proc. 2020;95:1865–76.
27. Essa H, Dobson R, Wright D, Lip GYH. Hypertension management in cardio-oncology. J Hum Hypertens. 2020;34:673–81.
28. Cascella M. Preoperative cardiac evaluation and anesthetic considerations for cancer patients who underwent chemotherapy. Trends Anaesthesia Crit Care. 2017;14:9–18.
29. Huynh TTT, Pisimisis GT, Broadbent KC, Mehran RJ. Carotid artery disease in patients with cancer. In: Yusuf S, Banchs J, editors. Cancer and cardiovascular disease. Cham: Springer; 2018.
30. Keyhani S, Madden E, Cheng EM, et al. Risk prediction tools to improve patient selection for carotid endarterectomy among patients with asymptomatic carotid stenosis. JAMA Surg. 2019;154:336–44.
31. Valdes E. Metastatic and paraneoplastic cardiomyopathy. Jpn Heart J. 1973;14:548–53.
32. Desai A, Noor A, Joshi S, Kim AS. Takotsubo cardiomyopathy in cancer patients. Cardiooncology. 2019;5:7.
33. Burgdorf C, Kurowski V, Bonnemeier H, Schunkert H, Radke PW. Long-term prognosis of the transient left ventricular dysfunction syndrome (Tako-Tsubo cardiomyopathy): focus on malignancies. Eur J Heart Fail. 2008;10:1015–9.
34. Kyaw H, Shaikh AZ, Ayala-Rodriguez C, Deepika M. Paraneoplastic cardiac involvement in renal cell carcinoma with dermatomyositis sine dermatitis. Ochsner J. 2017;17:421–5.
35. Kermani TA, Warrington KJ, Amin S. Malignancy risk in vasculitis. Ther Adv Musculoskelet Dis. 2011;3:55–63.
36. Solans-Laqué R, Bosch-Gil JA, Pérez-Bocanegra C, Selva-O'Callaghan A, Simeón-Aznar CP, Vilardell-Tarres M. Paraneoplastic vasculitis in patients with solid tumors: report of 15 cases. J Rheumatol. 2008;35:294–304.
37. Park HJ, Ranganathan P. Neoplastic and paraneoplastic vasculitis, vasculopathy, and hypercoagulability. Rheum Dis Clin N Am. 2011;37:593–606.
38. Burazor I, Aviel-Ronen S, Imazio M, Goitein O, Perelman M, Shelestovich N, et al. Metastatic cardiac tumors: from clinical presentation through diagnosis to treatment. BMC Cancer. 2018;18:202.
39. Goldberg AD, Blankstein R, Padera RF. Tumors metastatic to the heart. Circulation. 2013;128:1790–4.
40. Cardonick E, Dougherty R, Grana G, Gilmandyar D, Ghaffar S, Usmani A. Breast cancer during pregnancy: maternal and fetal outcomes. Cancer J. 2010;16:76–82.
41. Scheede-Bergdahl C, Minnella EM, Carli F. Multi-modal prehabilitation: addressing the why, when, what, how, who and where next? Anaesthesia. 2019;74(Suppl 1):20–6.
42. Chockalingam P, Rajaram A, Maiya A, Contractor A. A multicentre retrospective study on quality and outcomes of cardiac rehabilitation programs in India. Indian Heart J. 2020;72:55–7.
43. Sayed N, Ameen M, Wu JC. Personalized medicine in cardio-oncology: the role of induced pluripotent stem cell. Cardiovasc Res. 2019;115:949–59.
44. Scott E, Hasbullah JS, Ross CJD, Carleton BC. Reducing anthracycline-induced cardiotoxicity through pharmacogenetics. Pharmacogenomics. 2018;19:1147–50.
45. Dreyfuss AD, Bravo PE, Koumenis C, Ky B. Precision cardio-oncology. J Nucl Med. 2019;60:443–50.

Respiratory Prehabilitation in Cancer Surgery

4

Eunice Kok, Remadevi, and Ashokka Balakrishnan

Abbreviations

6MWT	6-minute walk test
ABG	Arterial blood gas
ARDS	Acute respiratory distress syndrome
BAL	Bronchoalveolar lavage
COPD	Chronic obstructive pulmonary disease
CT	Computed tomography
CTCAE	Common Terminology Criteria for Adverse Events
CXR	Chest X-ray
DLCO	Diffuse capacity for carbon monoxide
DNA	Deoxyribonucleic acid
FBC	Full blood count
FEV1	Forced expiratory volume in first second
FRC	Functional residual capacity
FVC	Forced vital capacity
GOLD	Global Initiative for Chronic Obstructive Lung Disease
ICS	Inhaled corticosteroid
ICU	Intensive care unit
LABA	Long-acting beta-agonist
LAMA	Long-acting muscarinic antagonist
MLD	Mean lung dose
NICE	National Institute for Health and Care Excellence

E. Kok (✉) · A. Balakrishnan
Department of Anaesthesia, National University Health System, Singapore, Singapore

Remadevi
Department of Anaesthesia, Indira Gandhi Medical College and Research Institute, Pondicherry, India

A. Chakraborty, A. Balakrishnan (eds.), *Prehabilitation for Cancer Surgery*,
https://doi.org/10.1007/978-981-16-6494-6_4

RILI	Radiation-induced lung injury
RON	Reactive nitrogen species
ROS	Reactive oxygen species
RTOG	Radiation Therapy Oncology Group
SWOG	Southwest Oncology Group
TLC	Total lung capacity
V20	Volume of normal lung
VO_2max	Maximal oxygen uptake

4.1 Introduction

Pulmonary rehabilitation has been an established concept since the 1970s. It has been defined as "a multidimensional continuum of services directed to persons with pulmonary disease and their families, usually by an interdisciplinary team of specialists, with the goal of achieving and maintaining the individual's maximum level of independence and functioning in the community" [1]. Prehabilitation has been shown to improve physiological reserves, lead to lower post-operative complication rate, and facilitate earlier restoration of premorbid function [2–5]. Pulmonary rehabilitation is a major aspect of prehabilitation, involving the optimization of medical conditions, physical intervention and nutritional optimization. The duration of preoperative pulmonary rehabilitation remains deeply contested among experts, as it poses a challenge to balance the urgency of surgery to prevent disease progression, and prehabilitation to optimize outcomes post-surgery. Current literature generally suggests a duration of 2–6 weeks for preoperative pulmonary rehabilitation.

4.2 Respiratory Diseases and Risk Factor Optimization

4.2.1 Smoking

The deleterious effects of smoking on the respiratory system are well established. Smoking causes reduced oxygen delivery to tissues, increased secretion of mucus, mucociliary dysfunction and impairment of tracheobronchial clearance [6].

Smoking cessation would lead to improved closing volume and small airway function, reduced secretions and better tracheobronchial clearance, thereby enhancing the respiratory function during the peri-anaesthesia period and minimizing post-operative pulmonary complications. The ideal duration of smoking cessation is controversial—a minimum of 6–8 weeks prior to surgery is generally recommended; however, a randomized trial on perioperative smoking cessation found that a preoperative smoking cessation period of 4 weeks already significantly reduces the risk of post-operative complications [7]. The timing of smoking cessation and benefits are elaborated upon in Table 4.1, which is adapted from the Australian and New Zealand College of Anaesthetists guidelines on smoking cessation [8].

Table 4.1 Timing of smoking cessation prior to surgery and the corresponding benefits

Time of smoking cessation prior to surgery	Benefits
1 day	• Reduced carboxyhaemoglobin and nicotine levels • Improved tissue oxygen delivery
3 weeks	• Improved wound healing
6–8 weeks	• Sputum volumes reduced to the level of non-smokers • Improved pulmonary function
6 months	• Significant recovery in immune function

There are various types of interventions that can facilitate smoking cessation. Non-pharmacological interventions include smoking cessation counselling, cognitive therapy to learn adjustment techniques, as well as support groups. Pharmacological interventions include nicotine replacement therapy (e.g. patch, inhaler, nasal spray), bupropion and varenicline.

4.2.2 Chronic Obstructive Pulmonary Disease (COPD)

Pulmonary rehabilitation in both stable disease and acute exacerbations of chronic obstructive pulmonary disease (COPD) have shown to improve the functional status in patients. The National Institute for Health and Care Excellence (NICE) guidelines for COPD recommends a course of pulmonary rehabilitation for patients with COPD before undergoing surgery, if time permits. Patients with severe COPD are at an elevated risk of serious post-operative pulmonary complications as compared to patients with mild or no disease [9]. Pulmonary rehabilitation in COPD patients has been shown to have numerous benefits physiologically—these include increased lung volumes, maintenance of small airways patency, strengthened respiratory muscles and increased efficiency of breathing. It also reduces symptoms and minimizes the disease exacerbation rate [10].

Given this multitude of physiological benefits, the role of pulmonary rehabilitation in the preoperative setting should be emphasized. A multidisciplinary approach—including various stakeholders such as respiratory physicians, specialty nurses, dieticians, and anaesthetists—should be adopted in the execution of preoperative pulmonary rehabilitation.

A suggested framework for pulmonary prehabilitation and preoperative optimization of COPD patients is described below.

4.2.2.1 Patient Education

There are various aspects to patient education in COPD. Patients should be counselled on the correct inhaler techniques, medication compliance, and side effects of the medications. Additionally, patients may be taught methods of energy conservation and simplification of work of breathing, including special breathing techniques for COPD such as pursed lip and diaphragmatic breathing. An illustration of pursed lip breathing is shown below (Fig. 4.1).

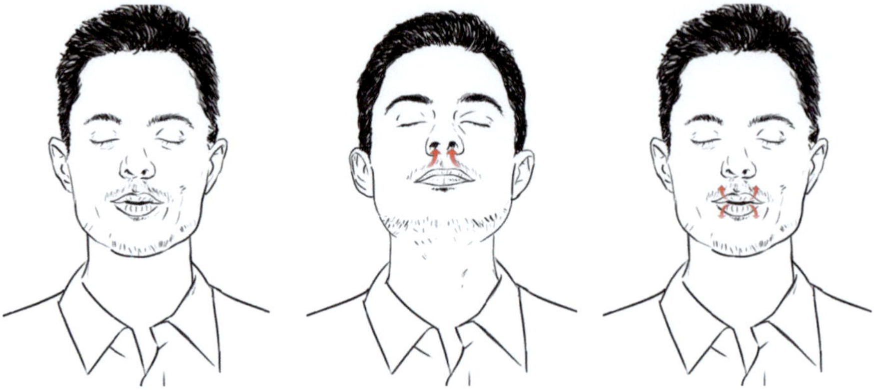

Fig. 4.1 Pursed lip breathing

Table 4.2 Initial pharmacological treatment for COPD according to GOLD guidelines 2020

GOLD A	GOLD B	GOLD C	GOLD D
Bronchodilator	Long-acting bronchodilator (LABA or LAMA)	LAMA	1. LAMA or 2. LAMA + LABA or 3. ICS + LABA

4.2.2.2 Pharmacological Optimization of Disease Control

This typically starts with an assessment of the stage of COPD according to the Global Initiative for Chronic Obstructive Lung Disease (GOLD) classification. Initial pharmacological therapy would then be dependent on the stage of disease. This typically includes a combination of bronchodilators (long-acting or short-acting beta-agonists and muscarinic antagonists) and inhaled corticosteroids. Table 4.2, adapted from the GOLD guidelines, shows the recommended treatment for each stage of COPD.

4.2.2.3 Physiotherapy

Preoperative exercise and chest physiotherapy can improve respiratory status and effort tolerance. Some benefits include improvements in lung mechanics, lung parenchyma function and cardiopulmonary reserves. This will be further elaborated upon in Sect. 4.3 on physical intervention, as well in Chap. 8.

Asthma is another type of obstructive lung disease. However, unlike COPD, the routine referral of patients with asthma to pulmonary rehabilitation is generally not recommended according to the British Thoracic Society guidelines.

4.2.3 Pneumonia

Preoperative pneumonia has been found to contribute to adverse post-operative outcomes including respiratory failure, prolonged intubation and mechanical ventilation, deep vein thrombosis, pulmonary embolism, sepsis, blood transfusions, hospital and ICU length of stay. In particular, general, orthopaedic, thoracic and vascular surgeries were associated with increased mortality in patients with preoperative pneumonia [11]. The severity of the pneumonia was also shown to be associated with a corresponding increase in 1-year mortality risk [12].

A retrospective database study found that preoperative pneumonia was associated with increased morbidity and mortality in both emergency and elective surgeries; however, the extent of increase in mortality was higher in elective than in emergency surgeries. The authors consequently recommended that elective surgery be delayed until the preoperative pneumonia resolves [11].

The treatment of pneumonia typically includes antibiotic therapy, chest physiotherapy and supportive treatment such as supplemental oxygen and mechanical ventilation in severe cases. A retrospective study done on geriatric patients undergoing hip fracture surgery revealed that treatment of preoperative pneumonia resulted in 81.7% of patients having improvements on their chest radiographs. Further analysis illustrated that patients with preoperative pneumonia who were treated and showed radiographic improvement had a higher survival rate than those who did not show radiographic improvement [12].

In light of the above evidence, when faced with preoperative pneumonia, it is prudent to ensure adequate treatment of the pneumonia preoperatively, and strongly consider postponing elective surgeries until the pneumonia resolves, so as to reduce the risk of adverse post-operative outcomes.

4.2.4 Pleural Effusion

Pleural effusion has significant physiological effects on the respiratory system. Firstly, it causes a restrictive ventilatory defect, characterized by a global reduction in lung volumes including forced vital capacity, functional residual capacity and total lung capacity. This restrictive ventilatory defect results in reduced lung compliance. Secondly, the accumulation of fluid in the pleural space leads to an increase in chest wall volume, consequently decreasing the length of inspiratory respiratory muscles and hence impairing their function. Thirdly, hypoxemia often develops due to ventilation/perfusion mismatch. Large pleural effusions may impair right heart filling and decrease cardiac output, further exacerbating the ventilation/perfusion mismatch [13].

Among the many causes of pleural effusions, the most commonly encountered ones are infective (parapneumonic effusion, empyema), heart failure, malignant and protein deficiency. Malignant pleural effusions are most prevalent in lung cancer, breast cancer, lymphoma, gynaecological cancers and malignant mesothelioma [14]. The broad principles of management of pleural effusions include: (1) supportive treatment (supplemental oxygen), (2) treating the underlying condition (e.g. antibiotic therapy for pneumonia, diuretics for heart failure), (3) therapeutic drainage of pleural effusion. In special causes such as malignant pleural effusions, surgical treatment such as pleurodesis may be a consideration. Ultimately, it is imperative to be aware of the physiological changes that pleural effusions cause, and to treat pleural effusions adequately in the preoperative period in order to maximize the respiratory function for surgery.

4.2.5 Pulmonary Fibrosis and Interstitial Lung Disease

Pulmonary fibrosis and interstitial lung disease can cause significant restrictions in gas exchange in the lungs resulting in reduction in functional reserves and functional capacity. Pulmonary fibrosis can present as an independent lung comorbidity in patients with cancer or it could be an independent risk factor for increased incidence of lung cancer. It also noted in association with smoking, COPD, emphysema and chronic bronchiectasis. Lung fibrosis is also common with previous history of lung infections (e.g. Tuberculosis), radiation exposure or chemotherapy-induced lung injury.

Irrespective of the aetiopathology, the primary presenting symptoms are decreased exercise tolerance, breathlessness and easy fatiguability. Clinical investigations include a chest radiograph and a CT thorax that can identify the extent and severity of zones affected, lung function tests that quantify presence of restrictive lung disease and coexisting obstructive pathology of the lungs. Subjective measures of lung function include dyspnoea scores and exercise capacity measured by anaerobic thresholds. Diffusion capacity of carbon monoxide (DLCO) stratifies the degree of parenchymal disease.

Prehabilitation for patient with lung fibrosis includes the recognition and stratification of presence of restrictive lung disease per se or its co-presentations with obstructive lung diseases. The prehabilitative process in the presence of lung cancer is more complex and includes general prehabilitative measures for systemic prehabilitation in addition to pulmonary prehabilitation (Fig. 4.2).

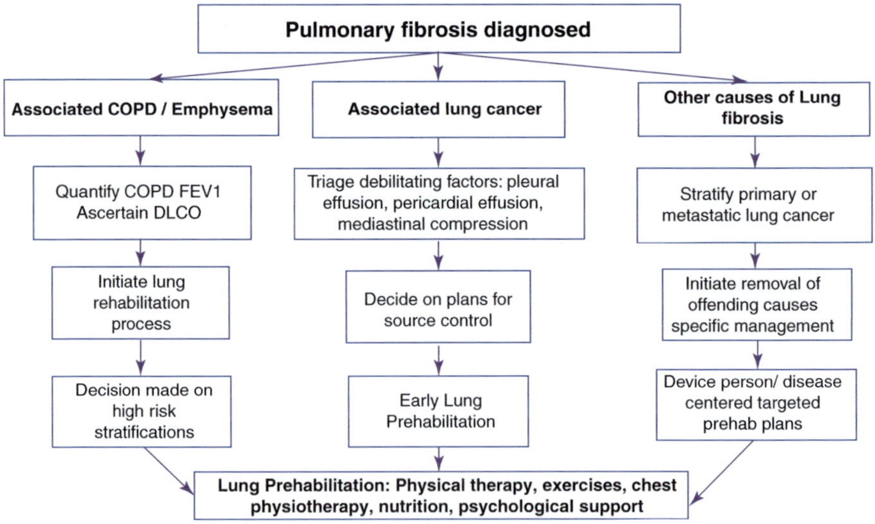

Fig. 4.2 Proposed workflow for evaluation and management of pulmonary fibrosis in the preoperative period

The reader is referred to Chap. 8 (Physiotherapy in cancer prehabilitation) for details on structured physical therapy for prehabilitation in cancer patients. Lung recruitment manoeuvres and chest physiotherapy are described in Sect. 4.3.2 in this chapter.

4.2.6 Pulmonary Metastases

Metastatic lung diseases include both synchronous and metachronous tumours. Synchronous metastasis refers to lung tumour diagnosed during tumour workup or within first 3 months after diagnosis; metachronous tumours refer to diagnosis of metastasis after 3 months of diagnosis, usually tend to be after primary surgical resection. Patients with metachronous metastatic lung disease have 50% lesser survival rates compared to patients with synchronous metastasis [15].

Common presentations include breathlessness, cough, weight loss, pleuritic chest pain and cachexia. Majority of lung metastases are incidental diagnoses and are not picked up early in the presentation. Clinical presentations might vary with pleural versus parenchymal metastatic diseases and could have more advanced systemic disease when paraneoplastic features are present such as hypercalcemia, hormone secreting features and procoagulant states resulting in thromboembolic diseases.

Patients with pulmonary metastases can present with breathlessness for a variety of reasons loss of active participatory lung surface for gas exchange, obstruction or restriction resulting in the reduction in air entry (shunts) from treatment induced lung injury (including chemotherapy- or radiation-induced lung injury), or from pleural effusions and reduction of lung volume. Breathlessness and fatiguability are also precipitated by the presence of severe anaemia from poor nutritional status or from reduced production of red cells.

Common investigations that guide the diagnosis, staging and further management include chest radiographs, CT thorax scans, cytologic examinations of pleural fluid or sputum, bronchoscopy studies and sampling, mediastinoscopy, needle or surgical biopsy of the lung.

Chemotherapy is usually the main treatment of choice. Radiation therapy, and palliative placement of airway stents or laser ablation therapy are other modalities of treatment. The range of surgeries planned for patients with metastatic tumours range from lung surgeries planned for management of the metastasis (minimally invasive video assisted thoracoscopic surgeries, lobectomy, etc.) or for management of the primary tumours (colon, uro-gynaecological, germ cell tumours) or for other distant metastasis (spine surgeries, liver resection).

Prehabilitation and preparation for surgery would include the management of systemic therapy such as nutrition, physical therapy, psychological support, and corrections of specific altered physiological states due to debilitation from cancer (electrolyte derangements, sarcopenia, etc.), extensive spread of cancer (spine metastases and immobility, pleural and pericardial effusion, malignant ascites, brain metastasis), or from the side effects of medications (nausea, vomiting, loss of appetite and taste). Specific pulmonary rehabilitation depends on the degree of functional capacity and amount of pulmonary reserves. Preoperative testing (pulmonary function tests, exercise testing and anaerobic threshold measurements) can help to quantify the functional status and will help to guide the strategies.

Pulmonary prehabilitation in metastatic lung cancer will include improvement in lung reserve through incentive spirometry, cough mechanics and lung volumes, postural drainage of consolidation and inspissated secretions from partially obstructed small airway, hydration and nutritional support.

While prehabilitation might provide improvements in quality of life and physical well-being of patients, the cost-benefit and resources management rationale of it is not well ascertained for metastatic cancer disease [16]. There are reports to state the possibilities of inoperable high-risk patient. About half the number of metastatic lung cancer patients are inoperable at presentations and early palliative care might improve patient satisfaction, minimize futility and guide appropriate allocation of facilities in resource limited settings.

4.2.7 Chemotherapy-Induced Lung Injury

Neoadjuvant chemotherapy is a mainstay of treatment for many cancers, including lung cancer, gastrointestinal cancers and breast cancer. It plays the critical roles of downstaging cancers and improving resectability of tumours. However, many chemotherapeutic agents are notorious for causing pulmonary toxicity, which can be detrimental in the population undergoing neoadjuvant chemotherapy as the impaired pulmonary function may result in greater post-operative respiratory complications.

4.2.7.1 Mechanisms of Lung Injury

Chemotherapeutic agents may cause pulmonary toxicity through a variety of mechanisms. Some common chemotherapeutic agents with their possible mechanisms of pulmonary toxicity are detailed in Table 4.3 below.

Despite the different mechanisms of injury, chemotherapeutic agents generally share the same final common pathway which begins from the inflammatory infiltration that occurs in the alveoli and pulmonary interstitium. This inflammatory process results in increased diffusion distance, damaged pulmonary capillary bed and reduced diffusion area. These changes are manifested in both clinical presentation and on the pulmonary function test. Patients with chemotherapy-induced lung injury may present with interstitial pneumonia or pneumonitis, pulmonary fibrosis or hypersensitivity syndrome [17, 18]. There is a reduction in diffusion capacity for carbon monoxide (DLCO). The trend of DLCO after high-dose chemotherapy has also been shown, in a study of breast cancer patients [19], to be a predictor for chemotherapy-related pneumonitis.

Table 4.3 Classes of chemotherapeutic agents and their mechanisms of action

Class of chemotherapeutic drug	Mechanism of lung injury
Cytotoxic agents	
Bleomycin	Oxidative damage Release of inflammatory mediators—cytokines, lipid metabolites, oxygen radicals
Mitomycin	Oxidative damage
Anthracyclines (e.g. doxorubicin, epirubicin)	Do not cause direct pulmonary toxicity, but may increase toxicity of other agents when used in combination
Alkylating agents	
Cyclophosphamide	Reactive oxidative moieties
Busulphan	Direct toxicity to epithelial lining cells Severe desquamation of injured epithelial cells into alveolar spaces results in diffuse alveolar damage
Antimetabolites	
Methotrexate	Hypersensitivity Direct toxicity
Cytarabine	Unknown
Nitrosoureas	
Carmustine	Oxidative effect
Miscellaneous	
Procarbazine	Hypersensitivity
Vinca alkaloids (e.g. vinclastine, vinorelbine)	Unknown
Molecular agents	
Checkpoint-inhibitor immunotherapy	Unintended dysregulation of immune system and T-cell activation
Anti-epidermal growth factor receptors agents	Impaired alveolar repair mechanisms

4.2.7.2 Clinical Presentation

Chemotherapy-induced lung diseases may present in a multitude of syndromes. Table 4.4 below describes the various clinical manifestations and the usual offending chemotherapeutic agents associated with each presentation.

4.2.7.3 Diagnosis

The diagnosis of chemotherapy-induced lung injury is difficult to confirm, as the radiographical and histopathological features are typically seen in a wide variety of clinical contexts and are not specific to chemotherapy-induced lung diseases.

The evaluation of possible chemotherapy-induced lung injury commonly includes the following as shown in Table 4.5 below.

Evidently, investigations yield highly non-specific findings and there is a lack of pathognomonic findings for the diagnosis of chemotherapy-induced lung diseases. The diagnosis is usually made with a combination of (1) a compatible clinical pattern, (2) a suspected offending drug, (3) the temporal relationship between administration of chemotherapy and onset of lung injury and (4) the exclusion of other potential causes such as infection or metastatic disease [20].

Table 4.4 Clinical syndromes of chemotherapy-induced lung

Syndrome	Clinical features	Investigations	Offending agents
Hypersensitivity pneumonitis (type IV delayed hypersensitivity reaction)	• Dyspnoea • Cough • Rashes • Angioedema • Fever	• CXR: normal/ pulmonary opacities/ ground-glass opacities/ reticular infiltrates • FBC: may have eosinophilia • Lung biopsy: chronic inflammation with predominantly lymphocytes and plasma cells, may include eosinophils/ neutrophils/mast cells, poorly circumscribed granulomas	Bleomycin Methotrexate Cytarabine Dactinomycin
Interstitial pneumonitis	• Non-productive cough • Progressive dyspnoea • Low-grade fever • Fine crepitations	• CXR: diffuse or focal opacities (e.g. septal thickening, ground-glass opacities, consolidation) • Bronchoalveolar lavage (BAL): non-specific findings—lymphocytosis, neutrophilia	Bleomycin Mitomycin Methotrexate Cyclophosphamide Gemcitabine Tyrosine kinase inhibitors Taxanes
Pulmonary fibrosis	• Progressive dyspnoea, markedly worse on exertion • Chronic non-productive cough • Fine crepitations	• CXR/CT thorax: reticular or ground-glass opacities • Pulmonary function tests: restrictive lung disease pattern (reduced FEV1, reduced FVC, normal or slightly increased FEV1/FVC), reduced DLCO	Bleomycin Mitomycin Methotrexate Busulfan Carmustine
Acute bronchoconstriction	• Dyspnoea • Wheezing • Desaturation • Scattered rhonchi • Prolonged expiratory phase	• Spirometry: reduced FEV1, reduced FEV1/ FVC with bronchodilator response	Carboplatin Cyclophosphamide Paclitaxel Rituximab Vinorelbine

Table 4.4 (continued)

Syndrome	Clinical features	Investigations	Offending agents
Alveolar haemorrhage	• Dyspnoea • Haemoptysis • Desaturation	• CXR: patchy or diffuse opacities • CT thorax: ground-glass opacities, consolidation (usually diffuse and bilateral, more central than peripheral) • BAL: lavage aliquots progressively more haemorrhagic, haemosiderin-laden macrophages • Pulmonary function test: increased DLCO	Docetaxel Gemcitabine Bevacizumab Sorafenib
Non-cardiogenic pulmonary Oedema	• Dyspnoea • Wheezing • Desaturation • Widespread coarse crepitations	• CXR: alveolar oedema, Kerley B lines, upper lobe diversion, pleural effusion	Mitomycin Cytarabine Gemcitabine Interleukin-2
Adult respiratory distress syndrome (ARDS)	• Dyspnoea • Tachypnoea • Desaturation • Fever • Coarse crepitations	• CXR: bilateral opacities • ABG: respiratory failure (reduced pO_2 ± increased pCO_2), reduced PaO_2/FiO_2 ratio	Dactinomycin Bleomycin Cytarabine Gemcitabine Mitomycin
Pulmonary veno-occlusive disease	• Dyspnoea • Desaturation	• CT thorax: diffuse or mosaic ground-glass opacities, septal lines, pulmonary artery enlargement, mediastinal adenopathy	Bleomycin Carmustine Cisplatin Cyclophosphamide Gemcitabine Mitomycin

4.2.7.1 Management

Management of chemotherapy-induced lung injury comprises:

1. Discontinuing the offending drug
2. Supportive treatment

   Supportive treatment is usually based on the clinical syndrome. It may include supplemental oxygen, bronchodilators, diuretics and mechanical ventilation.
3. Corticosteroid therapy

   The use of corticosteroids for chemotherapy-induced lung diseases is controversial; available literature suggests that it could play a role in severe disease, although the effect may be modest or transient [19].

Table 4.5 Investigations to evaluate for possible chemotherapy-induced lung injury

Test	Findings
Pulmonary function test	• Reduced DLCO • Restrictive pattern—reduced TLC, reduced FVC
Imaging	CXR: • Patchy unilateral/bilateral reticular markings, ground-glass opacities, consolidations • Pleural effusion High resolution CT thorax: • Pulmonary fibrosis – Bibasilar subpleural reticular and ground-glass opacification with volume loss and blunting of costophrenic angles – Fine nodular densities – Progressive consolidation and honeycombing • Pulmonary veno-occlusive disease – Enlarged central arteries – Centrilobular ground-glass opacities – Septal thickening – Pleural effusion
Bronchoscopy and bronchoalveolar lavage (BAL)	• BAL fluid count: lymphocytosis, neutrophilia, +/− eosinophilia • Main role is to exclude infection (especially opportunistic organisms) or recurrent malignancy
Lung biopsy (histopathology)	• Interstitial pneumonitis • Eosinophilic pneumonia • Diffuse alveolar damage • Alveolar haemorrhage

4. Rechallenge

   The decision to rechallenge a suspected culprit drug should come after careful consideration of several factors: the level of suspicion of the culprit drug, the severity of the reaction, the availability of alternative therapies.

4.2.7.5 Implications for Surgery

Neoadjuvant chemotherapy causes a significant reduction in physical fitness and preoperative peak oxygen uptake (VO_2max) through a host of factors—pulmonary toxicity (reduction in diffusion capacity), cardiotoxicity and skeletal muscle toxicity. Low VO_2max and reduced DLCO have both been associated with an increased rate of post-operative pulmonary complications, such as acute respiratory failure, adult respiratory distress syndrome, pneumonia (compounded by poor response to antibiotics due to immunosuppression from chemotherapy), atelectasis, and pulmonary oedema [21]. Lower baseline fitness has also been associated with increased post-cancer surgery morbidity [22] and mortality [23].

This poses a conundrum—neoadjuvant chemotherapy has been shown to effectively downstage cancers and convert certain non-resectable tumours to become resectable, but often at the expense of the overall physical fitness of patients which can lead to higher rates of post-operative complications. The solution lies in prehabilitation. Preoperative aerobic training in these patients have been shown to improve VO_2max, consequently reducing the risk of post-operative pulmonary complications. A randomized trial done on patients undergoing neoadjuvant chemotherapy revealed a 13% increase in VO_2max in the group who underwent preoperative aerobic training, as compared to a 8% decrease in VO_2max in the group who did not undergo aerobic training [24].

4.2.8 Radiation-Induced Lung Injury (RILI)

4.2.8.1 Pathogenesis

The pathogenesis of RILI can be described using basic cellular processes—injury, inflammation and repair.

(1) **Injury**
Ionizing radiation generates reactive oxygen (ROS) and nitrogen (RON) species, which results in oxidative damage to DNA, lipids and proteins, and consequently cellular injury and death. These cellular injuries stimulate the recruitment of inflammatory cells to the site of injury to begin the repair process.

(2) **Inflammation**
Inflammatory cells such as leukocytes and macrophages are recruited to the site of injury. These cells stimulate the secretion of cytokines and growth factors that recruit and activate more cells that are involved in wound repair, setting off an inflammatory cascade. In RILI, the inflammatory response is dysregulated, resulting in chronic inflammation and cellular loss.

(3) **Repair**
In the repair process, inflammation coupled with tissue remodelling ultimately leads to a change in the composition of the lung. Pulmonary fibrosis is a common outcome of ionizing radiation. Tissue growth factors promote the chemoattraction of fibroblasts and their conversion to myofibroblasts, eventually resulting in changes in lung architecture.

There are many factors which influence the development of RILI. The most pertinent factors are the volume of irradiated lung, the dose of radiation, fractionation and the presence of concurrent chemotherapy.

The risk of RILI is directly proportional to the volume of irradiated lung as well as the dose of radiation. V20, defined as the volume of normal lung (total lung volume—target volume for radiotherapy) that receives more than 20 Gy of radiation, is a critical predictor of the risk of RILI. Mean lung dose, defined as the average radiation dose in the lung volume irradiated defined by CT, is used as a quantitative measurement for the dose of radiation. A V20 of less than 30–35% and a MLD of less than 20–23 Gy was found to reduce the risk of pneumonitis to less than 20% [25].

Fractionation is the division of total radiation dose into fractions. A larger dose for each fraction would entail a shorter exposure time. Larger doses per fraction is associated with a higher risk of more severe RILI [26].

Several chemotherapeutic drugs are known sensitizers to radiotherapy, and can cause an increased risk of RILI. These include bleomycin, doxorubicin, dactinomycin, cyclophosphamide, mitomycin C and gemcitabine. A meta-analysis in 2012 showed an increased odds ratio of radiation pneumonitis in patients who underwent concurrent chemotherapy as compared to sequential chemotherapy [27].

4.2.8.2 Clinical Presentation

The clinical manifestations of RILI may be classified by an early onset process (radiation pneumonitis) or a late onset process (radiation fibrosis). These are detailed in Table 4.6.

There are several scores that have been established to grade the severity of RILI. The most commonly used scores are the Common Terminology Criteria for Adverse Events (CTCAE) 5.0, the Radiation Therapy Oncology Group (RTOG) and the Southwest Oncology Group (SWOG) criteria (Table 4.7).

4.2.8.3 Investigations

The evaluation for possible RILI typically includes radiological and pulmonary function tests.

On a chest radiograph, diffuse infiltrates in the areas of the irradiated lung, which may coalesce to form a relatively sharp edge corresponding to the shape and size of

Table 4.6 Clinical presentations of RILI

Early onset (radiation pneumonitis)	Late onset (radiation fibrosis)
1–3 months	6–24 months
• Dyspnoea • Non-productive cough • Low-grade fever • Acute respiratory failure	• Dyspnoea • Fine crepitations • Chronic respiratory failure • Pulmonary hypertension, cor pulmonale

Table 4.7 Various scores for grading the severity of RILI

Criteria/Grade	CTCAE 5.0	RTOG	SWOG
0	No changes	No changes	Normal
1	Asymptomatic/only radiological findings	Asymptomatic or mild symptoms	Radiographic changes, does not require steroids
2	Symptomatic, does not interfere with daily activities	Moderate symptoms, radiographic changes	Require steroids or drainage of pleural effusion
3	Symptomatic, interferes with daily activities, requires oxygen	Severe symptoms, dense radiographic changes	Requires oxygen
4	Life-threatening, requires mechanical ventilation support	Symptoms of severe respiratory failure requiring assisted ventilation or continuous oxygen	Requires assisted ventilation
5	Death	Death	–

the radiation field may be observed. There may also be a mediastinal shift towards the ipsilateral irradiated side, and an elevated hemidiaphragm on the ipsilateral irradiated side. Additionally, pleural effusions may be present.

Post-radiotherapy pulmonary function test most commonly reveals a reduction in DLCO, presumably a result of radiation-induced pulmonary fibrosis. An improvement in forced expiratory volume in the first second (FEV1) is occasionally seen as radiotherapy assists in tumour reduction and reduced airway obstruction. The forced vital capacity, however, is usually reduced—concordant with a restrictive pattern of pulmonary disease.

4.2.8.4 Management

Several pharmacological agents have been described in literature for the prevention and treatment of RILI (Table 4.8).

4.2.8.5 Implications for Surgery

RILI often causes a reduction in DLCO and a restrictive pattern (reduced FVC and FEV1) on post-radiotherapy pulmonary function tests. These have been found to have an impact on post-operative pulmonary complications, such as pneumonia, ARDS, respiratory failure, prolonged intubation and mechanical ventilation [30, 31]. Pulmonary prehabilitation can help to improve and optimize the respiratory status post-radiotherapy and preoperatively. A retrospective study done on lung cancer patients who had received induction chemoradiotherapy prior to lung resection surgery found that patients who underwent pulmonary prehabilitation (which was carried out during neoadjuvant chemoradiotherapy) were associated with a significantly greater increase in preoperative FVC and FEV1, as compared to those who did not undergo prehabilitation [32].

4.2.9 Superior Vena Cava Syndrome

Superior vena cava syndrome when present can be life-threatening when not attended in the right time frame. It results from extrinsic compression of the veins

Table 4.8 Pharmacological agents for prevention and treatment of RILI

Drug	Mechanism of action
Amifostine	• Phosphorylated aminothiol • Acts as free radical scavenger • Repairs DNA via selective cytoprotective mechanism
Captopril	• Thiol group functions as free radical scavenger and exhibits superoxide dismutase like activity
Pentoxifylline	• Xanthine derivative • Inhibits platelet aggregation, enhances microvascular blood flow, inhibits tumour necrosis factor
Corticosteroids	• Anti-inflammatory • Recommended dose [28, 29]: 1 mg/kg/day for several weeks, then tapered down over weeks to months

of the thoracic inlet with or without symptoms suggestive of airway oedema and cerebral oedema. The most common symptom is dyspnoea [33]. The lung tumours represent most causes; while it can also be from venous thrombosis from indwelling catheter triggered thrombus or from mediastinal tumour producing extrinsic compression of right atrial inflow (e.g. lymphomas) [34]. Chest radiographs can show mediastinal widening. However, the definitive imaging modality is a CT venography [35].

Management has shifted from emergency radiation therapy to endovascular stents that achieve early revascularization and improvement in symptoms. Presence of airway compromise might need careful attention when preoperative staging mediastinoscopy or minimally invasive biopsies are planned. Haemodynamic compromise when present could mean the possibility of cardiac involvement like mediastinal compression or pericardial effusion.

Prehabilitation would involve decision making of actual optimization of symptoms, prevention of catastrophe like airway and haemodynamic compromise and identification and initiation of non-surgical primary tumour management. This could involve glucocorticoids for steroid responsive lymphomas, chemotherapeutic agents for chemoresponsive small cell tumours and use of antibiotics when additional causes such as mediastinitis are present. The overall survival rates of patients who present with SVC syndromes is 6 months; hence careful patient selection; prompt initiation of definitive management and preparation for surgery is important when planned.

Table 4.9 is a summary of important respiratory conditions (in terms of clinical presentation, investigations and management) to consider during preoperative evaluation and optimization.

4.3 Physical Intervention

Physical intervention is a cornerstone in pulmonary prehabilitation, with the goals of improving the functional and respiratory status in patients undergoing surgery.

4.3.1 Physical Exercise

Exercise prescription may be guided by the FIIT principle: frequency, intensity, time and type of exercise [36]. Current literature for prehabilitation generally recommends a minimum duration of 150 min of exercise a week, which may be divided across a total of 5 sessions of 20–30 min of exercise in a week. This frequency and duration may be increased as tolerated by the patient. A combination of aerobic or endurance, and strength or resistance exercises are recommended. Aerobic exercises include walking, cycling, jogging and swimming. Optimization of exercise intensity is commonly based on heart rate (Karvonen formula), and/or the Borg

Table 4.9 Summary of major respiratory conditions

	COPD	Consolidation	Collapse	Effusion	Fibrosis
Symptoms	• Dyspnoea (progressive, exertional) • Chronic cough and sputum production • Wheezing • Chest tightness	• Dyspnoea • Cough (may have productive sputum) • Pleuritic chest pain • Fever, chills, rigours	• Dyspnoea	• Dyspnoea • Pleuritic chest pain	• Dyspnoea (worse on exertion) • Chronic cough (dry, non-productive) • Loss of appetite and weight • Chronic fatigue/ malaise
Signs	• Barrel chest • Pursed lip breathing • Hoover's sign • Bilateral reduced chest excursion • Hyperresonant percussion note • Prolonged expiratory phase • Expiratory rhonchi	• Respiratory distress • Febrile • Crepitations • Bronchial breath sounds • Increased vocal resonance	• Unilateral reduced chest excursion • Dull percussion note • Reduced breath sounds • Reduced vocal resonance • Tracheal deviation to affected side	• Unilateral reduced chest excursion • Stony dull percussion note • Reduced breath sounds • Reduced vocal resonance • Tracheal deviation away from affected side	• Bilateral reduced chest excursion • Fine end-inspiratory crepitations • Clubbing
Investigations					
CXR	• Hyperinflation • Flat hemidiaphragms • Tubular mediastinum/ elongated cardiac silhouette • Horizontalization of ribs • Bullae	• Opacity—lobar or bronchial pattern • May have associated parapneumonic effusion	• Opacity over affected zone • Tracheal/ mediastinal deviation to affected side	• Blunting of costophrenic angle • Opacity over affected zone • Tracheal/ mediastinal deviation away from affected side	• Reticulonodular shadowing

(continued)

Table 4.9 (continued)

	COPD	Consolidation	Collapse	Effusion	Fibrosis
ABG	• May have chronic respiratory acidosis • May have acute-on-chronic respiratory acidosis and type 2 respiratory failure in acute exacerbations	• Acute respiratory acidosis or alkalosis • Respiratory failure (type 1/type 2)	Hypoxemia	• Hypoxemia	• Hypercapnia • Hypoxemia
Spirometry	• Obstructive pattern: FEV1/FVC <0.7 • Reduced FEV1/FVC ratio not reversible with bronchodilators • Post-bronchodilator FEV1 predicts severity of COPD	–	–	• Restrictive pattern: reduced FEV1/FVC/TLC, preserved FEV1/FVC ratio (>0.7)	• Restrictive pattern: reduced FEV1/FVC/TLC, preserved FEV1/FVC ratio (>0.7)
DLCO	Unchanged	–	–	–	Reduced

Management	• Pharmacological – Bronchodilator – ICS • Non-pharmacological. – Smoking cessation. – Supplemental oxygen (including long-term oxygen therapy) – Chest physiotherapy	• Antibiotic therapy (refer to institutional guidelines on choice of antibiotics). • Supportive treatment. – Supplemental oxygen – Chest physiotherapy	• Treatment of underlying cause (mucus plugging, foreign body, infection, tumour, enlarged lymph nodes)	• Treatment of underlying cause (pneumonia, heart failure, malignancy) • Therapeutic drainage for symptomatic pleural effusions • Pleurodesis for malignant pleural effusions	• Supportive treatment. – Supplemental oxygen – Smoking cessation – Pulmonary rehabilitation (chest physiotherapy, regular pulmonary toileting) • Anti-fibrotics for idiopathic pulmonary fibrosis (e.g. pirfenidone, nintedanib) • Treatment of underlying cause (connective tissue disease, drug-induced fibrosis)

scale. The Borg scale is a subjective rating scale of perceived exertion. The patient rates his perceived exercise intensity on a numerical scale (refer to Fig. 4.3). The exercise intensity would need to be adjusted accordingly to target 12–16 in the prehabilitation setting. The Borg scale has been shown to correlate well with heart rate, respiratory rate, serum lactate and VO_2max.

The outcomes of pulmonary prehabilitation can be measured in various ways. The 6-minute walk test (6MWT) evaluates the capacity to maintain a moderate level of walking and reflects the capacity to perform activities of daily living. This entails having the patient walk along a 30-m stretch of unimpeded walkway as many times as possible at his/her own pace. The total distance walked in 6 min is then recorded. Prehabilitation has been shown to improve 6MWT distances in several randomized controlled trials [3, 37, 38]. Greater distances achieved in the preoperative 6WMT is suggestive of a higher functional capacity and is associated with reduced postoperative complications. The maximum oxygen uptake, VO_2max, is another frequently used parameter to measure pulmonary prehabilitation outcomes. It is a yardstick for anaerobic threshold as it measures the plateau of oxygen uptake as exercise intensity increases. Several randomized controlled trials have illustrated an increase in VO_2max in the prehabilitation groups [39–41]. Finally, pulmonary prehabilitation has resulted in improvements in FEV1, most markedly in patients with poorer baseline pulmonary functions.

Chapter 8 expounds on the concepts introduced here.

Fig. 4.3 Borg scale of perceived exertion

Rating	Perceived exertion
6	No exertion
7	Extremely light
8	
9	Very light
10	
11	Fairly light
12	
13	Somewhat hard
14	
15	Hard
16	
17	Very hard
18	
19	Extremely hard
20	Maximal exertion

4.3.2 Chest Physiotherapy and Pulmonary Rehabilitation

Chest physiotherapy includes methods for improving the clearance of secretions and enhancing the scope of improved gas exchange. This is achieved through systemic measures such as improved hydration to make secretions thin, pharmacotherapy to liquify the secretions, and methods to improve the strength and quality of cough.

Lung recruitment manoeuvres include deep breathing exercises and methods to expand specific regions of the lung through selective expansion of the areas of the lung.

The use of an incentive spirometer helps in enabling the use of inspiratory measures of lung volume and guide markers placed to help patients outperform their previous best. Simple bedside techniques such as blowing a balloon have also been described but with inconsistent results.

An important aspect of chest physiotherapy is the postural drainage of secretions. This entails positioning the patient in a posture that allows the flow of secretions and mucus from smaller airways to larger airways so that they can be coughed up more readily. A combination of chest percussion and vibration is used for this purpose. Chest percussion may be performed by giving alternate taps to a patient's chest wall using cupped hands, at an acceptable force that does not cause overt pain or too much discomfort to the patient. The duration of percussions can be in the range of 15–30 min, repeated two to three times a day, or more often as required. This process is labour intensive and can be influenced by provider fatigue and patient cooperation especially when patients are frail with cancer cachexia or have local tenderness in the chest wall. Vibration therapy may be used to complement chest percussion. It entails placing a flat hand placed on top of a particular lung segment that is targeted for mucus drainage, and then applying light pressure to achieve a rapid shaking movement that results in a vibratory effect. These techniques may occasionally be performed after pre-dosing with analgesics as necessary.

Other more efficient and consistent methods for provision of chest physiotherapy include the use of automated motorized vibratory belts that provide scope of agitation of the secretions and displacement for patient to propel to cough out [42]. The devices are designed with various range of pressures and frequency based on the clinical needs. High frequency chest oscillations have been trialled and found to have successful results, and are applied when the resources enable such affordances [43].

Once the secretions are displaced by manoeuvres such as chest percussion and vibration, they need to be assisted to reach the main airways to enable them to be coughed out. The migration of secretions can be enhanced by gravity and there are the specific manoeuvres for postural drainage. The direction of the flow of secretions should match the lobar and bronchopulmonary segments and their bronchiolar arrangements. Each posture is maintained to a safe maximum of 2–4 h after which the patient is turned to an alternate posture to prevent soiling of the healthy lung from the secretions. Table 4.10 illustrates the various positions for postural drainage of secretions that are commonly performed during chest physiotherapy.

Table 4.10 Various positions for postural drainage

Region of lung	Position	Location of therapy
Upper lobe, apical segment	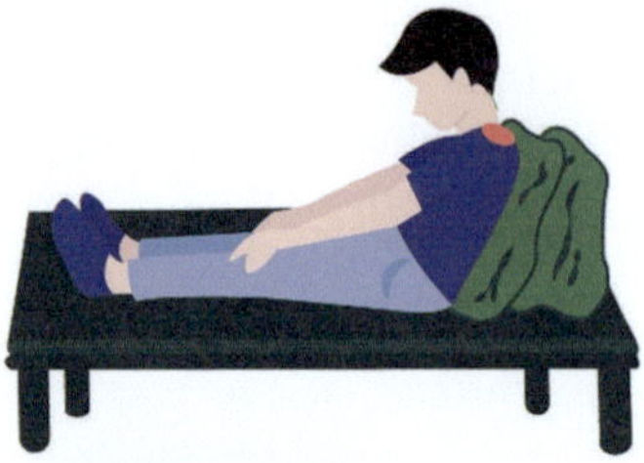	Area between clavicle and scapula
Upper lobe, posterior segment	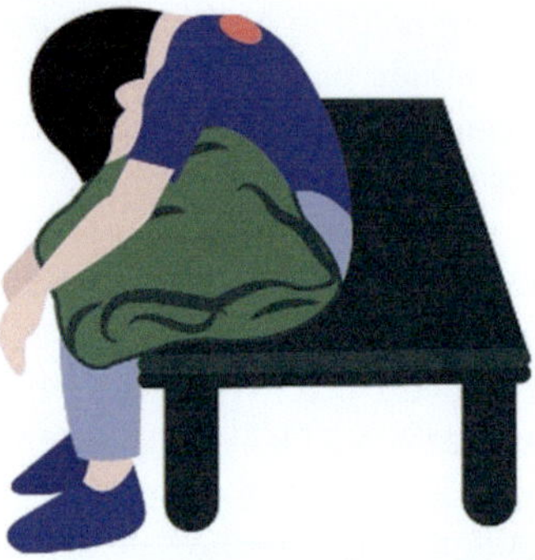	Upper back
Upper lobe, anterior segment	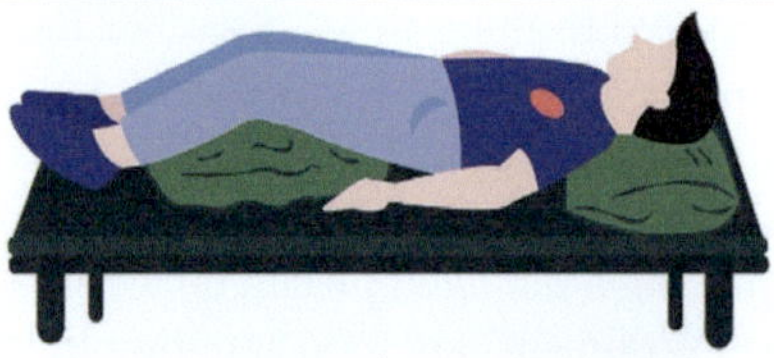	Upper aspect of anterior chest (between clavicle and nipple)
Lingula	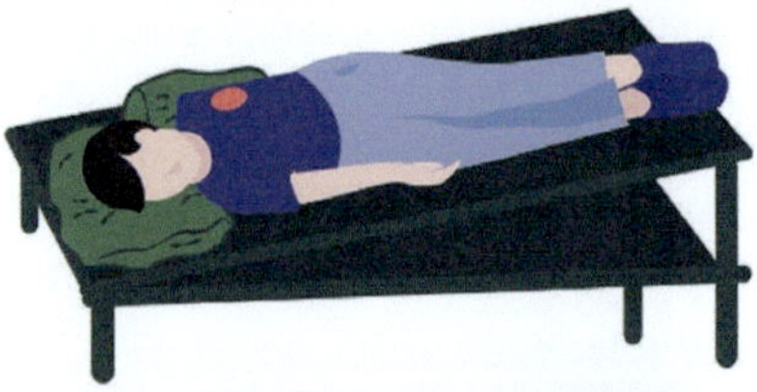	Lateral to nipple
Middle lobe	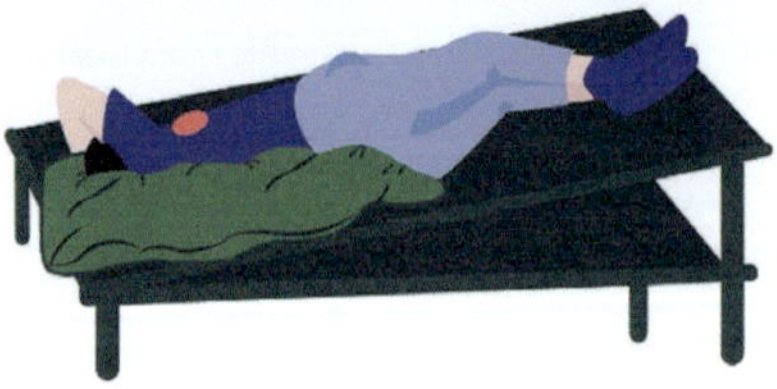	Lateral to right nipple

Table 4.10 (continued)

Region of lung	Position	Location of therapy
Lower lobe, anterior basal segment	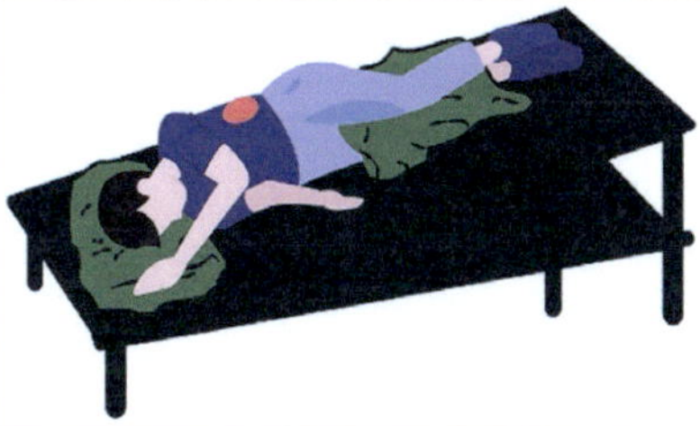	Lower lateral chest wall
Lower lobe, posterior basal segment	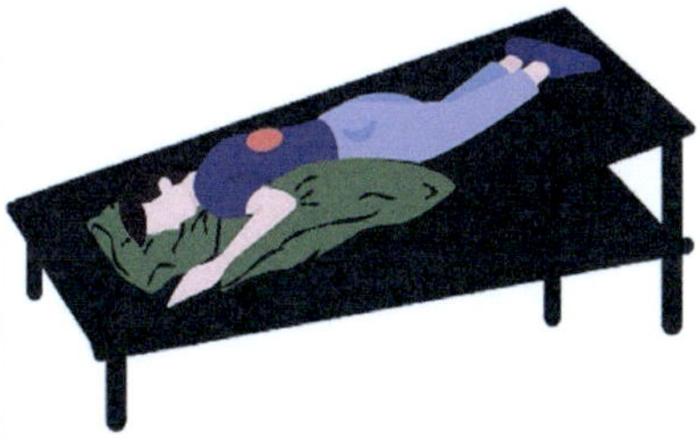	Midback (corresponding to lower lobes of lungs)
Lower lobe, lateral basal segment	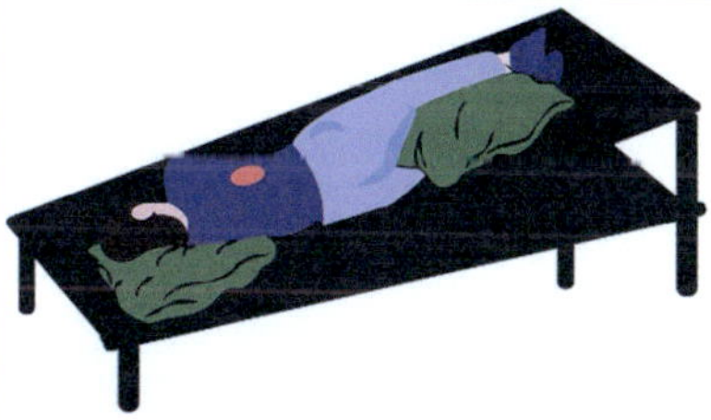	Lower lateral chest wall
Lower lobe, superior segment	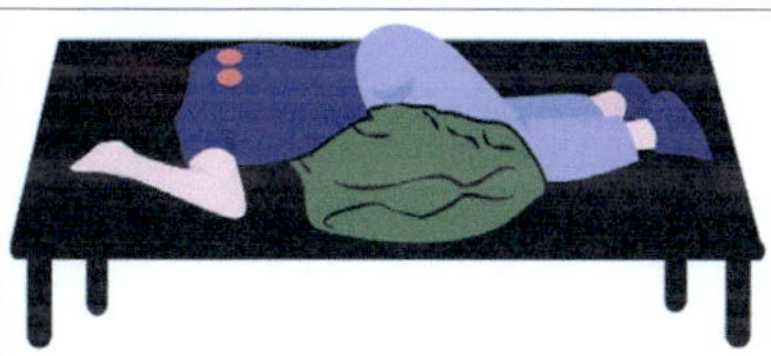	Below scapula

Modern ways of providing chest physiotherapy include enhanced systematic airway clearance techniques. These include stratification of location of area of concern into proximal and peripheral locations. Proximal clearance is achieved by flow acceleration techniques (expiratory flow acceleration) and cough augmentation methods (manual assisted breathing, lung volume recruitment bags, non-invasive ventilation, intermittent positive pressure ventilation). Peripheral clearance techniques include conventional techniques (positioning, postural drainage), breathing exercises (autogenic drainage, active cycle of breathing techniques), provision of positive expiratory pressure (devices and valves) and wall oscillatory devices (High Frequency Chest Wall Oscillation) [42].

References

1. Fishman AP. Pulmonary rehabilitation research. Am J Respir Crit Care Med. 1994;149:825–33.
2. Barberan-Garcia A, Ubré M, Roca J, Lacy AM, Burgos F, Risco R, et al. Personalised prehabilitation in high-risk patients undergoing elective major abdominal surgery: a randomised blinded controlled trial. Ann Surg. 2018;267(1):50–6.
3. Gillis C, Li C, Lee L, Awasthi R, Augustin B, Gamsa A, et al. Prehabilitation versus rehabilitation: a randomized control trial in patients undergoing colorectal resection for cancer. Anesthesiology. 2014;121(5):937–47.
4. Li T, Yang M, Tseng AH, Lee HH. Prehabilitation and rehabilitation for surgically treated lung cancer patients. J Cancer Res Pract. 2017;4(3):89–94.
5. Sebio Garcia R, Yáñez Brage MI, Giménez Moolhuyzen E, Granger CL, Denehy L. Functional and postoperative outcomes after preoperative exercise training in patients with lung cancer: a systematic review and meta-analysis. Interact Cardiovasc Thorac Surg. 2016;23(3):486–97.
6. Egan TD, Wong KC. Perioperative smoking cessation and anesthesia: a review. J Clin Anesth. 1992;4(1):63–72.
7. Lindstrom D, Azodi OS, Wladis A, Tonnesen H, Linder S, Nasell H, et al. Effects of a perioperative smoking cessation intervention on postoperative complications: a randomized trial. Ann Surg. 2008;248(5):739–45.
8. Guideline on smoking as related to the perioperative period [Internet]. Melbourne (AU): Australian and New Zealand College of Anaesthetists; 2014 [cited 3 June 2021]. Available from: https://www.anzca.edu.au/getattachment/a3591188-1d7d-41cf-807a-b3b2f0226109/PS12BP-Guideline-on-smoking-as-related-to-the-perioperative-period-Background-Paper
9. Grichnik KP, Hill SE. The perioperative management of patients with severe emphysema. J Cardiothorac Vasc Anesth. 2003;17(3):364–87.
10. Vagvolgyi A, Rozgonyi Z, Kerti M, Vadasz P, Varga J. Effectiveness of perioperative pulmonary rehabilitation in thoracic surgery. J Thorac Dis. 2017;9(6):1584–91.
11. Jamali S, Dagher M, Bilani N, Mailhac A, Habbal M, Zeineldine S, et al. The effect of preoperative pneumonia on postsurgical mortality and morbidity: a NSQIP analysis. World J Surg. 2018;42(9):2763–72.
12. Shen J, Zhang P, An Y, Jiang B. Prognostic implications of preoperative pneumonia for geriatric patients undergoing hip fracture surgery or arthroplasty. Orthop Surg. 2020;12(6):1890–9.
13. Mitrouska I, Klimathianaki M, Siafakas NM. Effects of pleural effusion on respiratory function. Can Respir J. 2004;11(7):499–503.
14. Skok K, Hladnik G, Grm A, Crnjac A. Malignant pleural effusion and its current management: a review. Medicina. 2019;55(8):490.
15. Mitry E, Guiu B, Cosconea S, Jooste V, Faivre J, Bouvier A-M. Epidemiology, management and prognosis of colorectal cancer with lung metastases: a 30-year population-based study. Gut. 2011;59(10):1383–8.

16. Temel JS, Greer JA, Muzikansky A, Gallagher ER, Admane S, Jackson VA, et al. Early palliative care for patients with metastatic non-small-cell lung cancer. N Engl J Med. 2010;363:733–42.
17. Higenbottam T, Kuwano K, Nemery B, Fujita Y. Understanding the mechanism of drug-associated interstitial lung disease. Br J Cancer. 2004;91(S2):S31–7.
18. Camus P, Kudoh S, Ebina M. Interstitial lung disease associated with drug therapy. Br J Cancer. 2004;91(S2):S18–23.
19. Lind PA, Marks LB, Jamieson TA, Carter DL, Vredenburgh JJ, Folz RJ, et al. Predictors for pneumonitis during locoregional radiotherapy in high-risk patients with breast carcinoma treated with high-dose chemotherapy and stem-cell rescue. Cancer. 2002;94(11):2821–9.
20. Ryu JH. Chemotherapy-induced pulmonary toxicity in lung cancer patients. J Thorac Oncol. 2010;5(9):1313–4.
21. Leo F, Solli P, Spaggiari L, Veronesi G, de Braud F, Leon ME, et al. Respiratory function changes after chemotherapy: an additional risk for postoperative respiratory complications. Ann Thorac Surg. 2004;77(1):260–5.
22. West MA, Loughney L, Barben CP, Sripadam R, Kemp GJ, Grocott MPW, et al. The effects of neoadjuvant chemotherapy on physical fitness and morbidity in rectal cancer surgery patients. Eur J Surg Oncol. 2014;40(11):1421–8.
23. Jack S, West MA, Raw D, Marwood S, Ambler G, Cope TM, et al. The effect of neoadjuvant chemotherapy on physical fitness and survival in patients undergoing oesophagogastric cancer surgery. Eur J Surg Oncol. 2014;40(10):1313–20.
24. Hornsby WE, Douglas PS, West MJ, Kenjale AA, Lane AR, Schwitzer ER, et al. Safety and efficacy of aerobic training in operable breast cancer patients receiving neoadjuvant chemotherapy: a phase II randomized trial. Acta Oncol. 2013;53(1):65–74.
25. Marks LB, Bentzen SM, Deasy JO, Kong FM, Bradley JD, Vogelius IS, et al. Radiation dose-volume effects in the lung. Int J Radiat Oncol Biol Phys. 2010;76(3):S70–6.
26. Arroyo-Hernández M, Maldonado F, Lozano-Ruiz F, Munoz-Montano W, Nunez-Baez M, Arrieta O. Radiation-induced lung injury: current evidence. BMC Pulm Med. 2021;21(1):1–12.
27. Vogelius IR, Bentzen SM. A literature-based meta-analysis of clinical risk factors for development of radiation induced pneumonitis. Acta Oncol. 2012;51(8):975–83.
28. Gross NJ. Pulmonary Effects of Radiation Therapy. Ann Intern Med. 1977;86(1):81–92.
29. Lopez Rodriguez M, Cerezo PL. Toxicity associated to radiotherapy treatment in lung cancer patients. Clin Transl Oncol. 2007;9(8):506–12.
30. Elliott JA, O'Byrne L, Foley G, Murphy CF, Doyle SL, King S, et al. Effect of neoadjuvant chemoradiation on preoperative pulmonary physiology, postoperative respiratory complications and quality of life in patients with oesophageal cancer. Br J Surg. 2019;106(10):1341–51.
31. Abou-Jawde RM, Mekhail T, Adelstein DJ, Rybicki LA, Mazzone LA, Caroll PJ, et al. Impact of induction concurrent chemoradiotherapy on pulmonary function and postoperative acute respiratory complications in esophageal cancer. Chest. 2005;128(1):250–5.
32. Tarumi S, Yokomise H, Gotoh M, Kasai Y, Matsuura N, Chang SS, et al. Pulmonary rehabilitation during induction chemoradiotherapy for lung cancer improves pulmonary function. J Thorac Cardiovasc Surg. 2015;149(2):569–73.
33. Lepper PM, Ott SR, Hoppe H, Schumann C, Stammberger U, Bugalho A, et al. Superior vena cava syndrome in thoracic malignancies. Respir Care. 2011;56(5):653–66.
34. Wilson LD, Detterbeck FC, Yahalom J. Superior vena cava syndrome with malignant causes. N Engl J Med. 2007;356(18):1862–9.
35. Drews RE, Rabkin DJ. Malignancy-related superior vena cava syndrome [Internet]. Waltham, MA: UpToDate; 2021 [cited 2021 May 30] Available from: https://www.uptodate.com/contents/malignancy-related-superior-vena-cava-syndrome?search=Drews,%20R.%20E.,%20Rabkin,%20D.%20J.,%20Eidt,%20J.%20F.,%20%26%20Collins,%20K %20A.%20(2016).%20Malignancy-related%20superior%20vena%20cava%20syndrome.%20UpToDate,%20Waltham,%20MA.&source=search_result&selectedTitle=1~150&usage_type=default&display_rank=1
36. Scheede-Bergdahl C, Minnella EM, Carli F. Multi-modal prehabilitation: addressing the why, when, what, how, who and where next? Anaesthesia. 2019;74:20–6.

37. Carli F, Charlebois P, Stein B, Feldman L, Zavorsky G, Kim DJ, et al. Randomized clinical trial of prehabilitation in colorectal surgery. Br J Surg. 2010;97(8):1187–97.
38. Jensen BT, Petersen AK, Jensen JB, Lausten S, Borre M. Efficacy of a multiprofessional rehabilitation programme in radical cystectomy pathways: a prospective randomized controlled trial. Scand J Urol. 2014;49(2):133–41.
39. Dunne D, Jones R, Lythgoe D, Malik H, Poston GJ, Jack S, et al. Prehabilitation before liver surgery. Eur J Surg Oncol. 2014;40(11):S52.
40. Banerjee S, Manley K, Thomas L, Shaw B, Saxton J, Mills R, et al. O2 Preoperative exercise protocol to aid recovery of radical cystectomy: results of a feasibility study. Eur Urol Suppl. 2013;12(6):125.
41. West MA, Loughney L, Lythgoe D, Barben CP, Cripadam R, Kemp GJ, et al. Effect of prehabilitation on objectively measured physical fitness after neoadjuvant treatment in preoperative rectal cancer patients: a blinded interventional pilot study. Br J Anaesth. 2015;114(2):244–51.
42. Belli S, Prince I, Savio G, Paracchini E, Cattaneo D, Bianchi M, et al. Airway clearance techniques: the right choice for the right patient. Front Med. 2021;8:73.
43. Kuyrukluyildiz U, Binici O, Kupeli I, Ertuk N, Gulhan B, Akyol F, et al. What is the best pulmonary physiotherapy method in ICU? Can Respir J. 2016:1–5.

Endocrine Prehabilitation 5

Joel Lau, James Lee, Anirban Sinha, and Rajeev Parameswaran

Abbreviations

ACTH	Adrenocorticotropic hormone
ALP	Alkaline phosphatase
CRH	Corticotropin-releasing hormone
CT	Computer tomography
CVA	Cardiovascular accident
CVS	Cardiovascular system
DIT	Diiodotyrosine
ECG	Electrocardiogram
ECMO	Extracorporeal membrane oxygenation
GIS	Gastrointestinal system
HPA	Hypothalamic-pituitary-adrenal
ICU	Intensive care unit
IHD	Ischaemic heart disease
IONM	Intra-operative nerve monitoring

J. Lau · J. Lee
Endocrine Surgery, National University Health System, Singapore, Singapore

A. Sinha
Department of Endocrinology, Medical College Kolkata, Kolkata, India

R. Parameswaran (✉)
Endocrine Surgery, National University Health System, Singapore, Singapore

Department of Surgery, Yong Loo Lin School of Medicine, National University of Singapore, Singapore, Singapore

National Cancer Institute of Singapore, National University Hospital, Singapore, Singapore

Alexandra Hospital, Singapore, Singapore
e-mail: rajeev_parameswaran@nuhs.edu.sg

A. Chakraborty, A. Balakrishnan (eds.), *Prehabilitation for Cancer Surgery*,
https://doi.org/10.1007/978-981-16-6494-6_5

IOPTH	Intra-operative parathyroid hormone
MEN	Multiple endocrine neoplasia
MIT	Monoiodotyrosine
MRI	Magnetic resonance imaging
PTH	Parathyroid hormone
PTU	Propylthiouracil
SCSI	Subcutaneous soluble insulin sliding scale
SNS	Sympathetic nervous system
T3	Triiodothyronine
T4	Thyroxine
TFT	Thyroid function test
TRAb	Thyroid receptor autoantibody
TRH	Thyrotropin releasing hormone
TSH	Thyroid stimulating hormone
VIP	Vasoactive intestinal peptide

5.1 Introduction

In this modern age of surgery, patients are becoming increasingly complex with multiple underlying comorbidities. The outcomes of surgery are not solely dependent on the surgery but also on psychological and physical well-being including quality of life. There is evidence in the literature to suggest that following major surgeries, nearly half of the patients continue to show some degree of disability downstream [1]. There has been a major shift in clinical practice to optimize the patient before surgery to improve outcomes through the strategy called *Prehabilitation.*

The concept of prehabilitation is essentially 4 pronged as shown in Fig. 5.1. It is not uncommon to see patients with comorbidities especially in the elderly and includes conditions such as diabetes, hypertension, renal impairment and thyroid dysfunction. Other issues seen are fraility, poor respiratory reserve, anaemia, anxiety, depression and poor nutritional status which are some of the modifiable risks that can be addressed before surgery [2]. While the first 3 prongs of prehabilitation are essential for any patients undergoing surgery, medical prehabilitation which addresses all the medical issues is more important in the context of endocrine surgical patients.

Endocrinopathies such as diabetes mellitus, thyroid disorders and endocrine hypertension are becoming more commonplace and adequate perioperative optimization is essential for a successful surgery. While most thyroid and parathyroid surgery can be performed with short stay in hospital, cancer surgery especially adrenal cancer, parathyroid cancer and invasive cancers of the thyroid are associated with significant medical problems. These conditions commonly present with electrolyte abnormalities, hypertension and rarely even present with crises that may even be fatal. Overproduction or underproduction of hormones can have life-threatening

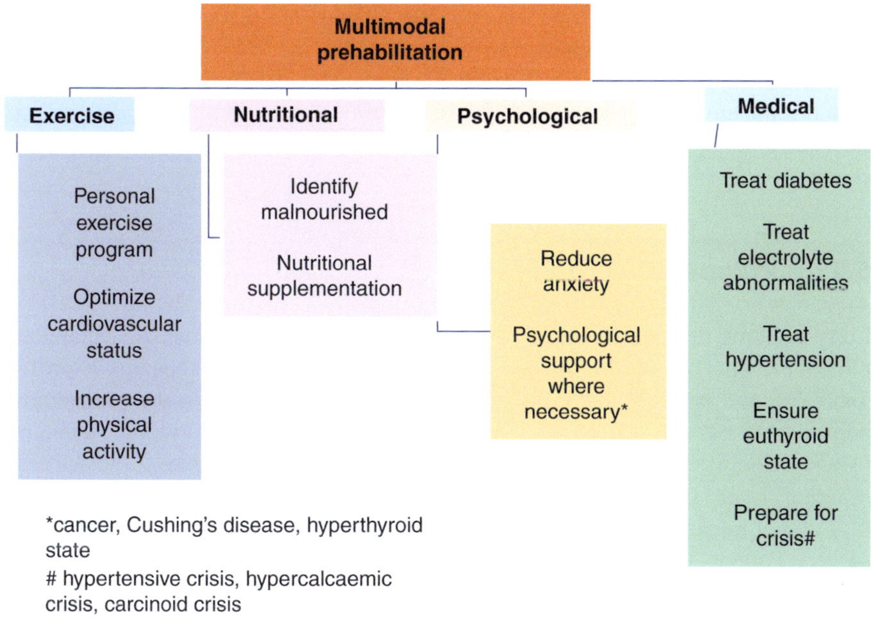

Fig. 5.1 The 4 pillars of prehabilitation in endocrine surgery

consequences and affect the anaesthetic management of such patients. This chapter aims to discuss the perioperative management and prehabilitation of conditions affecting the main endocrine organs—pancreas, thyroid, parathyroid and adrenal glands.

5.1.1 Diabetes and Glucose Control

Diabetes is a common disorder that affects millions of people around the world with a rising incidence year on year. Diabetes is diagnosed when the fasting plasma glucose is greater than 126 mg/dl (7.0 mmol/L) or with a haemoglobin A1c concentration (HbA1c) reading of >6.5%. Many patients are diagnosed diabetic during routine screening in the preoperative period. There are a significant number of patients of known type 2 diabetes who had poor glycaemic control on routine screening preoperatively. These patients have an increased risk of perioperative wound infections and cardiovascular complications.

Surgery and general anaesthesia lead to an acute stress response with activation of both the hypothalamic-pituitary-adrenal (HPA) axis and sympathetic nervous system (SNS). The stress response results in increased release of norepinephrine, epinephrine, cortisol and proinflammatory cytokines (i.e. IL-1, IL-6, TNF-alpha). This stimulates hepatic gluconeogenesis, glycogenolysis and insulin resistance which results in stress hyperglycaemia [3]. Studies have shown that new-onset stress hyperglycaemia has a poorer outcome than known diabetic patients in post-operative ICU settings. In addition to the neuroendocrine stress response, perioperative diabetic control involves the holistic management of multiple factors. This includes the anticipated duration of fasting, timing of the operative procedure, sepsis management, type of diabetes, diabetic medications and pre-existing diabetic control.

5.2 Preoperative Evaluation

Long-standing diabetes is known to lead to macrovascular and microvascular complications. The common problems seen in association with diabetes is shown in Table 5.1 and needs to be addressed before elective surgery. In the preoperative period, these patients should be screened for cardiovascular comorbidities including hypertension, ischaemic heart disease and congestive cardiac failure. An electrocardiogram should be obtained preoperatively and if necessary, an echocardiogram or myocardial perfusion scan should be obtained to help risk-stratify patients before surgery. Patients with diabetes have an increased risk of silent myocardial infarction, while asymptomatic, these patients are at higher risk of cardiovascular morbidity.

Table 5.1 Common problems seen in patients with diabetes mellitus and risk posed at anaesthesia

System	Pre-op issues	Intra-operative risks	Post-operative risks
CVS	Hypertension Silent IHD CVA MI Cardiomyopathy autonomic neuropathy	Tachycardia bradycardia Postural hypotension	Tachycardia Bradycardia MI Hypotension
Renal	Microalbuminuria Hypertension IHD	Hypotension Electrolyte abnormalities	Renal failure Hypotension
Respiratory	Poor respiratory reserve	Poor oxygenation and ventilation (especially obese)	Chest infections
GI	Reflux Hyperacidity Poor gastric emptying	Aspiration (at induction)	Stress ulcers Worsening of reflux Chest infection (if aspiration)
Airway	Thickening of soft tissues Intubation may be difficult (difficult mouth opening)	Intubation may be difficult (difficult mouth opening) Neck extension may be difficult (thyroid and parathyroid surgery)	Neck pain (if hyperextension)

Also, routine blood tests should be taken to evaluate for chronic renal impairment. Nearly one-third of diabetic patients have some form of renal impairment which can affect the anaesthesia and post-operative outcome. The Hba1c measurement indicates the patient's diabetic control in the preceding 3 months. Ideally, the patient's blood glucose should be optimized before the surgical intervention to reduce the risk of post-operative wound infection. These patients should also be assessed for cerebrovascular disease and diabetic autonomic neuropathy.

5.3 Perioperative Management of Diabetes

In the preoperative period, it must be determined if the patient has type 1 or type 2 diabetes as this has a consequence on the subsequent insulin management. There are many post-operative factors such as sepsis, hyperalimentation and glucocorticoid use. Patients with type 1 diabetes should be co-managed with the medical endocrine colleagues as these patients are at risk of having labile glycaemic control and can present with both extremes of hypoglycaemia and with diabetic ketoacidosis. These patients should be put on GIK (glucose insulin potassium) infusion from the time of fasting before surgery.

The perioperative glycaemic control aims to avoid hypoglycaemia, marked hyperglycaemia or crisis states such as diabetic ketoacidosis or hyperosmolar hyperglycaemic non-ketoacidosis states. As a general guide, blood glucose levels should be kept under 180 mg/dL (10.0 mmol/L). For patients at risk of hypoglycaemia, a less stringent glucose target is acceptable.

Patients with type 2 diabetes can be categorized into those on diet control, on oral hypoglycaemic agents and insulin-dependent. For patients on diet control, no special measures are required, and patients should have their blood glucose checked before surgery.

For patients on oral hypoglycaemic agents or insulin, patients will be required to have frequent point-of-care blood glucose monitoring every 4 h while waiting for surgery. The subcutaneous sliding scale should not be used as it causes significant fluctuation of glycaemia. Dextrose-containing drip with added soluble insulin can also be administered for patients with long fasting duration. For a more prolonged duration of operation, an insulin infusion can be considered especially in cases of brittle diabetes or type 1 diabetes. Patients with poorly controlled glycaemic control with blood glucose levels >14 mmol/L on 2 or more readings should be started on a basal insulin regimen (Table 5.2).

Most patients who are on oral antidiabetic agents who undergo short-duration surgery may continue with the same medications if glycaemic control is acceptable. We need to avoid sulfonylurea on the day of surgery to avoid hypoglycaemia. SGLT2 inhibitors need to be stopped 4 days before surgery to avoid dehydration perioperatively. Metformin preferably is stopped 24 h before surgery if there is a risk of acidosis or renal hypoperfusion before surgery.

Table 5.2 Adjusting of basal insulin dose

Current regimen		Suggested titration
No previous basal insulin		Starting dose of 0.2 units/kg body weight given as SC NPH in 2 divided doses
Long-acting basal insulin (glargine/detemir)	50% basal: 50% prandial	Continue current basal insulin dosage
	Disproportionately more basal than prandial insulin	Add total daily dose and give half as basal long-acting insulin
Intermediate acting basal insulin (NPH)		Decrease dose to 50% on morning of surgery
Pre-mixed insulin (i.e. 70/30 NPH/regular)		Decrease dose to 50% of pre-mixed insulin and keep patient on dextrose-containing drip

Patients who are on basal insulin especially on larger doses need to continue the same with a slight reduction of dose by 10–20% on the night before admission. We need to avoid any prandial insulin when NPM starts.

5.4 Post-operative Management of Diabetes

Post-operatively, the patient's blood sugar level must be regularly monitored every 2–4 h before resuming oral intake. Corrective short-acting insulin may be given in case of hyperglycaemia reported. For patients who develop hypoglycaemia, oral carbohydrates or intravenous dextrose (25–50 cc of 50% dextrose) can be administered with a repeat blood glucose measurement at 15 min. In the context of endocrine surgery, bilateral adrenalectomy or unilateral adrenalectomy for Cushing's syndrome or pheochromocytoma can lead to glucose instability. These patients will also be routinely started on glucocorticoid therapy post-operatively which can precipitate steroid-induced hyperglycaemia. The insulin dose needs to be frequently evaluated and titrated based on the steroid dose use and the blood glucose level.

5.4.1 Thyroid Disorders

5.4.1.1 Thyroid Hormone Physiology

Thyroid hormone synthesis is based on the Thyrotropin Releasing Hormone (TRH) and Thyroid Stimulating Hormone (TSH) pathway. TRH from hypothalamus stimulates TSH from the anterior pituitary which in turn stimulates the thyroid follicular cells to synthesize Triiodothyronine (T3) & Thyroxine (T4). Iodine is absorbed by the gastrointestinal tract and converted to iodide ion. TSH receptors bound to TSH stimulate iodide transport into the thyroid gland by the sodium iodide symporter. In the thyroid gland, iodide is oxidized and bound to tyrosine in the thyroglobulin to form iodotyrosine (MIT and DIT). MIT and DIT couple to form the hormonally active iodothyronines, T4 and T3. T3 is the active form which influences the individual's metabolic rate.

For all patients undergoing thyroid surgery, evaluation of the airway, cardiac function and biochemical evaluation of the thyroid status is mandatory. A clinical history assessing for hyper- and hypothyroidism symptoms, thyroid compressive symptoms (i.e. dysphagia, dyspnoea) and a recent change of voice will provide guidance on the preoperative anaesthesia management for these patients.

5.4.1.2 Hyperthyroidism and Hypothyroidism

Hyperthyroidism commonly manifests with symptoms of weight loss, heat intolerance, diarrhoea, proximal muscle weakness and anxiety. In addition, palpitations, new-onset atrial fibrillation, fine tremors, sweaty palms and presence of exophthalmos suggest excess thyroid hormones. The diagnosis of hyperthyroidism can be confirmed with a preoperative thyroid function test (TFT) consisting of T4 and TSH. Most commonly, this is caused by uncontrolled or newly diagnosed Graves' disease or patients with toxic multinodular goitre.

For patients suspected of Graves' disease, a thyroid receptor autoantibody (TRAb) can be measured to confirm the diagnosis. Preoperative control of hyperthyroidism is paramount before surgery. Cardiovascular changes lead to tachycardia, decreased systemic vascular resistance, increased myocardial oxygen consumption, everything leading to cardiovascular instability. These patients are more prone to arrhythmias and cardiac ischaemia. Patients with hyperthyroidism usually have increased anaesthetic requirements, mostly to control blood pressure and heart rate. Hyperthyroid patients have increased sensitivity to catecholamines, and hypotension. Respiratory muscle weakness occurs with hyperthyroidism, which may warrant mechanical ventilation increasingly in the post-operative period. Use of antithyroid drugs such as propylthiouracil (PTU), methimazole or carbimazole should be started with a consultation with an endocrinologist. For patients with arrhythmias the use of beta-blockers should also be considered judiciously. Lastly, some endocrine surgeons will routinely start patients on Lugol's iodine 14 days prior to surgery to decrease thyroid gland vascularity. This should only be started once the patient becomes euthyroid.

Patients should be euthyroid prior to surgery. Uncorrected hyperthyroidism or hypothyroidism may lead to increased risk of cardiovascular and respiratory complications. For patients with hyperthyroidism, they are at risk of thyroid storm which will manifest as severe tachycardia, arrhythmias, new onset AF, hyperthermia and cardiac dysfunction. This can occur intra-operatively or in the immediate post-operative period, usually within the first 6–24 h. The use of the Burch and Wartofsky Scoring System (Table 5.3) can give an indicator of the likelihood of overt thyroid storm [4]. Intra-operatively, thyroid storm can mimic malignant hyperthermia; however, thyroid storm is not associated with muscle rigidity and elevated creatine kinase. Patients presenting with thyroid storm represents a medical emergency and acute management involves intravenous fluids, cooling measures, correcting of electrolytes and glucose levels. A non-cardio selective beta blocker (i.e. propranolol) is the first-line drug of choice followed by thionamide (i.e.

Table 5.3 Burch and Wartofsky scoring system

Diagnostic parameters	Scoring points[a]	
Temperature	37.2–37.7	5
	37.8–38.2	10
	38.3–38.8	15
	38.9–39.4	20
	39.4–39.9	25
	>40.0	30
Tachycardia	99–109	5
	110–119	10
	120–129	15
	130–139	20
	>140	25
CNS effects	Mild (agitation)	10
	Moderate (delirium/psychosis)	20
	Severe (seizure/coma)	30
Gastrointestinal and hepatic dysfunction	Moderate (diarrhoea)	10
	Severe (jaundice)	20
Congestive heart failure	Mild	5
	Moderate	10
	Severe	15
Atrial fibrillation	Absent	0
	Present	10
Precipitant history	Absent	0
	Present	10

[a]Scoring Points: ≥45 = highly suggestive, 25–44 = supports dx, <25 = unlikely

propylthiouracil). Lugol's iodine can be administered but only 1 h after propylthiouracil to prevent iodine from being used as a substrate for new hormone synthesis. Excess iodine administration transiently inhibits thyroid iodide organification also known as the Wolff–Chaikoff effect. Also, high dose intravenous glucocorticoid (i.e. hydrocortisone) is recommended to reduce the T4–T3 conversion.

Patients who are hypothyroid before surgery, present with different set of challenges. Clinical manifestation of hypothyroidism includes lethargy, weight gain despite a decrease in appetite, cold intolerance, constipation, bradycardia, decreased myocardial contractility and decreased cardiac output. Biochemically, primary hypothyroidism is diagnosed by an elevated TSH with a decrease in T4. This should be distinguished from euthyroid sick syndrome where TSH is normal while T3 is low and T4 is normal or low. In euthyroid sick syndrome, thyroid hormone replacement is not required [5].

Patients with hypothyroidism can also be categorized to having subclinical hypothyroidism (elevated TSH with normal T4), moderate hypothyroidism (elevated TSH, low T4) or severe hypothyroidism (elevated TSH, low T4 with severe clinical symptoms). In patients with moderate or severe hypothyroidism, they are at risk for cardiovascular complications. These patients have decreased intravascular volume, decreased preload, decreased cardiac output and blunted baroreceptor reflexes.

Anaesthetic agents will take longer to wear off and patients may have vasopressor-resistant hypotension. Hypothyroid patients may have a lesser response to alpha- and beta-adrenergic agents, leading to higher requirement of vasopressor agents. In addition to cardiovascular complications, these patients are at risk for ventilatory dysfunction due to respiratory muscle weakness, hyponatremia, decreased clearance of drugs due to decreased renal perfusion, anaemia and hypothermia. Obstructive sleep apnoea is detected more commonly and should be suspected in patients with hypothyroidism before operative intervention. Coagulation abnormality is also common in this population.

Patients should be rendered euthyroid before elective surgery to minimize perioperative morbidity. This can be done by starting patients on levothyroxine (T_4) starting at a dose of 50 μg daily and titrated over several weeks after liaising with an endocrinologist. A dreaded complication from hypothyroid patients undergoing surgery is myxoedema coma where patients present with altered mental status, hypothermia, hypopnoea, bradycardia, congestive heart failure and hyponatremia. However, if emergency surgery is required liothyronine (T_3) may be given at a dose of 10–50 μg slowly intravenously with ECG monitoring and may be followed by 8-hourly replacement. As iv levothyroxine or liothyronine is not available in all countries, the oral/NGT route of LT4 (100–150 μg) can be an equally effective alternative as it did not alter the mortality in a small observational study. For patients with refractory hypotension, the diagnosis of concurrent adrenal insufficiency should be considered and patients started on IV glucocorticoid.

5.5 Retrosternal Goitre

In addition to the common predictors of difficult endotracheal intubation [6], assessment of the extent of the thyroid goitre is important. For patients with substernal goitres or having compressive symptoms, further imaging with contrasted computer tomography (CT) or magnetic resonance imaging (MRI) of the neck and thorax will be recommended. In the majority of patients with substernal goitre, trachea compression and deviation occur distally without supraglottic compromise. These patients can usually be intubated routinely without the need for awake fibre-optic intubation [7]. Some of the factors that are predictive of difficult intubation in thyroid surgery include decreased cervical joint mobility precluding neck extension, short thyromental distance and inter-incisor gap and increasing age [6, 8].

Rarely one may encounter a retrosternal goitre that may present with an airway crisis as shown in Fig. 5.2 and these cases can be quite challenging and require a multidisciplinary input. There are significant variations in clinical practice in difficult airway scenarios, with some preferring to do awake intubation, some with advanced techniques such as jet ventilation, and most experiences cited were from personal series of cases. The difficult airway society has proposed an algorithm for challenging cases such as these [9] (Fig. 5.3). Rarely, an emergent tracheostomy may be needed but even this may not be possible due to the highly vascular thyroid tissue and the situation may require an emergent salvage with ECMO.

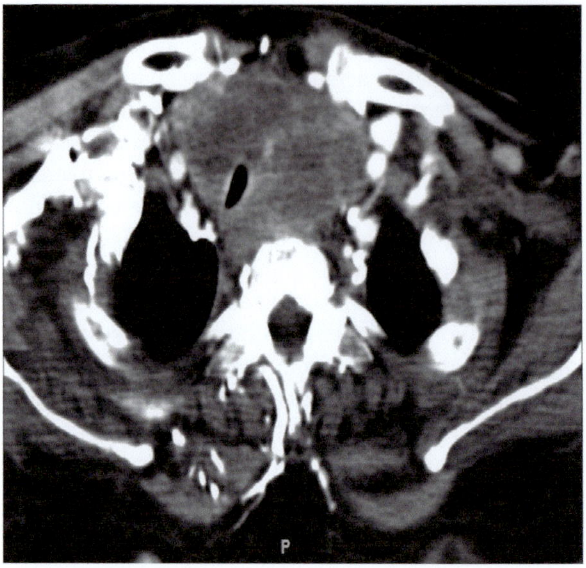

Fig. 5.2 Axial CT scan showing the presence of a retrosternal goitre with significant tracheal compression

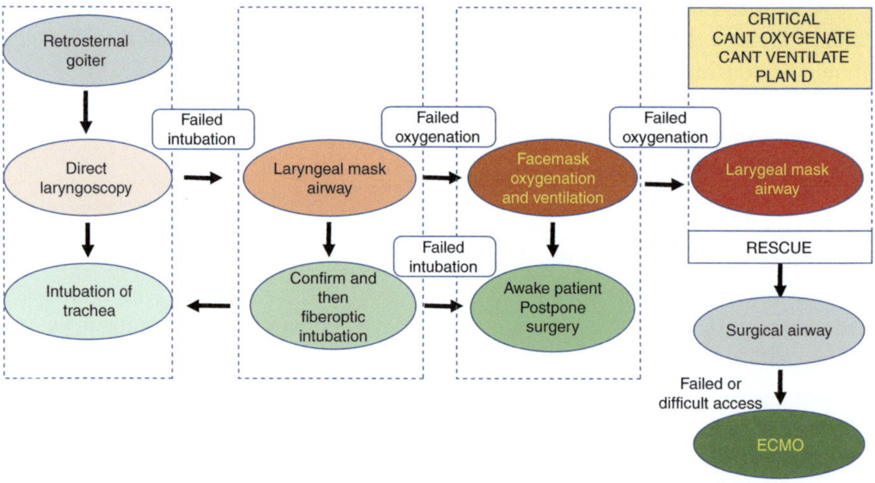

Fig. 5.3 Strategies for difficult airway in retrosternal goitre

5.6 Recurrent Laryngeal Nerve and Intra-operative Nerve Monitoring

Patients with preoperative voice changes or undergoing repeat thyroid operation should have their vocal cords evaluated via video nasendoscopy before surgery. Pre-existing immobility of one side of the vocal cord puts the patients at higher risk of bilateral recurrent laryngeal nerve injury post-operatively which may make extubating challenging.

Modern-day thyroid surgery often employs the use of intra-operative nerve monitoring (IONM) to ensure the functional integrity of the vagus and recurrent laryngeal nerve intra-operatively. The use of IONM is gaining acceptance as the standard of care in thyroid surgery. Most commonly, the use of endotracheal tube-based surface electrodes remains the most popular approach. The anaesthetist should be familiar with the placement and location of the electrode on the endotracheal tube. Intubation when performed with video laryngoscopy allows for accurate placement for the electrode to be in contact with the mucosa of the vocal cord. Tube placement should be verified again after patient positioning with neck extension before the commencement of surgery to minimize failure risk of IONM. Malposition of the endotracheal tube remains the most common cause of equipment failure [10].

Intubation should be performed with non-depolarizing neuromuscular blockade agents. The use of neuromuscular blockade decreases laryngeal injury [10]. However, the operating surgeon must be aware of the possibility of false-negative responses from the IONM during the initial phase of the surgery. It is suggested that patients be dosed with one effective dose of rocuronium (0.3 mg/kg) as this was associated with a lower false-negative response as compared to patients dosed with two effective doses (0.6 mg/kg) during the early phase of surgery [11]. Maintenance of anaesthesia is usually with propofol, remifentanil and fentanyl.

In the event where a unilateral recurrent laryngeal nerve injury is documented on IONM, careful consideration should be made before embarking on surgical resection of the contralateral thyroid lobe. Bilateral recurrent laryngeal nerve injury can potentially result in airway compromise with failure to extubate the patient post-operatively. These patients may require ICU care and may potentially require tracheostomy in event of prolonged intubation.

5.7 Post-operative Complication

In the immediate post-operative period, the anaesthetist should be wary of the development of a neck haematoma with resultant acute airway distress. If a rapidly enlarging neck haematoma is noted during patient reversal (before extubating), urgent surgical evaluation should be made and extubation withheld. The patient may require an urgent re-exploration of the neck wound, evacuation of haematoma and repeat surgical haemostasis. If the neck haematoma occurs after extubation has occurred, tracheal compression and laryngopharyngeal oedema will make re-intubation difficult. Immediate treatment involves opening of the neck wound with a horizontal incision through the platysma muscle and then a vertical incision between the strap muscles to allow for haematoma evacuation. Airway protection with awake fibre-optic intubation may be required as the neck haematoma may distort the airway.

In thyroid surgery, bleeding with resultant acute expanding neck haematoma is an uncommon complication. To minimize the risk of post-operative bleeding, meticulous haemostasis and intra-operative application of Valsalva manoeuvre at 40 mmHg can help to identify potential venous bleeding sites.

5.7.1 Parathyroid and Disorders of Calcium Homeostasis

For patients undergoing parathyroid surgery, an understanding of the underlying aetiology is important in planning the anaesthetic approach. Hyperparathyroidism is a biochemical diagnosis and patients' electrolytes should be corrected before surgery. For patients with secondary or tertiary hyperparathyroidism secondary to renal failure, preoperative intravascular access is important especially for patients who are anticipated to require intravascular calcium infusion post-operatively.

5.8 Calcium Homeostasis

Calcium plays many functions including being a mediator of intracellular signal, regulating cell membrane permeability, being involved in neuromuscular transmission, smooth and skeletal muscle contraction, coagulation, bone formation and regulating the secretion of parathyroid hormone and calcitonin. Calcium is regulated mainly by three different hormones, parathyroid, calcitonin and vitamin D.

The parathyroid hormones which are secreted by the parathyroid glands located posterior to the thyroid parenchyma acts on the bone, kidney and gastrointestinal system to regulate serum ionized calcium. The parathyroid hormone increases skeletal osteoclastic activity, increases calcium reabsorption from the distal convoluted tubules of the kidney and enhances 1-hydroxylation of 25-hydroxyvitamin D which increases intestinal absorption of calcium. Parathyroid also increases urinary phosphate excretion. Calcitonin which is produced by the parafollicular C cells opposes the effect of PTH on calcium homeostasis.

5.9 Primary Hyperparathyroidism

Diagnosis for primary hyperparathyroidism is biochemical [12, 13]. Primary hyperparathyroidism which is commonly due to a hyperfunctioning parathyroid adenoma can present with hyperglycaemic crisis (cCA > 3.5 mmol/L) which must be stabilized before surgery to minimize cardiovascular complications. These patients should be managed with an endocrinologist. Intravascular normal saline administration to ensure adequate hydration should be the first step. Loop diuretics, calcitonin and bisphosphonate may be considered to ensure that calcium levels are stabilized. Elevated calcium levels can result in cardiac arrhythmias.

Long-standing primary hyperparathyroidism can also lead to chronic renal impairment, osteoporosis and neuropsychiatric complications. Primary hyperparathyroidism can be resolved with the surgical removal of the offending adenoma with improvement in renal function, bone density and reduction in cardiovascular events. Localized parathyroid surgery may be performed under GA or under local anaesthesia and sedation safely. However, patients with non-localized surgery or parathyroid cancer or those with inherited disorders such as MEN-1 related parathyroid disease require surgery under GA and at times can last for about 3–4 h.

Intra-operatively, the use of intra-operatively PTH (IoPTH) measurement with a rapid assay can guide the operating surgeon on the success of the parathyroid excision [14]. The IoPTH measurement can be drawn from a peripheral vein (i.e. lower limb plug), arterial catheter or internal jugular vein. Both pre- and post-excision IoPTH have to be drawn from the same location. The IoPTH should decrease by more than 50% and be in the normal range 10 min after the parathyroid adenoma is excised [14].

5.10 Secondary/Renal Hyperparathyroidism

Secondary hyperparathyroidism also commonly referred to as renal hyperparathyroidism poses a different set of challenges to the anaesthetic team. These patients are commonly high-risk surgical candidates with multiple comorbidities, secondary to long-standing renal failure. Preoperatively, these patients must undergo a thorough anaesthetic evaluation with referral to cardiology, respiratory, reanal and endocrinology physicians as appropriate.

Before undergoing operation following points should be followed in the preparatory phase:

- Preferably avoid situations that aggravate hypercalcaemia if possible, mostly thiazide diuretic and lithium therapy, volume depletion, high-calcium diet (>1000 mg/day), prolonged bed rest, or inactivity.
- Promote physical activity to minimize bone loss.
- Promote adequate hydration (6–8 glasses of water per day) to reduce the risk of renal stone.
- Promote a moderate calcium intake (1000–1500 mg/day). A low calcium diet may lead to stimulation of PTH secretion and could aggravate bone involvement, so moderate calcium restriction (e.g. <800 mg/day) is probably warranted when the serum calcitriol concentration is elevated.
- We should promote moderate vitamin D intake (400–800 international units daily) to maintain (25[OH]D) levels of at least 20 or 30 ng/mL (50 or 75 mmol/L).

Surgery for hyperparathyroidism is often planned months in advance to allow time for optimization. Indications for surgery include symptomatic hyperparathyroidism such as bone pain, calciphylaxis, bone fracture or pruritus or in patients with severe hyperparathyroidism who have failed medical therapy [15]. Severe hyperparathyroidism is defined as a PTH value greater than 9 times the upper limit for the assay. In people whose primary indication for surgery is symptomatic and/or severe hypercalcaemia (for whom bone density is normal), cinacalcet rather than bisphosphonates is preferred.

Preoperatively, the alkaline phosphate (ALP) value prognosticates which patients would experience post-operatively hypocalcaemia. Protocols should be in place for pre-loading of calcium and Vitamin D before surgery. Non-calcium-based bisphosphonates and cinacalcet should also be stopped 1–2 weeks before the surgery date. Usually, this will be performed after discussion with the endocrine surgery team and nephrologist. Patients must also be adequately dialyzed before surgery.

Often, patients with secondary hyperparathyroidism being planned for parathyroidectomy have long-standing renal failure and will have venous access complications. Insertion of a central venous line is more complicated in these patients as many of them will have central venous stenosis which makes line insertion difficult. These patients should be identified preoperatively and be planned for radiological guided line insertion under fluoroscopy on the morning of the surgery. Intra-operatively, once all four parathyroids have been identified and removed, intravenous calcium infusion should be commenced via the central line. There should be a standardized protocol to guide the dilution of calcium and the rate of calcium infusion.

Post-operatively, due to the rapid decrease in PTH, this will lead to an osteoblastic influx of calcium into the bone which can lead to severe and prolonged hypocalcaemia, hypophosphatemia and hypomagnesemia. These patients who are at risk for hungry bone syndrome often will have preoperative bone disease due to chronic osteoclastic bone resorption from elevated PTH. Prognostic factors that predict for post-parathyroidectomy hungry bone syndrome include older age, high ALP and preoperative radiological evidence of bone disease (like subperiosteal erosions, lytic lesions, pathological fractures, browns tumours, osteitis fibrosa cystica). Patients with hypocalcaemia will commonly present with perioral or peripheral numbness. Classical clinical manifestations of hypocalcaemia such as Chvostek sign (twitching of facial muscles on tapping over the facial nerve) and Trousseau sign (carpal spasm following inflation of the blood pressure cuff over the arm) can also be seen.

For patients with post-operative hypocalcaemia IV calcium (1 or 2 g of calcium gluconate, equivalent to 90 or 180 mg elemental calcium, in 50 mL of 5% dextrose or normal saline) can be infused over 10–20 min for immediate treatment. For maintenance therapy of hungry bone syndrome, an IV solution containing 1 mg/mL of elemental calcium is prepared by adding 11 g of calcium gluconate (equivalent to 1000 mg elemental calcium) to normal saline or 5% dextrose water of 1000 mL. Patients are usually given 0.5–1.5 mg/kg of elemental calcium per hour.

In our local practice, we minimize the occurrence of symptomatic hypocalcaemia by using protocolized preoperative calcium loading and post-operative calcium infusion. Patients' blood calcium levels are checked 6–8 hourly post-operatively to guide the calcium infusion rates.

5.10.1 Adrenal Disorders and Endocrine Hypertension

The adrenal gland is divided into the adrenal cortex and medulla. The adrenal cortex has three zones, the zona glomerulosa produces mineralocorticoid, the zona fasciculata produces glucocorticoid, and the zona reticularis produces sex hormones. The adrenal medulla contains chromaffin cells which produce catecholamines from tyrosine.

5.10.1.1 Conn's Syndrome

Conn's Syndrome is related to an overproduction of aldosterone which is usually secondary to an adrenal adenoma. Aldosterone acts on the renal tubules to increase reabsorption of water, it also increases reabsorption of sodium in exchange for potassium and hydrogen ions. These patients commonly present with sustained hypertension (i.e. >140/90 on multiple readings), difficult to manage hypertension (i.e. >140/90 resistant to three conventional antihypertensive), controlled hypertension but with use of four or more antihypertensive agents or hypertension with hypokalaemia. Diagnosis involves biochemical screening with plasma renin and aldosterone. Localization tests can be performed with CT adrenal and use of adrenal vein sampling. Surgery is curative only in patients with unilateral aldosterone-producing tumour.

Preoperatively, these patients should be managed with spironolactone, an aldosterone antagonist for at least 2–3 weeks before surgery. Potassium levels should be normalized before surgery.

Post-operatively, all antihypertensive and potassium replacement should be stopped. An undetectable plasma aldosterone concentration confirms correct preoperative adenoma localization and long-term cure. If the post-operative plasma aldosterone concentration is >5 ng/dL, the patient needs to be followed closely by monitoring daily home blood pressure measurements and at least weekly serum potassium concentrations. Normalization of potassium is expected in almost all patients while hypertension is cured in 42% of patients [16]. Males, older age, longer duration of hypertension, and the greater number of antihypertensive agents used portends a poor prognostic factor for cure [16]. Most patients with Conn's syndrome, despite not achieving a cure, benefit from a decrease in pill burden. Patients should be monitored closely for hyperkalaemia post-operatively, which may result from transient hypoaldosteronism due to chronic suppression of renal renin release. Post-operatively we may need to discontinue drugs like ACE or ARB to avoid hyperkalaemia.

5.10.1.2 Cushing's Syndrome

Cushing syndrome is related to an overproduction of cortisol by the zona fasciculata within the adrenal cortex. The excess cortisol would normally lead to negative feedback on the hypothalamic-pituitary-adrenal axis which downregulates the corticotropin-releasing hormone (CRH) and adrenocorticotropic hormone (ACTH). Excess cortisol production over a prolonged period can lead to a myriad of clinical manifestations. Patients presenting with supraclavicular fat pads, central obesity with wasting of the extremities, rounded facies, spontaneous bruising, proximal myopathy, purple striae and glucose intolerance should be suspected for Cushing [17]

Cushing's syndrome can be classified into ACTH dependent or ACTH independent. The most common cause of ACTH-dependent hypercortisolism is due to Cushing's disease which is usually caused by an ACTH secreting adenoma of the pituitary gland. Other causes include paraneoplastic syndrome associated with ectopic ACTH secretion. ACTH independent hypercortisolism can be caused by adrenal cortical neoplasm or bilateral adrenal hyperplasia.

Preoperative evaluation involves optimization of cortisol-dependent comorbidities. This includes optimization of electrolytes as patients can present with hypokalaemic metabolic alkalosis from the mineralocorticoid activity of glucocorticoid.

Strict glycaemic control with the use of either oral hypoglycaemic agents or subcutaneous insulin is also essential before surgery. Patients should be screened for psychiatric disorders, hypertension, hyperlipidaemia and osteoporosis [17]. Due to the presence of proximal myopathy, patients can be reviewed by physiotherapists perioperatively to undergo intense muscle training.

Before surgical intervention, perioperative steroid replacement should be given as the patient's adrenal gland may not be able to respond to perioperative stress. However, preoperative glucocorticoid replacement is not essential unless cortisol production has been blocked completely by adrenal enzyme inhibitors. Patients are also at risk for infective complications, venous thromboembolism and adrenal insufficiency in the post-operative period [17]. The current recommendation from the endocrine society suggests for age-appropriate vaccination with influenza, herpes zoster and pneumococcal before surgery for patients [17]. The risk of venous thromboembolism is highest within the first 4 weeks after surgery, current consensus suggests post-operative prophylaxis for 4 weeks with early mobilization. Post-operative stress ulcer prophylaxis with proton pump inhibitors should also be started. Post-operatively, glucocorticoids must be stopped for 24 h before serum cortisol can be measured to assess cure. Glucocorticoid replacement can be continued for a few days, with careful monitoring for the development of adrenal insufficiency. Patients with successful surgery may require stress coverage with cortisol replacement up to 12 months post-surgery. Diabetes insipidus can develop up to 20% of patients post pituitary surgery in pituitary Cushing's disease which requires regular monitoring and management of hyponatremia.

In general, patients with macroadenomas have lower cure rates. All patients should be regularly screened annually for several years and less frequently thereafter. This is important in those who had initial intermittent hypersecretion of cortisol.

For patients who underwent bilateral adrenalectomy, they will require lifelong glucocorticoid and mineralocorticoid replacement. These patients must be issued an emergency card stating the need for stress dose of glucocorticoid during future emergency admission.

5.10.1.3 Pheochromocytoma

Pheochromocytoma is a catecholamine-secreting tumour that arises from chromaffin cells. Classically, symptoms include episodic headache, palpitations, diaphoresis, pallor and anxiety. Patients also have either persistent or paroxysmal hypertension. The variability of symptoms is due to the episodic nature of the catecholamines secreted. Different clinical phenotypes exist depending on the secretory profile of the tumour [18]. Pheochromocytoma can involve tumours that predominantly secrete norepinephrine, epinephrine or dopamine. The risk of sustained hypertension is highest in norepinephrine secreting tumours owing to alpha-1, alpha-2 and beta-1 stimulation. Tumours can also be biochemically silent or secrete catecholamines only when stimulated (i.e. from surgical manipulation).

Pheochromocytoma surgery is usually associated with haemodynamic instability due to inadequate preoperative hypertensive control or associated hypovolemia, and both of these can contribute to significant mortality. Surgical mortality rates are increased due to lethal hypertensive crises, malignant arrhythmias and multiorgan failure. It is therefore imperative that these factors be addressed before surgery with optimization of blood pressure, tachycardia and restoration of intravascular volume before surgery. There are no randomized trials which have compared the efficacy of various antihypertensive regimes to control hypertension preoperatively. The commonly used drugs are a combination of alpha-adrenergic receptor antagonists, beta-adrenergic receptor antagonists and calcium channel blockers. The catecholamine synthetic pathway and the receptors they act on, is shown in Fig. 5.4.

Patients diagnosed with pheochromocytoma should be instituted on alpha-adrenergic blockade at least 1–2 weeks before surgery [19]. Phenoxybenzamine, a long-acting, non-competitive, irreversible alpha antagonist is commonly used for blood

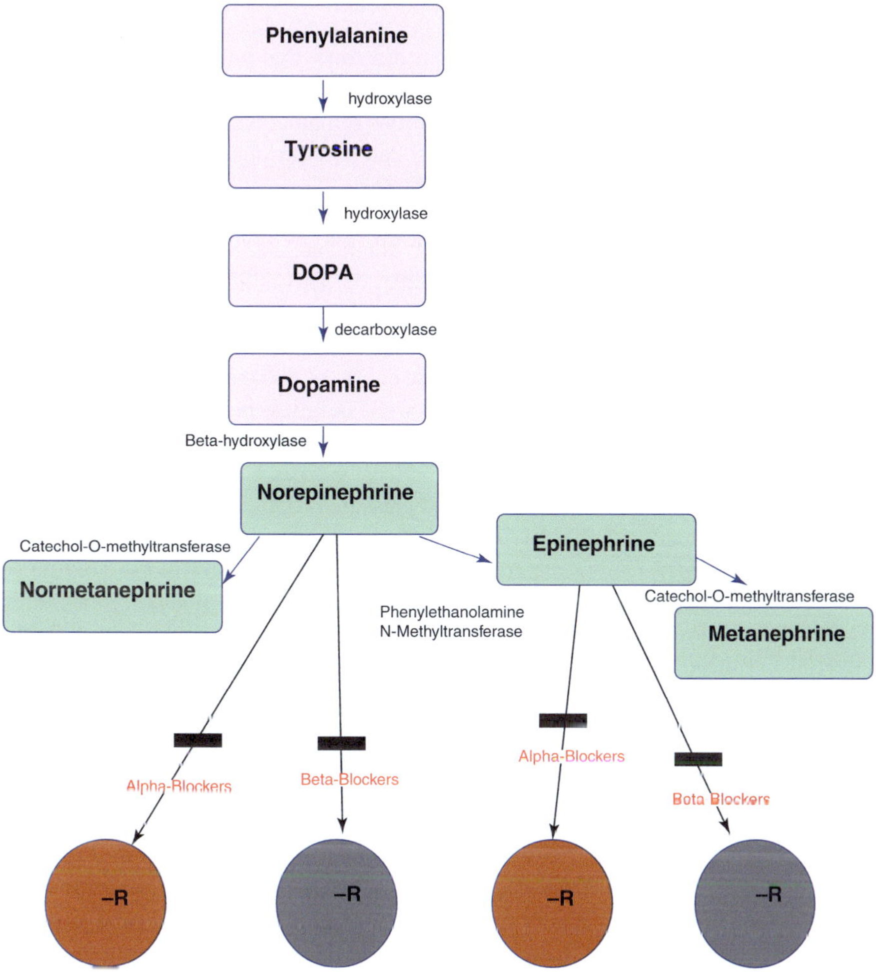

Fig. 5.4 Synthetic pathway of catecholamines and the action of antihypertensive medications

Table 5.4 Roizen criteria

1	No in-hospital blood pressure > 160/90 mmHg for 24 h prior to surgery
2	No orthostatic hypotension with blood pressure < 80/45 mmHg
3	No ST or T wave changes for 1 week prior to surgery
4	No more than 5 premature ventricular contractions per minute.

pressure control and prevention of arrhythmias. The medication is initiated at 10 mg twice a day and titrated with an eventual daily dose of between 40 and 120 mg/day [20]. Another alternative alpha-blocker is doxazosin which is a selective and competitive α1-adrenergic receptor blocker with a maximum daily dose of 24 mg twice daily. Both of these drugs were compared in a randomized clinical trial which noted no difference in blood pressure control preoperatively between these two alpha blockade agents [21]. The PESCRIPT trial did show that phenoxybenzamine was more effective in preventing intra-operative haemodynamic instability; however, the clinical impact on cardiovascular complications remained similar [21]. Before surgery, the use of Roizen criteria (Table 5.4) can give an objective indicator of the adequacy of the preoperative alpha blockade [22].

Patients are encouraged to have a high salt diet (>5000 mg daily) and fluid intake 2–3 days after initiation of alpha-blockers to counteract catecholamine-induced volume contraction and postural hypotension [20, 23]. This much volume expansion is contraindicated in patients with congestive heart failure or renal insufficiency. Beta-blockers are started a few days before surgery to prevent cardiac arrhythmias. Adequate preoperative blockade involves blood pressure below 130/80 mmHg and a heart rate of 60–70 beats per minute. Beta-blockers must not be given before alpha-blockers in patients with pheochromocytoma to avoid unopposed alpha receptor-mediated vasoconstriction which can precipitate a fatal hypertensive crisis. Calcium channel blockers can be used as an additional therapy if blood pressure is not well controlled [23].

Patients are usually admitted 1–2 days before surgery with the initiation of intravenous crystalloids. This is aimed at restoration of circulating blood volume to minimize the risk of hypotension with the removal of the pheochromocytoma. Large-bore intravenous cannulas are placed to allow for rapid infusion of fluids. Arterial line insertion provides for real-time haemodynamic monitoring. If available, the use of a minimally invasive haemodynamic monitoring device (i.e. FloTrac) can be used to provide information on cardiac output, cardiac index, stroke volume and total systemic vascular resistance. Premedication may be given in the form of temazepam. The various steps that may be taken to ensure safe anaesthesia during the conduct of pheochromocytoma surgery are illustrated in Fig. 5.5.

The insertion of a central venous line can also be considered especially as patients tend to have labile blood pressure during the operation requiring vasopressors. Haemodynamic instability can occur at induction and intubation, surgical incision, pneumoperitoneum during the laparoscopic approach, tumour manipulation and most importantly during ligation of the adrenal vein. At this juncture, there is a risk of rapid and profound hypotension requiring the use of vasopressor. Norepinephrine and epinephrine are the usual drugs of choice.

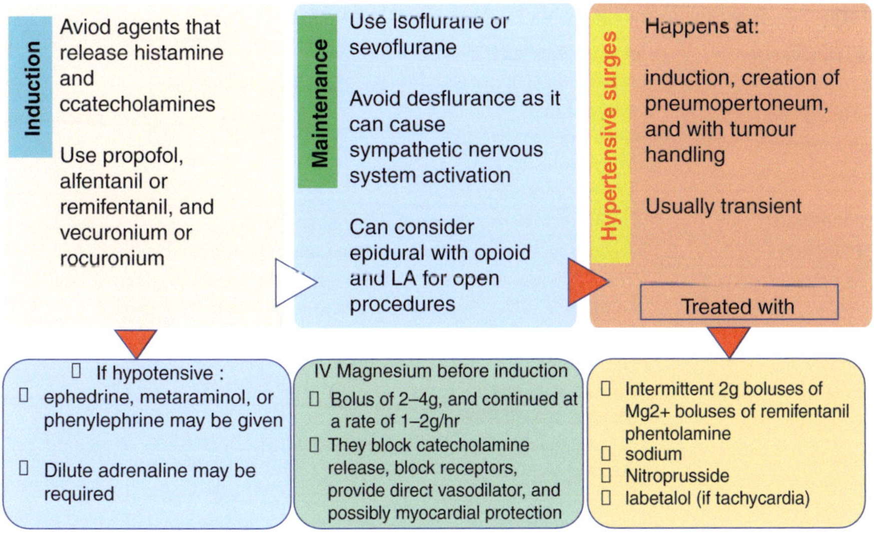

Fig. 5.5 Intra-operative anaesthetic management of pheochromocytoma

Post-operatively, patients are monitored in the high dependency unit as hypotension due to sudden decrease in circulating catecholamines can occur up to 48 h after surgery. Patients may also experience hypoglycaemia due to hyperinsulinemia from a sudden reduction in circulating catecholamines and increased peripheral glucose uptake. In up to 50% of patients, persistent hypertension can occur. Primary adrenal insufficiency mostly happens in patients treated with total adrenalectomy but only around 20% of patients underwent cortical-sparing adrenalectomy.

5.10.2 Carcinoid Tumours

Carcinoid tumours are neuroendocrine tumours arising in the gastrointestinal tract commonly, but can also arise in the bronchus and pancreas. Majority of these tumours are benign and about 25% of them are functional (hormone secreting). The most common vasoactive hormones secreted are serotonin, bradykinin, histamine, substance P, prostaglandins and vasoactive intestinal peptide (VIP). When these hormones are released into the systemic circulation, they can manifest as carcinoid syndrome, which is seen in about 10% of patients. Carcinoid tumours are usually asymptomatic and, in these patients, requiring surgery, anaesthesia is straightforward. However, when these tumours present with carcinoid syndrome, management can be quite challenging in the perioperative period.

Safe conduct of anaesthesia is important in the management of carcinoid tumours especially carcinoid syndrome and carcinoid heart disease as these patients present with complex symptoms that may be associated with significant morbidity and mortality [24]. Preoperative evaluation should be meticulous and evaluate the following: biochemistry which may correlate with tumour load, severity of symptoms,

Table 5.5 Anaesthetic management of carcinoid syndrome

Premedication	Anxiolytics such as benzodiazepine octreotide (100 μg (50–500 μg) SC 1 h preoperatively)
Monitoring	Arterial lines CVP line Monitor blood gases and glucose Transoesophageal ECHO
Analgesia	Epidural with low doses of local anaesthesia
Induction	Agents such as etomidate, fentanyl and vecuronium can be used
Maintenance	Total IV anaesthesia (TIVA) and inhalation techniques can be used Octreotide (10–20 μg boluses IV) to treat severe hypotension Avoid drugs that release histamine Use antihypertensives (labetalol, esmolol or ketanserin)
Post-operative care	Care in ICU or HDU Manage hypotension Manage analgesia with PCA with fentanyl or pethidine, or an epidural Wean octreotide after 7–10 days

assessment of potential triggers of crisis and risk factors such as pulmonary hypertension and right heart disease [25].

In the presence of symptoms such as diarrhoea, bronchospasm and dehydration treatments with antidiarrheals and bronchodilators is necessary along with correction of electrolyte imbalance and dehydration. The secretion of the vasoactive hormones can be prevented with octreotide given at a dose of 100 μg subcutaneously three times a day for 2 weeks prior to surgery and also at induction with 100 μg intravenously diluted to 10 μg/ml. Drugs that release histamine, such as atracurium need to be avoided along with other factors that may trigger a carcinoid crisis such as stress and anxiety. These patients should be managed in centres of excellence. A brief outline of the perioperative anaesthetic management is shown in Table 5.5. An algorithm for the safe conduct of anaesthesia in patients with carcinoid tumours and syndrome has been proposed by the Mount Sinai Group [24].

5.11 Conclusion

The concept of enhanced recovery and fast track surgery was to improve post-operative outcomes in surgical patients and has been in clinical practice for about 2 decades. Prehabilitation is where the functional capacity of the individual to withstand a stressful event such as surgery is enhanced using the 4 prongs of physical fitness, nutritional improvements, psychological support, and optimizing the medical problems commonly seen in endocrine disorders. Conditions affecting the thyroid, parathyroid, pancreas and adrenal glands are commonly seen in surgical practice and commonly associated with endocrine derangements. Endocrine prehabilitation is therefore important to reduce the morbidity and mortality associated with these conditions.

Appendix: Perioperative Management of Endocrine Disorders

Perioperative Management of Diabetes

Situation	Intervention
Hypoglycaemia	At risk: • Type 1 diabetes • Tight glycaemic control • Chronic renal disease • Past history of frequent hypoglycaemia • Known autonomic neuropathy Look for: • Tremor, palpitations, anxiety, sweating, hunger and paraesthesia unless under GA • Cognitive dysfunction Management: • Patient with a blood glucose of <70 mg/dL, administer IV dextrose (25 g) and repeat blood glucose measurements in 5–10 min • Put type 1 or labile glycaemic control on GIK infusion (prepared as a mixture of 500 mL 5% dextrose, 15 IU short-acting insulin and 10 mmol K (1 ampoule of 7.5% KCl) at rate started at 100 mL/h) then adjust insulin dose • Awake patient with a normal swallowing mechanism and gag reflex, 15 g of carbohydrates (glucose tablet, sweetened fruit juice)
Glycaemic target	• Avoid surgery if glycaemia >400 • Premeal target <140 mg/dl and random glucose <180 • Loose the target if hypoglycaemia is frequent
For surgery≥3 hrs	Most patients with type 1 diabetes should be using the insulin infusion rate starting roughly 0.5–1 U/h (mix 50 U short-acting insulin in 50 mL normal saline; i.e. 1 U = 1 mL), whereas infusion rates mostly increased in type 2 diabetics around 2–3 U/h or higher
Preoperative preparation	• Short surgery well controlled on oral agents – Continue same – Avoid sulfonylurea in the morning – Avoid SGLT2 inhibitor for 4 days prior to surgery – Avoid metformin for at least 12 h • On pre-mixed insulin – If well controlled, same can be continued with night before dose reduced by 20%. Morning dose can be withheld if FBG < 110 – If poorly controlled, shift to basal bolus regimen calculating the total dose and split it equally in basal and bolus insulin, then titrate • On basal bolus: Reduce the dose of basal insulin on the evening prior to surgery by 10–20% – Hold rapid acting dose in the morning – Start GIK infusion if required
Avoid subcutaneous sliding scale	Use i.v. insulin infusion algorithm if needed

Thyroid Disorders

Presentation	Intervention
Graves' disease	• Make euthyroid before operation • Look for arrhythmia and cardiac ischaemia • Hypotension should not be treated with catecholamine, as they have increased sensitivity to catecholamine • In arrhythmias the use of beta-blockers should also be started judiciously • Avoid Lugol's iodine before patient is euthyroid • Thyroid storm in OT requires intraveous fluids, cooling measures, correcting of electrolytes and glucose levels as well as steroids
Hypothyroidism	• Need to remember, anaesthetic agents will take longer to wear off and patients may have vasopressor-resistant hypotension • Obstructive sleep apnoea should be kept in mind • Make euthyroid at least for 2 weeks before surgery with starting dose of 1.8 μg/kg body wt. • Look for hypothermia, hypopnoea, bradycardia, congestive heart failure and manage accordingly • For short-duration preparation before surgery, need to keep the FT4 in range preoperatively as TSH take long to normalize
Recurrent laryngeal nerve injury	• Should have their vocal cords evaluated via video nasendoscopy before surgery • Modern-day thyroid surgery often employs the use of intra-operative nerve monitoring (IONM) to ensure the functional integrity of the vagus and recurrent laryngeal nerve intra-operatively • Need to be careful as bilateral recurrent laryngeal nerve injury can potentially result in airway compromise with failure to extubate the patient
Post-operative	• Avoid and be vigilant for neck haematoma • Document and take precaution for tracheomalacia

Hyperparathyroidism

Period	Intervention
Preoperative	• Preferably avoid situations that aggravate hypercalcaemia if possible, mostly thiazide diuretic and lithium therapy, volume depletion, high-calcium diet (>1000 mg/day), prolonged bed rest, or inactivity • Promote physical activity to minimize bone loss • Promote adequate hydration (6–8 glasses of water per day) to reduce the risk of renal stone • Promote a moderate calcium intake (1000 to 1500 mg/day). • We should promote moderate vitamin D intake • Non-calcium-based bisphosphonates and cinacalcet should also be stopped 1–2 weeks before the surgery

Period	Intervention
Post-operative	• Post-operatively, due to the rapid decrease in PTH, this will lead to an osteoblastic influx of calcium into the bone which can lead to severe and prolonged hypocalcaemia • Prognostic factors that predict for post-parathyroidectomy hungry bone syndrome include older age, high ALP, and preoperative radiological evidence of bone disease • For patients with post-operative hypocalcaemia IV calcium (1 or 2 g of calcium gluconate, equivalent to 90 or 180 mg elemental calcium, in 50 mL of 5% dextrose or normal saline) can be infused over 10–20 min for immediate treatment

Endocrine Hypertension

Situation	Intervention
Conn's syndrome	• Preoperatively, these patients should be managed with spironolactone, an aldosterone antagonist for at least 2–3 weeks before surgery. Potassium levels should be normalized before surgery • Post-operatively, all antihypertensive and potassium replacement should be stopped. An undetectable plasma aldosterone concentration confirms correct preoperative adenoma localization and long-term cure • Patients should be monitored closely for hyperkalaemia post-operatively, which may result from transient hypoaldosteronism due to chronic suppression of renal renin release • Post-operatively we may need to discontinue drugs like ACE or ARB to avoid hyperkalaemia
Cushing's syndrome	Preoperative • Optimization of electrolytes as patients can present with hypokalaemic metabolic alkalosis from the mineralocorticoid activity of glucocorticoid • Glycaemic control with the use of either oral hypoglycaemic agents or subcutaneous insulin • Should be screened for psychiatric disorders, hypertension, hyperlipidaemia and osteoporosis • Perioperative steroid replacement should be given as the patient's adrenal gland may not be able to respond to perioperative stress • Vaccination with influenza, herpes zoster and pneumococcal before surgery for patients Post operative: • Risk for infective complications, venous thromboembolism and adrenal insufficiency in the post operative period • Post-operatively, glucocorticoids must be stopped for 24 h before serum cortisol can be measured to assess cure • Glucocorticoid replacement can be continued for a few days, with careful monitoring for the development of adrenal insufficiency. Patients with successful surgery may require stress coverage with cortisol replacement up to 12 months post surgery • Diabetes insipidus can develop up to 20% patents post pituitary surgery in pituitary Cushing's disease

Situation	Intervention
Pheochromocytoma	Preoperative • Lethal hypertensive crises, malignant arrhythmias, and multiorgan failure with poor control have been documented • Optimization of blood pressure, tachycardia and restoration of intravascular volume before surgery • Should be instituted on alpha-adrenergic blockade at least 1–2 weeks before surgery • Before surgery, the use of Roizen criteria can give an objective indicator of the adequacy of the preoperative alpha blockade • Patients are encouraged to have high salt diet (>5000 mg daily) and fluid intake 2–3 days after initiation of alpha-blockers • Beta-blockers must not be given before alpha-blockers • Adequate preoperative blockade involves blood pressure below 130/80 mmHg and a heart rate of 60–70 beats per minute • Restoration of circulating blood volume to minimize the risk of hypotension with the removal of the pheochromocytoma Post-operative: • There is a risk of rapid and profound hypotension requiring the use of vasopressor. Norepinephrine and epinephrine are the usual drugs of choice • Hypotension due to sudden decrease in circulating catecholamines can occur up to 48 h after surgery • Patients may also experience hypoglycaemia due to hyperinsulinemia from a sudden reduction in circulating catecholamines

References

1. Barberan-Garcia A, et al. Personalised prehabilitation in high-risk patients undergoing elective major abdominal surgery: a randomized blinded controlled trial. Ann Surg. 2018;267(1):50–6.
2. Simcock R. Principles and guidance for prehabilitation within the management and support of people with cancer in partnership with acknowledgements. 2019.
3. Dungan KMMD, Braithwaite SSP, Preiser J-CP. Stress hyperglycaemia. Lancet. 2009;373(9677):1798–807.
4. Bahn RS, et al. Hyperthyroidism and other causes of thyrotoxicosis: management guidelines of the American Thyroid Association and American Association of Clinical Endocrinologists. Thyroid. 2011;21(6):593–646.
5. Himes CP, et al. Perioperative evaluation and management of endocrine disorders. Mayo Clin Proc. 2020;95(12):2760–74.
6. De Cassai A, et al. Prediction of difficult tracheal intubations in thyroid surgery. Predictive value of neck circumference to thyromental distance ratio. PLoS One. 2019;14(2):e0212976.
7. Hanson MA, Shaha AR, Wu JX. Surgical approach to the substernal goiter. Best Pract Res Clin Endocrinol Metab. 2019;33(4):101312.
8. Moon H-Y, et al. The causes of difficult tracheal intubation and preoperative assessments in different age groups. Korean J Anesthesiol. 2013;64(4):308–14.
9. Cook TM, Morgan PJ, Hersch PE. Equal and opposite expert opinion. Airway obstruction caused by a retrosternal thyroid mass: management and prospective international expert opinion. Anaesthesia. 2011;66(9):828–36.
10. Dionigi G, et al. Safety of neural monitoring in thyroid surgery. Int J Surg. 2013;11:S120–6.

11. Lu ICMD, et al. A comparative study between 1 and 2 effective doses of rocuronium for intraoperative neuromonitoring during thyroid surgery. Surgery. 2011;149(4):543–8.
12. Bilezikian JP. Primary hyperparathyroidism. J Clin Endocrinol Metab. 2018;103(11):3993–4004.
13. Insogna KL. Primary hyperparathyroidism. N Engl J Med. 2018;379(11):1050–9.
14. Shawky M, et al. Impact of intraoperative parathyroid hormone monitoring on the management of patients with primary hyperparathyroidism. Clin Endocrinol (Oxford). 2019;90(2):277–84.
15. Wang AY-M, et al. 2017 kidney disease: improving global outcomes (KDIGO) chronic kidney disease–mineral and bone disorder (CKD-MBD) guideline update implementation: Asia summit conference report. Kidney Int Rep. 2019;4(11):1523–37.
16. Muth A, et al. Systematic review of surgery and outcomes in patients with primary aldosteronism. Br J Surg. 2015;102(4):307–17.
17. Schreiner F, Anand G, Beuschlein F. Perioperative Management of Endocrine Active Adrenal Tumors. Exp Clin Endocrinol Diabetes. 2019;127(2/03):137–46.
18. Isaacs M, Lee P. Preoperative alpha-blockade in phaeochromocytoma and paraganglioma: is it always necessary? Clin Endocrinol. 2017;86(3):309–14.
19. Naranjo J, Dodd S, Martin YN. Perioperative Management of Pheochromocytoma. J Cardiothorac Vasc Anesth. 2017;31(4):1427–39.
20. Neumann HPH, Young WF, Eng C. Pheochromocytoma and Paraganglioma. N Engl J Med. 2019;381(6):552–65.
21. Buitenwerf E, et al. Efficacy of α-blockers on hemodynamic control during pheochromocytoma resection: a randomized controlled trial. J Clin Endocrinol Metab. 2020;105(7):2381–91.
22. Roizen MF, et al. The effect of alpha-adrenergic blockade on cardiac performance and tissue oxygen delivery during excision of pheochromocytoma. Surgery. 1983;94(6):941–5.
23. Challis BG, et al. Is there an optimal preoperative management strategy for phaeochromocytoma/paraganglioma? Clin Endocrinol. 2017;86(2):163–7.
24. Castillo J, Silvay G, Weiner M. Anesthetic Management of Patients with Carcinoid Syndrome and Carcinoid Heart Disease: the Mount Sinai algorithm. J Cardiothorac Vasc Anesth. 2018;32(2):1023–31.
25. Davar J, et al. Diagnosing and managing carcinoid heart disease in patients with neuroendocrine tumors: an expert statement. J Am Coll Cardiol. 2017;69(10):1288–304.

Haematological Prehabilitation 6

May Anne Cheong, Joshua Wei Sheng Loke, and Chandramouli Nagarajan

Abbreviations

ACD	Anaemia of chronic disease
aPTT	Activated partial thromboplastin time
CT-CAE	Common Terminology Criteria for Adverse Events
DIC	Disseminated intravascular coagulation
ESA	Erythropoiesis-stimulating agent
ECMO	Extracorporeal membrane oxygenation
HIT	Heparin-induced thrombocytopenia
IDA	Iron deficiency anaemia
ITP	Immune thrombocytopenic purpura
ISTH-BAT	International Society of Thrombosis and Haemostasis Bleeding Assessment Tool
PT	Prothrombin time
RBC	Red blood cell
RPI	Reticulocyte production index
TMA	Thrombotic microangiopathy
TEG	Thromboelastography
ROTEM	Rotational Thromboelastometry
TSAT	Transferrin saturation
TIBC	Total iron binding capacity
VTE	Venous thromboembolism
WHO	World Health Organization

M. A. Cheong (✉) · J. W. S. Loke · C. Nagarajan
Department of Haematology, Singapore General Hospital, Singapore General Hospital, Academia, Singapore, Singapore
e-mail: cheong.may.anne@singhealth.com.sg

A. Chakraborty, A. Balakrishnan (eds.), *Prehabilitation for Cancer Surgery*,
https://doi.org/10.1007/978-981-16-6494-6_6

6.1 Haematological Aspects of Oncological Surgery Prehabilitation

Patients undergoing oncological surgery often have concomitant haematological issues that would need careful consideration and management. This ranges from haemostatic challenges from profound bleeding to wide-spread thrombosis and the spectrum of these problems could be directly or indirectly related to the underlying cancer or may be entirely unrelated to it. Optimizing the condition of the patients, prior to surgery helps the patients to withstand the surgical insults and to reduce the risk of such haematological complications.

In this chapter we will review the Haematological issues in cancers and surgery: (1) Assessment and management of perioperative anaemia, (2) Assessment and management of perioperative cytopenias, (3) Assessment of haemostatic function and strategies to aid intraoperative haemostasis, (4) Venous thrombosis prevention and management and (5) Blood Transfusion Strategies in oncological patients.

6.2 Workup and Management of Perioperative Anaemia in the Cancer Patient

6.2.1 Overview of Cancer-Associated Anaemia

Anaemia is common in oncology patients [1]. Addressing anaemia in the preoperative setting is critical. Anaemia can impair the patient's functional status, diminish physiological reserve and result in delayed post-operative recovery [2]. Furthermore, anaemia is an independent predictor of poor prognosis in cancer patients [3, 4].

There are varying definitions of anaemia in the literature. The World Health Organization (WHO) definition for anaemia is based upon gender [5]. This can be further classified according to severity based on the Common Terminology Criteria for Adverse Events (CT-CAE) which grades severity based on haemoglobin levels [6]. Consolidating this allows for an anaemia grading system [7] (Table 6.1).

The pathogenesis of cancer-associated anaemia is complex. Often, multiple factors contribute to the development of anaemia. The mechanism of anaemia in patients with malignancy may be divided into blood loss, increased red blood cell

Table 6.1 Definition and criteria for grading cancer anaemia. (Adapted from Mclean et al. 2009, Gilreath et al. 2020) [5–7]

	CTCAE + WHO criteria	
Grade of anaemia	Women	Men
1	Hb 11.9–10.0 g/dL	Hb 12.9–10.0 g/dL
2	Hb 9.9–8.0 g/dL	
3	Hb < 7.9 g/dL	
4	Life-threatening consequences requiring urgent intervention, such as RBC transfusion	
5	Death	

Table 6.2 Mechanisms and causes contributing to anaemia in the oncosurgical patient

Mechanism causes	Blood loss	Increased red blood cell destruction	Decreased red blood cell production
Direct effect of neoplasm	Haemorrhage	Haemolysis	Bone marrow infiltration
Indirect or paraneoplastic manifestation	Haemostatic disorders e.g. Disseminated intravascular coagulopathy, factor deficiencies	Autoimmune, microangiopathic haemolytic anaemia Haemophagocytosis	Nutritional deficiencies e.g. Iron/B12 Anaemia of chronic disease Pure red cell aplasia
Effect of treatment	Perioperative blood loss Haemostatic disorders	Drug-induced haemolysis	Chemotherapy/ radiotherapy induced bone marrow toxicity

(RBC) destruction and decreased red blood cell production [8]. These may be as a result of the direct effect of the neoplasm, indirect or paraneoplastic effects or a consequence of cancer directed treatment (Table 6.2).

6.2.2 Assessment of Cancer-Associated Anaemia

The multifactorial nature of cancer-associated anaemia adds to the complexity of evaluation. An important starting point is recognizing that the patient has anaemia and to initiate further assessment at the earliest time point possible prior to planned surgery. Assessment should be guided based on a detailed history and physical examination and directed investigations. Common clinical manifestations include fatigue, dyspnoea and giddiness. Examination may reveal pallor. Often, these manifestations are not sensitive or specific to the type of anaemia. However, it is a useful reflection of the physiological and functional impact of anaemia on the patient. Further assessment for signs suggestive of contributing aetiology such as bleeding manifestations, jaundice and splenic enlargement should be performed.

There are 2 general approaches to investigate the cause of anaemia.

The **kinetic approach** addresses the mechanism resulting in anaemia and can be characterized based on decreased production or increased losses (due to haemolysis or haemorrhage).

The **morphologic approach** categorizes based on the red blood cell size measured by the/according to the mean corpuscular volume.

A comprehensive evaluation of the causes of anaemia often integrates both approaches and often it is a combination of factors (Fig. 6.1).

In the kinetic approach, calculation of reticulocyte production index (RPI) provides an indication of the bone marrow RBC production capacity [9] (Fig. 6.2). A normal RPI ranges between 1.0 and 2.0.

A **low RPI** (<2.0) suggest an inadequate bone marrow response for the degree of anaemia. This may be due to haematic deficiencies of iron, vitamin b12 or folate,

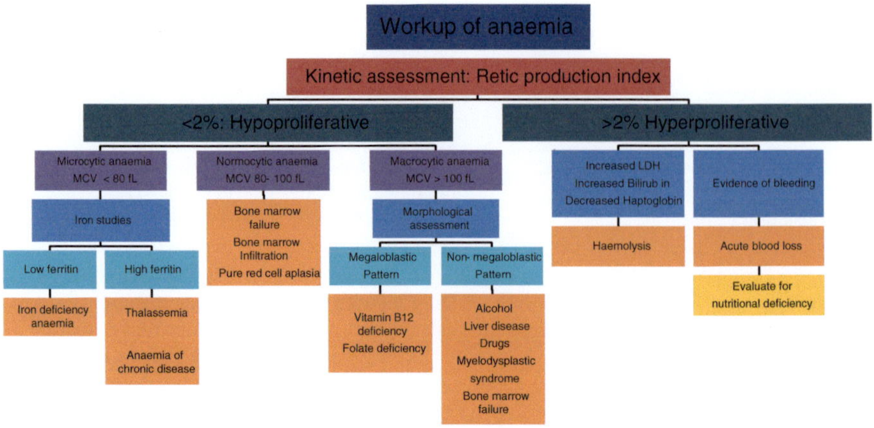

Fig. 6.1 Approach to the workup of anaemia. *MCV* mean corpuscular volume, *RPI* retic production index

An **RPI** >3 shows a normal marrow response to anaemia.
An **RPI** <2 is an inadequate response to anaemia

$$\text{Corrected retic} = \text{Retic (\%)} \times \frac{\text{Haematocrit (\%)}}{45}$$

$$\text{Retic Production Index} = \frac{\text{Corrected retic}}{\text{Maturation factor *}}$$

* Maturation factor: ≥35% = 1.0, 25 to <35% = 1.5, 20 to <25% = 2.0, <20% = 2.5
Maturation represents the maturation time of RBC (in days) at various levels of anaemia.

Fig. 6.2 Reticulocyte production index

bone marrow suppression due to chemotherapy or bone marrow infiltration of malignant neoplasm.

A **high RPI** (>2.0) suggests a normal or increased RBC production, indicative of blood loss or haemolysis.

In the morphological approach, classification is based on the average size of the RBC. A normal RBC has an approximate volume of 80–100 fL and the diameter of 7–8 microns, which is approximately the size of the nucleus of a small lymphocyte.

Microcytic anaemia (<80 fL) is usually associated with decreased RBC haemoglobin content resulting in a microcytic, hypochromic appearance. There are 3 most common causes of microcytosis: iron deficiency, thalassaemia and anaemia of chronic disease.

Macrocytic anaemia (>100 fL) may be due to increased reticulocytosis or impaired RBC maturation due to vitamin B12 and folate deficiencies or drug interference. An underlying haematological disorder, e.g. myelodysplastic syndrome or acute leukaemia, may also result in a macrocytic anaemia.

Normocytic anaemia (80–100 fL) has a long list of differentials including acute blood loss, haemolysis and anaemia of chronic disease. There may also be a combination of aetiologies. Often integrating the kinetic and morphological approach to determine the mechanism and cause of the anaemia is useful.

Additional Investigations are directed at evaluation of various aetiologies.

Iron deficiency: There are a number of tests available for the biochemical assessment of iron status. Serum ferritin is one of the more sensitive and specific tests used [10]. A cut-off level of less than 30 ng/mL is used to diagnose iron deficiency [11]. However, ferritin is an acute phase reactant and can be elevated regardless of iron status in conditions associated with inflammation, infection and malignancy [12]. As such, while a low ferritin level is diagnostic of iron deficiency, a relatively normal or elevated level may be a false normal result. In such cases, using other corroborative investigations such as transferrin saturation (TSAT), serum iron and total iron binding capacity (TIBC) should be used as indicators of the patient's iron status. TSAT is the ratio of serum iron to TIBC and a cut-off of below 20% is generally used to screen for iron deficiency (Table 6.3).

6.2.3 Management of Cancer-Associated Anaemia

In the management of anaemia, targeting the various underlying aetiologies is important. While there may be multiple factors contributing, there are specific therapies which can be instituted preoperatively to treat and optimize patients [13]. Management will also depend on the aetiology and severity of the anaemia, the type of surgical procedure and expected blood loss and the urgency of the procedure. Blood transfusion as a perioperative anaemia management is generally considered undesirable and transfusion is an independent risk factor for adverse outcomes [14]. Figure 6.3 details the overview of management of anaemia in the perioperative oncology patient. In addition, management of iron deficiency and the role of erythropoiesis-stimulating agents (ESAs) are detailed below.

6.2.3.1 Iron Deficiency

Patients with established iron deficiency should be treated with iron replacement [15]. Blood transfusions should generally be avoided. Most times the iron deficiency anaemia establishes itself over a long period of time and hence even patients that have fairly significant anaemia are tolerant of the low haemoglobin due to the

Table 6.3 Assessment of iron status and anaemia

	Ferritin	Serum Iron	TSAT	TIBC	Hepcidin
Iron deficiency	Decreased	Decreased	Decreased	Increased	Decreased
Functional iron deficiency	Normal to decreased	Normal to decreased	Decreased	Decreased	Decreased
Anaemia of chronic disease	Normal to increased	Normal to decreased	Normal to decreased	Decreased	Increased
Mixed anaemia (IDA + ACD)	Normal	Decreased	Normal to decreased	Decreased	Normal

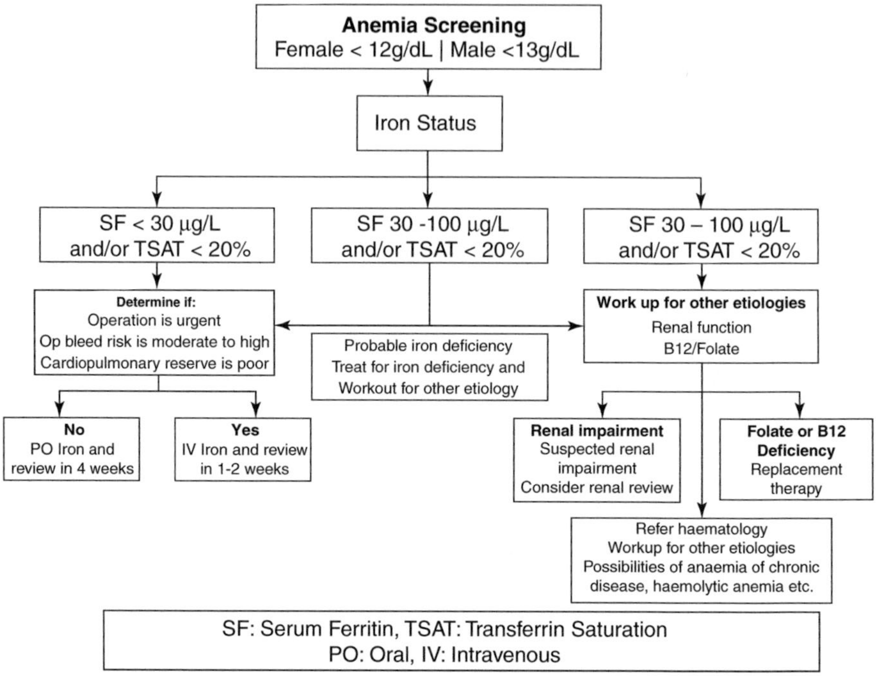

Fig. 6.3 Overview of management of anaemia in the perioperative oncosurgical patient

compensatory physiological changes and sudden especially larger volume transfusion is fraught with more problems than benefits—immune and non-immune immediate transfusion-related reactions, allo-immunization, transfusion-associated infections, circulatory overload to name a few. Further, in the perioperative setting surgical outcomes have been shown to be inferior with the use of transfusion [16]. Transfusion should only be considered if there is severe anaemia with a risk of organ ischaemia/ongoing significant blood loss or the surgical requirement in truly an emergency. The formulation of iron replacement is dependent on tolerance and time required for correction. Oral iron replacement usually requires 4–6 weeks for a response to be evident and will take longer to reach safe perioperative levels if the baseline is lower. In patients where the surgery is emergent, intravenous iron is a relatively quick and effective replacement therapy. It is also an option for patients who may have issues tolerating or absorbing oral iron [17]. All intravenous iron carries the risk of anaphylactoid reaction but newer formulations have significantly lesser incidence and severity of reactions [18].

6.2.3.2 Erythropoiesis-Stimulating Agents

Erythropoiesis-stimulating agents (ESAs) has a role in increasing red cell mass and improving haemoglobin levels [19]. The role of ESAs has been studied in cancer-associated anaemia. However, there are potential risk associated with therapy including the risk of venous thromboembolism and cancer progression [20]. The relative risk of venous thromboembolic events with the use of ESAs in patients with cancer is approximately 50% [21]. In addition to the commonly recognized risk factors for thromboembolism including immobilization, certain chemotherapy agents and surgery itself may compound the risk. Hence, while not contraindicated, there should be a caution exercised in the use of ESAs in the perioperative period especially for patients with multiple risk factors for thromboembolism with judicious use over a short period of time required to produce the meaningful desired response [22]. Findings from several controlled trials have suggested the use of ESAs to have negative survival outcomes in certain cancer patients [23, 24]. Multiple international and regional guidelines recommend the avoidance of ESAs when treatment is of a curative intent [22]. Despite the concerns, ESAs is still a possible management option for a selected group of patients. A careful risk-benefit analysis should be done in consultation with the patient. Epoetin alfa formulations are started 300–600 units/kg once weekly [25]. Supplemental iron to maintain transferrin saturation of ≥20% and serum ferritin of ≥100 ng/mL and thromboprophylaxis should be considered.

The reticulocyte production index (RPI) is an adjusted value used in the diagnosis of anaemia to evaluate the erythropoietic capacity of bone marrow.

The approach of the workup of anaemia integrating the kinetic and morphological approach.

An overview of the assessment and management of perioperative anemia is listed in Fig. 6.3.

6.3 The Approach to Perioperative Cytopenias

6.3.1 Approach to Thrombocytopenia

Thrombocytopenia (platelet count <150 × 10^9 L) remains a common perioperative clinical problem as platelet numbers and function remain key elements of haemostasis and therefore perturbations to platelet counts have been linked to adverse perioperative/post-operative outcomes (sepsis, renal and pulmonary complications, etc.) [26].

Nonetheless, the relationship between platelet count and bleeding risk is not linear as this is affected by other patient-specific variables and platelet function. Although there is a lack of high-quality data quantifying the bleeding risk in thrombocytopenic patients, it is accepted that functional platelet counts above 10 × 10^9 L are sufficient for thrombin generation and will prevent spontaneous bleeding. Table 6.4 summarizes the acceptable platelet counts and indications for platelet transfusions for thrombocytopenic patients having invasive procedures based on expert opinion and practice reviews [27].

6.3.1.1 Qualitative Platelet Dysfunction and Procedures

Acquired qualitative platelets defects can occur secondary to uraemia or medications (aspirin, non-steroidal anti-inflammatory drugs, P2Y12 adenosine

Table 6.4 Clinically significant platelet thresholds and targets. (Adapted from Nagrebetsky et al. 2019) [34]

Platelet count	Acceptable procedure
100	Brain or posterior eye surgery
50	Therapeutic enteroscopy, liver/kidney/transbronchial biopsy, non-neuraxial surgery
20	Central line insertion, diagnostic enteroscopy, bronchoscopy with lavage
10	Threshold for spontaneous bleeding

diphosphate receptor antagonists, dipyridamole, and glycoprotein IIb/IIIa antagonists, etc.). Interruption of these agents should be carefully considered before surgeries especially those that have a high risk for bleeding. This should be carefully weighed against the potential for precipitating thrombosis by the dose interruptions. Moreover, inherited platelets disorders (e.g. Bernard–Soulier syndrome, Hermansky–Pudlak syndrome, autosomal variant Glanzmann thrombasthenia) may also result in qualitative platelet dysfunction and these diagnoses need to be sought in appropriate clinical circumstances.

6.3.1.2 Evaluation of Unexplained Thrombocytopenia in the Post-Operative Patient

It is necessary to take a thorough medication history and a detailed bleeding history which includes previous responses to haemostatic challenges (e.g. previous surgeries and pregnancies). It would also be helpful to focus on the prior platelet count trends and to conduct an analysis of prior thrombocytopenic episodes.

The first step in the workup for unexplained thrombocytopenia is to rule out artifactual or spurious thrombocytopenia. This is seen in individuals who have clinically insignificant antibodies that promote clumping of platelets in the presence of EDTA. This results in falsely low enumeration of platelet counts in automated analyzers. Collecting peripheral blood in a citrated or heparinized tube will help minimize platelet clumping in most of these patients. Since this is an in-vitro phenomenon with no consequences to patients, it is important to identify this problem so that many unnecessary investigations and inappropriate interventions can be prevented. Notwithstanding the above, a small proportion of patients with genuine thrombocytopenia may also exhibit platelet clumping and further evaluation of this would need careful consideration of the individual clinical circumstances.

Once artifactual thrombocytopenia is excluded, causes of thrombocytopenia can be further classified based on the underlying mechanism (i.e. increased platelet destruction, decreased platelet production or platelet sequestration or dilution) (Table 6.5).

The peripheral blood film may suggest a number of possible aetiologies. Large platelets are suggestive of consumptive thrombocytopenia while fragmented red cells called schistocytes suggest thrombotic microangiopathy or destruction of red cells by endovascular devices.

Table 6.5 Typical causes of thrombocytopenia based on pathophysiologic mechanism. (Adapted from Nagrebetsky et al. 2019) [34]

Decreased platelet production	Increased platelet destruction	Platelet dilution or sequestration
Drug-related marrow suppression Liver disease (thrombopoietin deficiency)	Immune thrombocytopenia Drug-related platelet destruction Heparin-induced thrombocytopenia Thrombotic microangiopathy Extracorporeal membrane oxygenation (ECMO)	Large volume red blood cell transfusion Intravenous fluid administration Splenomegaly

Severe thrombocytopenia (often <10 × 109 L) following blood product transfusions may be secondary to post-transfusion purpura secondary to prior sensitization to foreign platelet glycoproteins.

A precipitous fall in platelet counts can be seen in the setting of infection or sepsis. This is due to neuraminidase secretion by certain bacteria or disseminated intravascular coagulation.

Drugs may cause thrombocytopenia via platelet activation (e.g. heparin), immune-related destruction (e.g. vancomycin), thrombotic microangiopathy (e.g. cyclosporine) or bone marrow suppression (e.g. Linezolid). Analysing the timing of drug initiation and occurrence of thrombocytopenia is crucial in arriving at a diagnosis of drug-induced thrombocytopenia. When the platelet count decreases to a point where bleeding is a concern, the likely offending drug(s) should be discontinued and in most patients that may be the only intervention required. Time taken for platelet count recovery after the cessation of offending drugs can be quite variable. In cases where the suspected drug is essential and cannot be suspended, platelets can be transfused as a temporary measure. However, its efficacy is limited if there is ongoing immune-mediated platelet destruction or platelet dysfunction. Unlike primary immune thrombocytopenic purpura (ITP), drug-induced ITP may not respond to corticosteroids. Intravenous immunoglobulin may be efficacious [28]. Recently, the use of thrombopoietin analogues for the management of thrombocytopenia peri-procedurally is being actively investigated with some promising results in clinical trials [28]. Figure 6.4 depicts an approach to thrombocytopenia.

6.3.1.3 Alternatives to Platelet Transfusion

Although platelet transfusion remains the most expeditious way of increasing platelet count, it subjects the patient to transfusion-related complications. Alternatives to platelet transfusion include non-specific haemostatic agents like desmopressin, antifibrinolytic agents (tranexamic acid) or procoagulant bypass agents (activated prothrombin complex concentrates and recombinant factor VIIa) when there is accompanying coagulopathy. Thrombopoietin receptor agonists (Eltrombopag, romiplostim, lusutrombopag and avatrombopag) can also raise platelet counts especially in Immune thrombocytopenia [29–31].

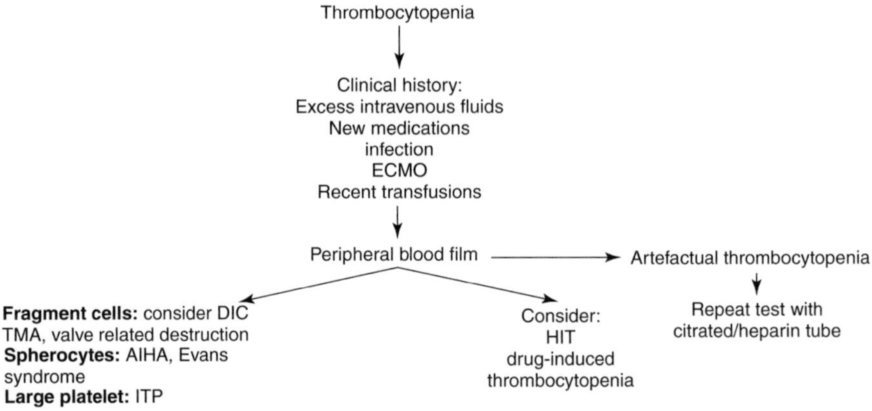

Fig. 6.4 Clinical approach to thrombocytopenia. (Adapted from Nagrebetsky et al. 2019) [34]. *DIC* disseminated intravascular coagulation, *ECMO* extracorporeal membrane oxygenation, *HIT* heparin-induced thrombocytopenia, *ITP* immune thrombocytopenic purpura, *TMA* thrombotic microangiopathy

6.3.2 Approach to Leukopenia

Mild transient leukopenia can be seen during or following common infections with various viruses. Though mostly inconsequential, at times even in an immunocompetent host post-viral leukopenia and neutropenia can be severe and certainly in oncological patients with compromised immune systems some of these viruses (e.g., cytomegalovirus, Epstein–Barr virus) can lead to profound cytopenias as well as additional complications. Drug-induced leukopenia is also not uncommon and can vary in severity from mild to severe. Neuropsychiatric drugs, antiepileptics and antithyroid medications can all cause leukopenia/agranulocytosis. Severe and persistent leukopenia is most commonly seen post-chemotherapy or if radiation therapy is administered to large areas of sites of active bone marrow proliferation. It can also be seen when the bone marrow is infiltrated by solid tumour malignancies.

Neutropenia is often diagnosed from a full blood count with accompanying white cell differential, where the absolute neutrophil count is <1500 μL for mild neutropenia, <1000 μL for moderate neutropenia and <500 μL for severe neutropenia. Patients with isolated neutropenia may or may not have any specific symptoms but a fever might be the first sign.

Many chemotherapy regimens for haematological malignancies and regimens for haematopoietic stem cell transplant are associated with a longer period of neutropenia as well as severity compared to those for solid tumour malignancies. During periods of neutropenia, patients can manifest fever which is often a sign of underlying infection—oncological emergency—that needs to be promptly managed according to neutropenic sepsis protocols. It is particularly important to note that in some groups of oncological patients the classical signs of sepsis like fever may not be apparent and the only symptoms or signs could be profound tiredness or hypotension (elderly/ongoing steroid therapy/some haematological cancers like myeloma).

Table 6.6 Diagnostic approach to leukopenia and their aetiologies. (Adapted from: Boxer 2012) [35]

Evaluation	Diagnoses
History • Acute or chronic leukopenia • General medical history • Drug history	Congenital syndromes Drug-associated neutropenia
Physical examination • Stomatitis, gingivitis, dental defects Splenomegaly	Congenital syndromes Hypersplenism
FBC with reticulocyte counts *ANC ≤ 1000 μL:* Acute onset neutropenia	Transient myelosuppression (e.g. viral infections) Drug-associated neutropenia Autoimmune neutropenia
ANC <500 μL on 3 separate tests Bone marrow aspiration with trephine and cytogenetics • Exocrine pancreatic enzymes • Skeletal radiographs	Congenital bone marrow aplasia: • SCN, Fanconi anaemia, Schwachman–diamond syndrome, cartilage-hair hypoplasia (see segment 3C)
ALC <1000 μL Repeat FBC in 4 weeks	Transient leukopenia (e.g. viral infections)
ALC <1000 μL on 3 separate tests Bone marrow aspiration with trephine and cytogenetics • HIV screen • Quantitative Igs (IgG, IgA and IgM) and lymphocyte subsets	HIV-1 infection Congenital or acquired immune function disorders
Pancytopenia • Folate, vitamin B12 levels • Bone marrow aspiration and trephine • Cytogenetics • Flow cytometry for phosphatidy-linositol-linked proteins • TCR rearrangement	Folate and vitamin B12 deficiencies BM replacement by malignancy, fibrosis, granulomata, storage cells Leukaemia, myelodysplasia Paroxysmal nocturnal haemoglobinuria Large granular lymphocytic leukaemia

The approach to cytopenia and their aetiologies (Table 6.6) begins with a targeted history, exploring any personal or family history of chronic leukopenia. The history may reveal a particular aetiology, for instance, viral infections, bone marrow malignancy, immune deficiencies, autoimmune disorders, etc. which can help direct further investigations.

Given that the infection risk is higher with longer durations of lymphopenia and neutropenia, whenever possible, non-emergency surgery should be postponed in these patients. Patients are also at higher risk of post-operative sepsis. Besides chemotherapy dose modification, initiation or neutropenia prophylaxis with granulocyte colony stimulating factors (GCSF) can aid in decreasing the duration of neutropenia and also the depth of absolute neutrophil count nadir. Even so, it would be wise to educate patients on neutropenic precaution. For instance, avoiding raw food and also minimizing exposure to plants and pets [32].

6.3.3 Approach to Bone Marrow Failures

Bone marrow failure refers to pancytopenia with associated bone marrow hypoplasia or aplasia. Table 6.7 summarizes the causes of bone marrow failure.

6.3.3.1 Clinical Evaluation of Marrow Failure

The urgency of clinical and bone marrow evaluation is guided by the depth of cytopenias and the clinical status. The history may help to elucidate the underlying aetiology (e.g. chemical/drug exposure, viral infections). A family history of cytopenias or dysmorphic features on examination may serve as a clue to inherited bone marrow failure syndromes.

Clinical examination should also entail a thorough examination for manifestations of inherited disorders (e.g. short stature, cutaneous, nail, eye, ear, skeletal or genitourinary abnormalities).

Serum chemistries with renal panel, liver function tests, folate and B12 assessment can help distinguish bone marrow failure from other causes of pancytopenia.

Table 6.7 Bone marrow failure aetiologies. (Adapted from Berliner et al. 2020; Shimamura 2009) [36, 37]

Organ system	Side effects	Culprit chemotherapy agents
Pulmonary	Radiation and inflammatory pneumonitis	Paclitaxel Procarbazine Methotrexate Mitomycin Bleomycin Busulphan
	Non-cardiogenic pulmonary oedema	Arabinoside Bleomycin
Cardiac	Cardiotoxicity- myocarditis, congestive cardiac failure, pericarditis	Daunorubicin Doxorubicin Epirubicin Cyclophosphamide Cisplatin
Hepatic	Hepatic veno-occlusion	Busulphan
	Gastrointestinal mucosal ulceration and denudation	Chlorambucil Cytarabine Dactinomycin
	Worsening of liver fibrosis	Mercaptopurine
	Hepatic necrosis	Mercaptopurine Methotrexate L-asparaginase
Renal	Renal impairment	Cisplatin and carboplatin Paclitaxel Cyclophosphamide Methotrexate
Neurology	Peripheral neuropathy	Vincristine Docetaxel

A bone marrow evaluation is required for the diagnosis of aplastic anaemia and to rule out other causes of pancytopenia.

While a detailed discussion on the evaluation of suspected aplastic anaemia and other marrow failure syndromes are beyond the scope of this chapter, it is imperative to be aware that specialized testing should be performed to detect co-existent disorders such as myelodysplastic syndrome, acute leukaemia or paroxysmal nocturnal haemoglobinuria. Flow cytometry, molecular and cytogenetic tests will also be essential for proper classification and for prognostic assessment. Genetic testing (chromosome breakage test, telomere length testing, etc.) can be performed if inherited bone marrow failure is suspected. Figure 6.5 depicts a general clinical approach to bone marrow failure.

6.3.4 Immunocompromised Host

Patients with most haematological cancers and those who have undergone haematopoietic stem cell transplant are immunocompromised. This is largely a contribution from the underlying disease, myelosuppression due to chemotherapy, drug-induced immunosuppression or recurrent infections post-chemotherapy. They are also at greater risk of malnutrition, organ dysfunction and anatomical distortions. In this age of multimodality cancer treatment, most patients presenting for surgery would have had a history of chemotherapeutic administration and radiotherapy and are hence immunocompromised.

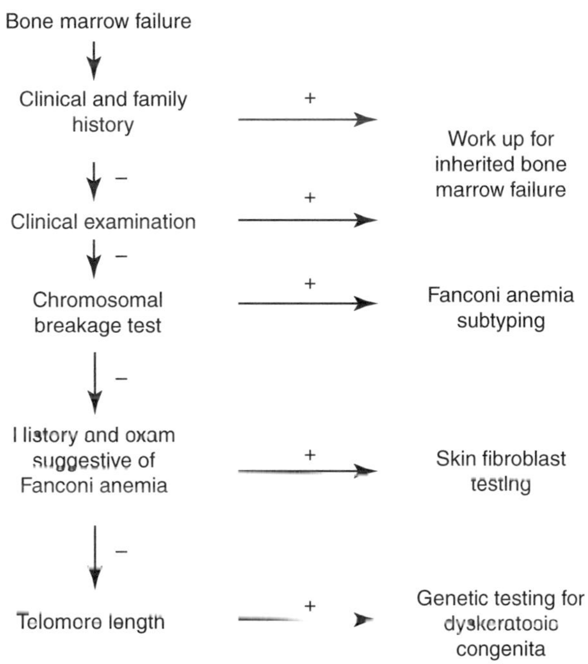

Fig. 6.5 A General approach for patients with marrow failure. (Adapted Shimamura 2009) [37]

There is a paucity of studies to guide the perioperative management of these individuals. Additionally, there is an expanding array of chemotherapeutic agents with an equally intimidating range of side effects adding to this management conundrum [33].

With such uncertainty, previously developed models of physiological reserve that have served clinicians well (e.g. with cardiovascular risk stratification) may not be well applied to cancer patients. Thus, the clinician needs to rely on basic principles, for instance ensuring that patients are meticulously treated for infection, optimizing their nutritional status and ensuring adequate analgesia for better perioperative optimisation.

It is to be hoped that further study in this field will lead to improved perioperative practice guidelines to benefit cancer patients.

6.4 Assessment of Haemostatic Function and Strategies to Aid Intraoperative Haemostasis

The preoperative assessment of the patient's haemostatic function is important to detect patients with abnormal bleeding caused by coagulation defects. Oncological surgery often also carries a higher bleeding risk with many patients requiring extensive surgical resection and haemorrhage from vascular tumours and tumour invasion to blood vessels. Early detection and management can prevent catastrophic bleeds during surgery. In addition, certain cancers are associated with distinctive coagulation defects. Some disorders, acquired haemophilia A, for example, are rare but can result in serious bleeding complications and require prompt diagnosis and management. A comprehensive understanding of the approach and management strategies will be important to mitigate the risk of complications in cancer patients.

6.4.1 Preoperative Clinical Assessment of Haemostatic Function

A good clinical assessment with history and physical examination is the foundation to the preoperative assessment. Consideration for further preoperative laboratory screening for coagulation disorders should be made on an individualized assessment.

The history should include the bleeding history of the patient, the circumstances surrounding the bleeds and history of bleeds after procedures, including dental procedures and major surgery. A medication history such as use of anti-platelet or anti-coagulation is important. Details of the family history of any bleeding tendencies should also be explored. Table 6.8 details the useful clinical features to note in evaluating a patient for a bleeding disorder. There are several standardized preoperative bleeding questionnaires to aid in this assessment such as the International Society of Thrombosis and Haemostasis Bleeding Assessment Tool (ISTH-BAT) [38].

While a good clinical history is critical in assessment, is it also important to recognize some of the difficulties. In patients with few previous haemostatic challenges, it may be difficult to differentiate mild bleeding disorders based on history

Table 6.8 Clinical features in evaluating a patient for a bleeding disorder

Bleeding history	Medication history
• Onset of bleeds: Neonates, childhood, adolescent or adult • Pattern of bleeding: Mucocutaneous bleeding or bleeding into muscles and joints • Bleeding after trauma: Assess if bleeding severity is proportionate • Bleeding after procedures including dental work and surgeries • For female: Menstrual history and bleeding during childbirth	• Drug history of anticoagulation, anti-platelet • Use of traditional and alternative medications **Family history** • Any family members with bleeding tendencies or disorders • A genogram if possible should be obtained

[39]. Furthermore, patients may over-report bleeding, often the symptoms of excessive nosebleed, gingival bleeding and easy bruising [40]. Hence, consideration for a consistent collection of bleeding symptoms, rather than a single symptom or event may be useful to suggest the presence of an underlying bleeding disorder.

The physical examination is focused on findings that might suggest underlying potential bleeding disorders and aetiologies. This includes examination of the skin for petechiae, ecchymosis or telangiectasias. A joint examination demonstrating joint deformities may suggest a history of haemarthrosis. Other systemic features may suggest chronic disease associated with bleeding tendencies such as chronic liver disease which will have a collection of physical stigmata that will serve as a clue to the underlying cause of the bleeding disorder.

6.4.2 Preoperative Coagulation Laboratory Testing

Indiscriminate preoperative coagulation testing to predict post-operative bleeding is not useful and is not recommended [41]. Patients planned for low bleeding risk procedures do not need additional laboratory testing if the clinical assessment do not suggest the presence of bleeding disorder [42]. The decision for further laboratory testing should be based on the clinical history and the procedural bleeding risk of the surgery. Table 6.9 details some of the common oncological procedures and operation and their bleeding risk.

It is important to recognize that there are a vast variety of bleeding disorders and no single coagulation test is able to identify all patients with such disorders [41]. Furthermore, coagulation cascade is a complex process and is an interplay of multiple components including the vascular, platelet, coagulation and fibrinolytic system. This cannot be accurately reproduced in the in-vivo setting hence there are limitations to coagulation testing. Understanding the principles of different coagulation assays and how to interpret and integrate it into a structured approach is critical. Figure 6.6 details a suggested approach to preoperative coagulation testing.

The screening coagulation tests routinely used are the activated partial thromboplastin time (aPTT) and the prothrombin time (PT). The aPTT is a test of the intrinsic and common coagulation pathway and prolongation would suggest deficiencies

Table 6.9 Common procedures and surgeries undergone by oncology patient and their procedural bleeding potential

Type of surgery	Bleeding potential		
	Minor	Moderate	High
General surgery	Excision biopsy OGD/colonoscopy Breast lump excision/mastectomy	Gastrectomy Anterior resection, hemicolectomy	Hepatectomy Whipple's surgery Esophagectomy Cytoreductive surgery APR/pelvic exenteration radical resections
ENT/ respiratory	Bronchoscopy	Thyroidectomy Tonsillectomy/ adenoidectomy Parotidectomy	Radical neck dissection Total laryngectomy pharyngectomy Mandibulectomy Glossectomy
Neuro		Burr hole Core needle brain biopsy Pituitary surgery	Craniectomy
O&G	Hysteroscopy	Ovarian cystectomy	Total hysterectomy and bilateral salpingo-ophorectomy Pelvic lymph node dissection
Ortho		Laminectomy Bone grafts Limb amputation	Spinal instrumentation and fusion Spinal decompression
CTS		Pericardial window VATS	Thoracotomy Pneumonectomy Thymectomy

OGD oesophago-gastro-duodenoscopy, *APR* abdominal perineal resection, *ENT* ear nose throat, neuro: neurosurgery, *O&G* obstetrics and gynaecology, *CTS* cardiothoracic surgery, *VATS* video-assisted thoracoscopic surgery

of factor VIII, IX and XI or inhibitors of the intrinsic and common pathway factors. PT is a test of the extrinsic and common coagulation pathway and prolongation would suggest deficiencies of factors II, V, VII and X or inhibitors of the extrinsic and common pathway factors. Table 6.10 shows the classification of bleeding disorders classified based on PT and aPTT abnormalities.

Evaluation of thrombocytopenia is discussed in the prior subsection.

The mixing studies for PT and APTT assays involve mixing a patient's plasma with normal plasma in a 1:1 ratio. This can help characterize a factor deficiency for which there will be correction of the assay based on the principle that 50% of normal factor activity is sufficient to achieve a normal clotting time. A non-correctable mixing study will suggest the presence of an inhibitor.

It is important to note that a normal PT and aPTT does not exclude a bleeding disorder. Furthermore, not all prolonged PT and aPTT will be associated with a condition which has a bleeding tendency. For example, Factor XII deficiency and the presence of a lupus anticoagulant are not associated with increased bleeding tendency despite prolonged aPTT. In the event of a diagnostic dilemma or planning for the perioperative plan for a patient with established haematological disorder, a haematological consult should be obtained early allowing enough time for evaluation that would guide appropriate management.

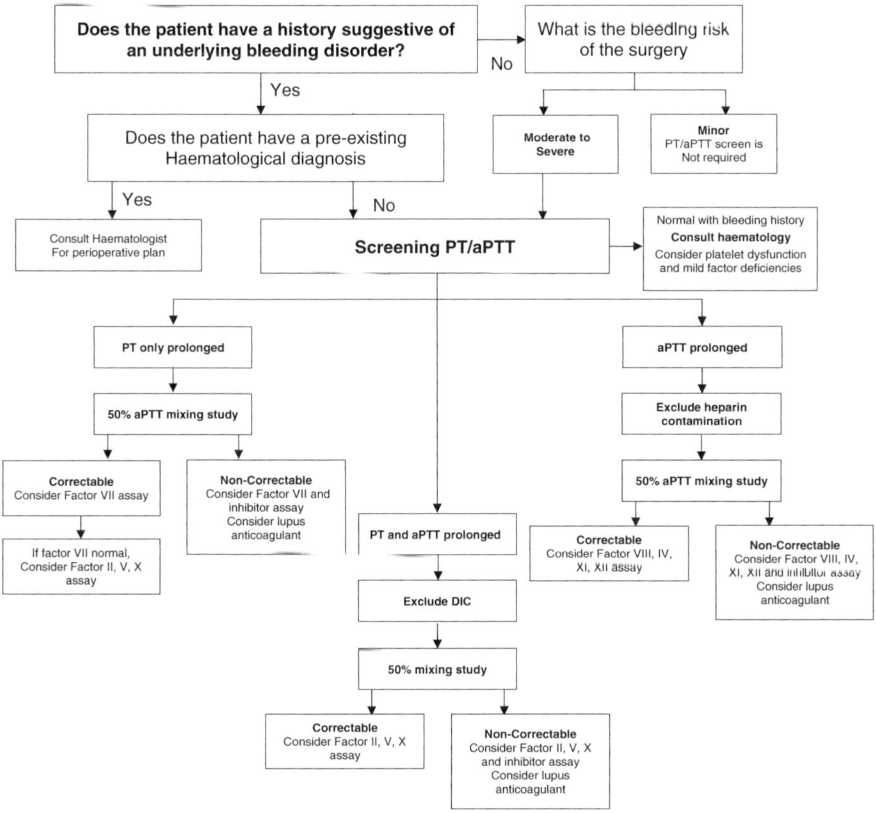

Fig. 6.6 Approach to preoperative coagulation testing

Table 6.10 Common bleeding disorders classified based on PT and aPTT abnormalities

Prolonged PT	Prolonged aPTT	Prolonged PT and aPTT	Normal PT and aPTT
FVII deficiencies Mild liver disease FVII inhibitor	Heparin use or contamination FVIII, IX, XI, XII deficiencies Von Willebrand disease FVIII, IX, XI, XII inhibitor Lupus anticoagulant	Vitamin K deficiency Warfarin Severe liver disease Disseminated intravascular Coagulopathy Factor II, V, X deficiencies Combined factor deficiency	F13 deficiency Mild vWD Mild factor deficiencies Platelet dysfunction Connective tissue disorder

It should be noted that this traditional view of the coagulation cascade with the intrinsic and extrinsic pathway may not be physiologically accurate. In addition, PT and aPTT tests were neither developed nor validated for the evaluation of predicting bleeding risk. The generation and amplification of thrombin is generally considered the primary contributor to clot propagation with the downstream thrombin mediated cleavage of fibrinogen to fibrin to form the fibrin clot [43]. Global coagulation assays may provide more information in the assessment of the perioperative patient especially given that they can happen in real time. Viscoelastic testing such as thromboelastography (TEG) and Rotational Thromboelastometry (ROTEM) are point-of-care tests which evaluate several parameters of clot formation dynamically in whole blood [44]. The utility in predicting bleeding in a preoperative setting has not been established [45]. However, there is demonstrated utility in the intraoperative haemostatic monitoring especially in the area of cardiac and hepatic surgery [44]. Exploring the availability of viscoelastic testing in high-risk oncological operations may be considered in the preoperative planning [46]. Other global coagulation assays which are under development are clot waveform analysis and thrombin generation assays [47].

6.4.3 Preoperative Management of Patients with Established Bleeding Disorders

For patients with established bleeding disorders such as haemophilia A and von Willebrand's disease, a comprehensive perioperative plan is required to ensure a safe procedure. This includes a multidisciplinary management between the surgeon, anaesthesiologist, haematologist and the patient [48]. As a general approach for patients with established factor deficiencies which result in increased bleeding risk, the preoperative assessment should include an assessment of the bleeding phenotype severity, inhibitor screen to identify newly developed inhibitor, determine the method and agents for factor replacement as well as the pre- and post-operative targets and duration taking into consideration bleeding and wound healing aspects [49].

6.4.4 Haemostatic Disorders in Cancer Patients

The haemostatic balance is often tipped in cancer patients. While the relationship between malignancy and thrombosis has been well established and described by Bouillaud and Trousseau in the nineteenth century, the association with bleeding disorders was less recognized [50]. There are various mechanisms which result in acquired bleeding disorders which is summarized in Table 6.11.

Disseminated intravascular coagulation can occur in cancer patients and can take an acute, subacute or chronic form. Commonly associated malignancies include acute promyelocytic leukaemia and adenocarcinomas [51]. The clinical presentation may be thrombosis or bleeding but can also happen concurrently. It is usually triggered by release of procoagulants from cancer cells resulting in activation of the coagulation cascade and intravascular coagulation and fibrinolysis. The balance between thrombosis and bleeding is dependent on the degree of microvascular thrombosis vs consumptive thrombocytopenia and hyperfibrinolysis. There is no single diagnostic test for disseminated intravascular coagulation. The clinical suspicion should be supported by investigations including platelet count, PT, aPTT,

Table 6.11 Acquired bleeding disorders associated with cancer

Platelet abnormalities
Thrombocytopenia: Cytotoxic chemotherapy, disseminated intravascular coagulation, bone marrow involvement, malignancy-associated thrombotic microangiopathy *Acquired platelet dysfunction*: Acquired Glanzmann syndrome
Coagulation factor abnormalities
Acquired factor inhibitor *Acquired von Willebrand syndrome* *Acquired factor deficiencies*: Liver failure, absorption of factors to tumour surface
Fibrinolytic abnormalities
Disseminated intravascular coagulation: Cancer associated

fibrinogen and D-Dimer [52]. Management is directed based on clinical presentation, in patients with disseminated intravascular coagulation with active bleeding, transfusion support with fresh frozen plasma and fibrinogen replacement should be done.

Acquired factor inhibitor is a rare coagulation disorder associated with malignancy, for which the most commonly affected factor is factor 8 [53]. The pathogenesis is the formation of neutralizing autoantibodies to the factor resulting in depletion of the factor. This could result in severe bleeding and pose a difficulty in preoperative management. Treatment principles are that of management of active bleeding with bypassing agents (FEIBA, recombinant activated factor seven) and eradication of inhibitors using immunosuppressive therapy. The treatment can be complicated as treatment of the cancer is required to stop the driver of inhibitor production; however, the presence of inhibitors results in extremely high bleeding risk for surgical intervention [54].

Acquired von Willebrand's syndrome may result from different mechanisms. The formation of autoantibodies to the von Willebrand factor protein is associated with monoclonal gammopathies and lymphoproliferative neoplasms [55]. Absorption of von Willebrand factor onto the cancer cell surface resulting in increased clearance is seen in Wilms tumours, multiple myeloma and Waldenström macroglobulinaemia [56, 57]. Treatment is targeted at the underlying mechanism of factor depletion and treating the underlying driver malignancy. Patients with autoantibodies may be treated with intravenous immunoglobulins, immunosuppressive therapy or plasmapheresis [58].

6.5 Venous Thrombosis Prevention and Management

Venous thromboembolism (VTE) has a close association with cancer and is a potentially fatal disease. It is the second highest cause of mortality in cancer patients [59]. It is also an independent risk factor of mortality, and patients with an established venous thromboembolism have a poorer overall prognosis compared to patients without a history [60]. In the case of the oncology patient undergoing a surgical procedure, a post-operative VTE is a poor prognostic factor [61].

Patients with cancer have a hypercoagulable state. This involves the interplay of many different variables including upregulation of tissue factors, increased cytokines and vascular venous stasis [62]. The risk is compounded by the venous thromboembolism risk factors contributed by surgery such as prolonged immobility. This contributes to the increased risk of post-operative thromboembolism and perioperative mortality [63, 64].

6.5.1 Risk Stratification for Venous Thromboembolism

The risk of venous thromboembolism is dependent on patient, tumour and perioperative factors as demonstrated in Fig. 6.7. An assessment of the risk helps to determine the thromboprophylaxis management in the perioperative period.

The absolute thromboembolism risk varies greatly in different types of surgery. The duration of surgery, site and technique (open versus laparoscopic) are all factors to be considered. Large resection and debulking surgeries have a very high risk of venous thromboembolism as contributed by the long operating times, venous compression by the tumour and extensive vascular injury as a result of tumour invasion and surgical dissection. Abdominal and pelvic surgery are generally associated with higher incidence of venous thromboembolism [65]. The perioperative thrombosis risk is also not static and may extend further to 30 days or more in the post-operative period [63].

There are various risk scores which can assist in stratification. A widely used model is the Modified Caprini Risk Assessment Model which has been validated in patients undergoing general and abdominal and pelvic surgery [66, 67] (Table 6.12). In the setting of oncology patients, the Khorana score risk stratifies based on clinical parameters such as site of primary tumour, hematologic parameters and body mass index [68] (Table 6.13).

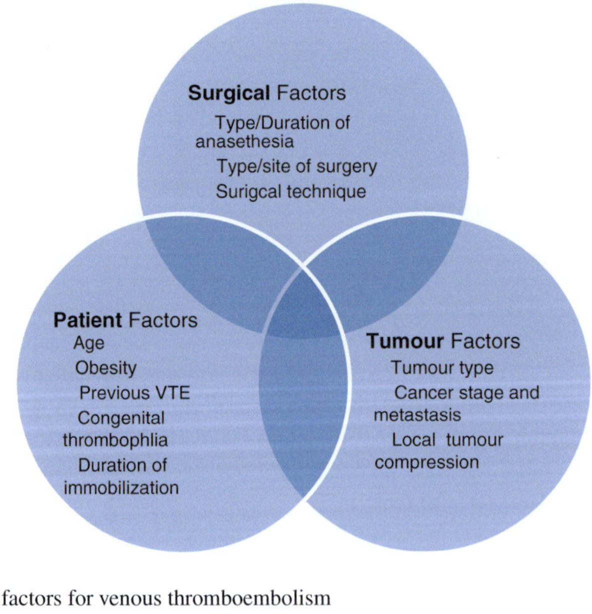

Fig. 6.7 Risk factors for venous thromboembolism

Table 6.12 Modified Caprini risk assessment model for VTE in general surgical patients. (Adapted from Gould et al. 2012)

Risk score			
1 Point	2 Point	3 Points	5 Points
Age 41–60 years	Age 61–74 years	Age ≥ 75 years	Stroke (<1 month)
Minor surgery	Arthroscopic surgery	History of VTE	Elective arthroplasty
BMI >25 kg/m^2	Major open surgery (>45 min)	Family history of VTE	Hip, pelvis, or leg fracture
Swollen legs	Laparoscopic surgery (>45 min)	Factor V Leiden	Acute spinal cord injury (<1 month)
Varicose veins	Malignancy	Prothrombin 20210A	
Pregnancy or postpartum	Confined to bed (>72 h)	Lupus anticoagulant	
History of unexplained or recurrent spontaneous abortion	Immobilizing plaster cast	Anticardiolipin antibodies	
Oral contraceptives or hormone replacement	Central venous access	Elevated serum homocysteine	
Sepsis (<1 month)	Age 61–74 years	Heparin-induced thrombocytopenia	
Serious lung disease, including pneumonia (<1 month)		Other congenital or acquired thrombophilia	
Abnormal pulmonary function			
Acute myocardial infarction			
Congestive heart failure (<1 month)			
History of inflammatory bowel disease			
Medical patient at bed rest			

Interpretation

Surgical risk category	Score	Estimated VTE risk in the absence of pharmacologic or mechanical prophylaxis (%)
Very low	0	<0.5
Low	1–2	1.5
Moderate	3–5	3.0
High	≥5	6.0

Table 6.13 Khorana score for Venous Thromboembolism in Cancer Patients. (Adapted from Khorana et al. 2008)

Cancer type	2 Point: Stomach, Pancreas 1 Point: Lung, Lymphoma, Gynaecologic, Bladder, Testicular 0 Point: Others	
Pre-chemotherapy platelet count $\geq 350 \times 10^9$ L	**1 Point:** Yes **0 Point:** No	
Haemoglobin level < 10 g/dL or using RBC growth factors	**1 Point:** Yes **0 Point:** No	
Pre-chemotherapy leukocyte count $>11 \times 10^9$ L	**1 Point:** Yes **0 Point:** No	
BMI $\geq$ 35 kg/m^2	**1 Point:** Yes **0 Point:** No	
Risk group	**Score**	**2.5 month rate of VTE**
Low	0	0.3–0.8%
Intermediate	1–2	1.8–2.0%
High	≥3	6.7–7.1%

6.5.2 The Role of Thromboprophylaxis

Thromboprophylaxis reduces the incidence of thrombotic events. There are various methods that are tailored based on the patient's profile and balanced to the patient's perioperative bleeding risk. Mechanical methods include the use of pneumatic compression and compression stockings. Pharmacological prophylaxis includes the use of anticoagulation at prophylactic doses. A combined regimen of pharmacologic and mechanical prophylaxis is usually deployed.

Mechanical methods for reducing thromboembolic events are usually complementary to pharmacological prophylaxis and particularly relevant in patients with high bleeding risk at critical sites such as the intracranial space. Data supporting use of intermittent pneumatic compression for the prevention of thromboembolism in the oncological setting are limited but there are some small studies in mixed surgical populations which demonstrate superiority to no prophylaxis and additional benefit to the use of low molecular weight heparin [69, 70]. Graduated compression stockings similar to intermittent pneumatic compression has some evidence for efficacy alone and when complemented with pharmacologic prophylaxis [71, 72]. Such intervention should be started before surgery and continued during the operation and in the post-operative setting.

There are several options for pharmacological thromboprophylaxis in the post-operative setting. Randomized controlled trials have shown prophylaxis with low molecular weight heparin, fondaparinux and unfractionated heparin reduce the risk of deep vein thrombosis and pulmonary embolism [73–75]. In general, low molecular weight heparin is the agent of choice. This is based on the ease of administration, large therapeutic window and lower risk of heparin-induced thrombocytopenia. There are various preparations of low molecular

Table 6.14 Overview of pharmacological thromboprophylaxis agents

Agents	Dosing/modifications
Enoxaparin	40 mg once daily: Starting 10–12 h preoperatively and continued post-operatively
Dalteparin	5000 U once daily: Starting 10–12 h preoperatively and continued post-operatively
Tinzaparin	3500 anti-Xa units once daily: Starting 2 h prior to surgery and continued post-operatively
Unfractionated heparin	5000 every 8 h: Starting 2–4 h preoperatively and continued every 8 h post-operatively
Fondaparinux	2.5 mg once daily: Starting 6–8 h post-operatively

weight heparin including enoxaparin, dalteparin and tinzaparin available currently. Low dose unfractionated heparin may be a preferred option for patients with impaired renal function. Table 6.14 details the dosing of the various agents. There is limited data for the use of direct oral anticoagulants such as rivaroxaban and apixaban in the setting of primary prophylaxis for oncological surgery. The main indications for such agents are currently in the setting of primary prophylaxis in ambulatory oncological patients with higher thromboembolic risk of a Khorana score of 2 or more [76, 77]. Thromboprophylaxis is not routinely recommended for all outpatients with cancer [76]. Most hospitalized patients with cancer and an acute medical condition require thromboprophylaxis throughout hospitalization [76].

The timing and duration of thromboprophylaxis is critical. Most international guidelines recommend that prophylaxis should be commenced preoperatively for patients undergoing major cancer surgeries [77]. The duration of pharmacologic thromboprophylaxis for patients undergoing major oncological surgery should be for at least 7–10 days. The patient's post-operative ambulatory status should be considered while deciding on the duration. It is important to consider that the thromboembolic risk extends beyond the post-operative hospital stay in patients undergoing oncological surgery [63]. Extended prophylaxis for up to 4 weeks should be considered for patients with abdominal/pelvic or major lower limb orthopaedic procedures with high-risk features such as extended immobility, obesity or history of venous thromboembolism [78, 79].

Patients with cancer should be periodically assessed for VTE risk factors that may emerge from time to time and their treating clinicians should provide patient education about the symptoms and signs of VTE such that if it occurs they can be identified early and managed promptly [76].

Prophylactic insertion of inferior vena cava filters for prophylaxis against post-operative thromboembolic events is to be avoided [80]. There is evidence to demonstrate that there may be a reduction in pulmonary embolism; however, the rate of post operative deep vein thrombosis is increased with no change in overall survival [81].

6.5.3 Management of Pre-Existing Venous Thromboembolism

The management of pre-existing venous thromboembolism and handling of anticoagulation in the perioperative period is a common but complex clinical scenario.

A clinical assessment of the balance between interrupting anticoagulation for a surgical procedure resulting in the increase in risk of thromboembolic progression versus the compounded operative bleeding risk which is increased by anticoagulants guides the management of such situations.

Approach to preoperative management involves balancing the risk of bleeding and thrombosis, taking into account the characteristics of the anticoagulation the patient is taking. Most of the time, plans will have to be individualized to the patient, but the decision making can be based on these basic considerations:

1. Estimation of the thromboembolic risk.
2. Estimation of the bleeding risk.
3. Determine the timing of anticoagulation interruption.
4. Determine the necessity of anticoagulation bridging.

6.5.3.1 Estimation of the Thromboembolic Risk

Most patients with active cancer would be classified to be at least a moderate risk for perioperative thromboembolism for most major cancer surgeries. This risk is further compounded by other disease characteristics which have been referenced above. Those with a recent thrombotic event, defined as within the past 3 months, have the greatest risk of progression or recurrence of thromboembolism (Table 6.15).

Often oncological patients have newly diagnosed cancer concurrently with the diagnosis of a venous thromboembolism. It is also at this point where planning for diagnostic or therapeutic surgical procedures may be made. With the thrombosis risk being the highest during this period, decision on timing of the operation where anticoagulation evidently will need to be held off is challenging. If the surgery is not emergently necessary, an approach to deter the operation for 3–4 weeks to allow for a duration of therapeutic anticoagulation will likely reduce the thromboembolic risk to some degree [82, 83].

Table 6.15 Perioperative thrombotic risk for venous thromboembolism. (Adapted from Douketis et al. 2011)

Risk	Condition
High	Recent (within 3 months) venous thromboembolism Severe thrombophilia (for example: Deficiency of protein C, protein S, or antithrombin; antiphospholipid antibodies; multiple abnormalities)
Moderate	Venous thromboembolism within the past 3–12 month Non-severe thrombophilia (for example: Heterozygous factor V Leiden or prothrombin gene mutation) Recurrent venous thromboembolism Active cancer (treated within 6 months or palliative)
Low	Venous thromboembolism of more than 12 months with no other risk factors

Table 6.16 Perioperative thrombotic risk for venous thromboembolism. (Adapted from Douketis et al. 2011)

High risk (2 day risk of major bleed: 2–4%)	Low risk (2 day risk of bleed: 0–2%)
Neurosurgical/urologic/head and neck/abdominal/breast cancer surgery Laminectomy Transurethral prostate resection Kidney biopsy Endoscopically guided fine-needle aspiration Any major operation (procedure duration >45 min)	Abdominal hysterectomy Gastrointestinal endoscopy ± biopsy, enteroscopy, biliary/pancreatic stent without sphincterotomy, endosonography without fine-needle aspiration Pacemaker Insertion Skin cancer excision Axillary node dissection Bronchoscopy ± biopsy Cutaneous and bladder/prostate/thyroid/breast/lymph node biopsies

Modified from Douketis et al. Including procedures commonly done for oncological patients

6.5.3.2 Estimation of the Bleeding Risk

The estimation of the bleeding risk is a combination of the intrinsic procedural and patient characteristics. The assessment of patient characteristics has already been discussed in the preceding section. The surgical procedure bleeding risk may be classified into high and low risk, based on the 2-day major bleeding risk (Table 6.16). There are multiple studies to classify bleeding risk based on operation type. The site of procedure is also important to consider based on the potential of bleeding and the critical sites such as the intracranial space, where bleeding may have devastating consequences.

6.5.3.3 Determine the Timing of Anticoagulation Interruption

The factors considered in the timing of anticoagulation interruption includes the surgical procedural bleeding risk and elimination half-life of the anticoagulation agent (Table 6.17). As all direct oral anticoagulants have a component of renal excretion, for patients with impaired kidney function, an additional day should be interrupted before low bleeding risk procedures and an additional 2 days for high bleeding risk procedures. Warfarin should be stopped 5 days prior to the surgical procedure with an INR check on the day of procedure to ensure an INR < 1.5 (Table 6.18).

6.5.3.4 Determine the Necessity of Anticoagulation Bridging

Bridging therapy involves the use of a shorter acting anticoagulation such as low molecular weight heparin when a longer acting anticoagulation like warfarin is interrupted. Bridging therapy in the setting of established thromboembolism in oncology patients is not often required, as warfarin is not the established anticoagulation of choice for management of cancer-associated thrombosis [77]. Warfarin is often given for primary or secondary stroke prophylaxis in patients with atrial fibrillation and in mechanical heart valves. In such cases, the approach should be guided by the stroke thrombosis risk, determined by the $CHADS_2$ score and valve thrombosis rates [84] (Table 6.19).

Table 6.17 Determining residual circulating anticoagulation based on elimination half-lives

Number of half-life	Percentage of dose	Agents	Half-life
1	50%	Apixaban	12 h
2	25%	Rivaroxaban	5–9 h
3	12.5%	Edoxaban	10–14 h
4	6.25%	Dabigatran	12–17 h
5	3.125%	Warfarin	20–60 h
6	1.6%		
Number of half-lives for which anticoagulation should be stopped based on bleeding risk			
Number of half-lives	Low bleeding risk: 4	High bleeding risk: 6	

Table 6.18 Perioperative management of anticoagulation

		Preoperative cessation		Post-operative resumption	
Drugs	Renal function	High bleed risk	Low bleed risk	High bleed risk	Low bleed risk
Apixaban 5 mg BD	Normal–Mild CrCl > 50 ml/min	3 days	2 days	Resume 48–72 h after surgery	Resume 24 h after surgery
	Moderate CrCl 30–50 ml/min	4 days	3 days		
Rivaroxaban 20 mg OM	Normal–Mild CrCl > 50 ml/min	3 days	2 days		
	Moderate CrCl 30–50 ml/min	4–5 days	3 days		
Edoxaban	60 mg daily Normal–Mild CrCl > 50 ml/min	3 days	2 days		
	30 mg daily Moderate CrCl < 50 ml/min				
Dabigatran 150 mg BiD	Normal–Mild CrCl > 50 ml/min	3 days	2 days		
	Moderate CrCl < 50 ml/min	4–5 days	3 days		
Warfarin	NA	5 days Consider bridging therapy		Resume if patient has no active bleeding issues	Resume 12–24 h after surgery

Table 6.19 When to consider bridging therapy. (Adapted from Douketis et al. 2015)

Conditions	Clinical scenarios to consider bridging therapy
Venous thromboembolism	Patients with a venous thromboembolism within the last 3 months
Atrial fibrillation	Patient with a previous stroke or transient ischaemic accident in the last 3 months Patients with a previous stroke and three or more of the following risk factors: • Congestive heart failure • Hypertension (>140/90 or on medication) • Age > 75 years • Diabetes mellitus
Mechanical heart valve	Patients other than those with a bi-leaflet aortic valve and no other risk factors

6.5.3.4.1 Consideration for Placement of Inferior Vena Cava Filters

While anticoagulation remains the mainstay for management of cancer-associated thrombosis, the perioperative periods with the associated bleeding risk may prohibit the use of anticoagulation. The role of preoperative placement of inferior vena cava filters as a means of mechanical thromboprophylaxis is hence sometimes considered. There is evidence to demonstrate filter insertion to decrease the incidence of pulmonary embolism [85]. However, the risk of filter insertion including the procedural risk, risk of filter thrombosis and need to remove the filters are all factors to consider. In addition, the placement of the filter does not negate the need to restart anticoagulation once haemostasis is achieved and it is safe to restart anticoagulation. This should be a multidisciplinary decision made in consultation with the patient.

6.6 Blood Transfusion Strategies in Oncological Patients

Patient blood management is the scientific use of safe and effective medical and surgical technologies to prevent anaemia and decrease bleeding to ensure that blood transfusion is administered only to those who will benefit from it [86]. It combines the prior tropics discussed including the investigation and management of preoperative management and workup and management of anaemia as well as haemostatic disorders.

Employment of patient blood management strategies has been shown to improve outcomes in surgical oncological patients [87]. Reducing blood transfusion is associated with reduced morbidity and mortality due to the adverse risk associated with transfusions. These risks include transfusion transmitted infections, transfusion-associated sepsis, transfusion-associated lung injury, transfusion-associated circulatory overload, anaphylaxis and haemolytic reactions [88]. Emerging evidence also suggests that blood transfusion is an independent predictor of morbidity and mortality in surgical patients, being associated with more ischaemic complications, organ dysfunction, infections, delayed wound healing and increased length of hospital stay [89]. Furthermore, blood transfusion may be associated with poorer outcomes postulated due to the immunogenic effects of transfusions [16].

The 3 pillars of patient blood management are: (1) Optimize red blood cell mass, (2) Minimize blood loss, (3) Manage anaemia (Table 6.20). This is a continuous progress during the patient's operative journey [90]. The prehabilitation process involves preoperative management to workup and treat the underlying anaemia, optimize cardiopulmonary function and manage the bleeding. Planning for the intraoperative and post-operative phases should also be considered such as adoption of restrictive transfusion strategies and planning for surgical techniques to reduce blood loss.

While the application of patient blood management principles is not exclusive to surgical oncology patients, it is a patient group with some unique challenges. The prevalence of anaemia is higher in this patient group than the standard preoperative patient due to bleeding from the tumour, nutritional deficiencies and anaemia of chronic inflammation. Often, transfusions are used as a modality for symptomatic relief and most clinicians may have a more liberal transfusion approach to such patients [91]. The safety concerns of erythropoietin stimulating agents due to the thrombosis risk and concerns on effects of overall survival also limit the strategies to manage anaemia [20]. The use of blood salvage methods such as cell-saver is also relatively contraindicated in oncological surgery due to the concerns of cancer metastasis [92]. Furthermore, most oncological surgeries are considered urgent and limit the time for optimization of anaemia and cardiovascular function in the preoperative setting.

Table 6.20 Patient blood management: A multidisciplinary team approach. (Adapted from Spahn et al. 2013)

	1. Optimize RBC mass	2. Minimize blood loss	3. Manage anaemia
PREOP	Identify, assess and treat anaemia Refer for further assessment if necessary	Identify and manage bleeding risk Review medications Minimize iatrogenic blood loss Preoperative embolization to reduce tumour vascularity Plan and practise procedure	Estimate patient tolerance for blood loss Evaluate and optimize patient's cardiopulmonary reserve Formulate patient-specific management plan
INTRAOP	Time surgery with optimization of red cell mass	Meticulous haemostasis and surgical techniques Blood-sparing surgical techniques Anaesthetic blood-conservation strategies Pharmacological and haemostatic agents Avoid coagulopathy	Optimize cardiac output Optimize ventilation and oxygenation Restrictive transfusion strategies
POSTOP	Manage nutritional or correctable anaemia Manage medications and potential drug interactions	Monitor and manage post-op bleeding Keep patient warm Minimize phlebotomy Management of haemostasis and anticoagulation	Maximize oxygen delivery Minimize oxygen consumption Treat infections Restrictive transfusion strategies

While there are many challenges in the management of transfusion strategies in oncological patients, what is critical is the development and implementation of a program which can result in reduced transfusion usage and improved outcome in these surgical patients. There are many successful programmes in various oncological cancers which serve as examples to be incorporated in the prehabilitation of the oncological surgical patient [93].

Take Home Points

1. Preoperative anaemia in the oncological patient often have multiple contributors and should be optimized prior to the surgical procedure.
2. It is difficult to predict the bleeding risk of a preoperative patient with thrombocytopenia. Diagnosis of the aetiology and determining the platelet threshold and preoperative optimization should be done.
3. A good clinical assessment with history and physical examination is the foundation to the preoperative assessment of haemostatic function.
4. Surgical oncology patients are at a higher thromboembolic risk, planning for thromboprophylaxis is important and should be initiated in the preoperative setting.
5. Employment of patient blood management strategies improves outcomes in surgical oncological patients.

We hope this chapter provides a guide to the haematological preoperative workup of the surgical oncology patient. Additional care in preoperative optimization serves to improve outcomes.

A pint of sweat saves a gallon of blood.

General George S. Patton.

References

1. Knight K, Wade S, Balducci L. Prevalence and outcomes of anemia in cancer: a systematic review of the literature. Am J Med. 2004;116(7 Suppl. 1):11–26.
2. Fowler AJ, Ahmad T, Phull MK, Allard S, Gillies MA, Pearse RM. Meta-analysis of the association between preoperative anaemia and mortality after surgery. Br J Surg. 2015;102(11):1314–24.
3. Wilson MJ, van Haaren M, Harlaar JJ, Park HC, Bonjer HJ, Jeekel J, et al. Long-term prognostic value of preoperative anemia in patients with colorectal cancer: a systematic review and meta-analysis. Surg Oncol. 2017;26(1):96–104.
4. Baumeister P, Canis M, Reiter M. Preoperative anemia and perioperative blood transfusion in head and neck squamous cell carcinoma. PLoS One. 2018;13(10)
5. McLean E, Cogswell M, Egli I, Wojdyla D, De Benoist B. Worldwide prevalence of anaemia, WHO vitamin and mineral nutrition information system, 1993 2005. Public Health Nutr. 2009;12(4):444–54.
6. Common Terminology Criteria for Adverse Events (CTCAE) [Internet]. [cited 2021 Jan 3]. https://ctep.cancer.gov/protocolDevelopment/templates_applications.htm
7. Gilreath JA, Rodgers GM. How I treat cancer anemia. Blood. 2020;136:801–13.

8. Schwartz RN. Anemia in patients with cancer: Incidence, causes, impact, management, and use of treatment guidelines and protocols. Am J Heal Pharm. 2007;64(3 Suppl. 2).
9. Poorana Priya P, Subhashree AR. Role of absolute reticulocyte count in evaluation of pancytopenia-a hospital based study. J Clin Diagnostic Res. 2014;8(8).
10. Cavill I. Iron status as measured by serum ferritin: the marker and its limitations. Am J Kidney Dis. 1999;34(4 Suppl. 2).
11. Mast AE, Blinder MA, Gronowski AM, Chumley C, Scott MG. Clinical utility of the soluble transferrin receptor and comparison with serum ferritin in several populations. Clin Chem. 1998;44(1):45–51.
12. Ruul A, Saar B. Anaemia of chronic disease. Eesti Arst. 2015;94(9):538–46.
13. Friedman BMT. Patient blood management in hematology and oncology. 2020:1–4.
14. Spahn DR, Goodnough LT. Alternatives to blood transfusion. Lancet. 2013;381(9880):1855–65.
15. Muñoz M, Acheson AG, Auerbach M, Besser M, Habler O, Kehlet H, et al. International consensus statement on the peri-operative management of anaemia and iron deficiency. Anaesthesia. 2017;72(2):233–47.
16. Acheson AG, Brookes MJ, Spahn DR. Effects of allogeneic red blood cell transfusions on clinical outcomes in patients undergoing colorectal cancer surgery: a systematic review and meta-analysis. Ann Surg. 2012;256(2):235–44.
17. Keeler BD, Dickson EA, Simpson JA, Ng O, Padmanabhan H, Brookes MJ, et al. The impact of pre-operative intravenous iron on quality of life after colorectal cancer surgery: outcomes from the intravenous iron in colorectal cancer-associated anaemia (IVICA) trial. Anaesthesia. 2019;74(6):714–25.
18. Tomer A, Amir B, Alon G, Hefziba G, Leonard L, Anat GG. The safety of intravenous iron preparations: systematic review and meta-analysis. Mayo Clin Proc. 2015;90(1):12–23.
19. Warner MA, Shore-Lesserson L, Shander A, Patel SY, Perelman SI, Guinn NR. Perioperative anemia: prevention, diagnosis, and management throughout the spectrum of perioperative care. Anesth Analg. 2020:1364–80.
20. Bohlius J, Schmidlin K, Brillant C, Schwarzer G, Trelle S, Seidenfeld J, et al. Recombinant human erythropoiesis-stimulating agents and mortality in patients with cancer: a meta-analysis of randomised trials. Lancet. 2009;373(9674):1532–42.
21. Tonia T, Mettler A, Robert N, Schwarzer G, Seidenfeld J, Weingart O, et al. Erythropoietin or darbepoetin for patients with cancer. Cochrane Database Syst Rev. 2012.
22. Bohlius J, Bohlke K, Castelli R, Djulbegovic B, Lustberg MB, Martino M, et al. Management of cancer-associated anemia with erythropoiesis-stimulating agents: ASCO/ASH clinical practice guideline update. J Clin Oncol. 2019;37(15):1336–51.
23. Henke M, Laszig R, Rübe C, Schäfer U, Haase KD, Schilcher B, et al. Erythropoietin to treat head and neck cancer patients with anaemia undergoing radiotherapy: randomised, double-blind, placebo-controlled trial. Lancet. 2003;362(9392):1255–60.
24. Leyland-Jones B, Semiglazov V, Pawlicki M, Pienkowski T, Tjulandin S, Manikhas G, et al. Maintaining normal hemoglobin levels with epoetin alfa in mainly nonanemic patients with metastatic breast cancer receiving first-line chemotherapy: a survival study. J Clin Oncol. 2005;23(25):5960–72.
25. https://www.accessdata.fda.gov/drugsatfda_docs/label/2008/103234s5196pi.pdf. [Internet]. [cited 2021 Jan 3]; http://library1.nida.ac.th/termpaper6/sd/2554/19755.pdf
26. Li Z, Yang F, Dunn S, Gross AK, Smyth SS. Platelets as immune mediators: their role in host defense responses and sepsis. Thromb Res. 2011;127(3):184–8.
27. Estcourt LJ, Birchall J, Allard S, Bassey SJ, Hersey P, Kerr JP, et al. Guidelines for the use of platelet transfusions. Br J Haematol. 2017;176(3):365–94.
28. Arnold DM, Heddle NM, Cook RJ, Hsia C, Blostein M, Jamula E, et al. Perioperative oral eltrombopag versus intravenous immunoglobulin in patients with immune thrombocytopenia: a non-inferiority, multicentre, randomised trial. Lancet Haematol. 2020;7(9):e640–8.
29. Al-Samkari H, Marshall AL, Goodarzi K, Kuter DJ. Romiplostim for the management of perioperative thrombocytopenia. Br J Haematol. 2018;182(1):106–13.

30. Peck-Radosavljevic M, Simon K, Iacobellis A, Hassanein T, Kayali Z, Tran A, et al. Lusutrombopag for the treatment of thrombocytopenia in patients with chronic liver disease undergoing invasive procedures (L-PLUS 2). Hepatology. 2019;70(4):1336–48.
31. Terrault N, Chen YC, Izumi N, Kayali Z, Mitrut P, Tak WY, et al. Avatrombopag before procedures reduces need for platelet transfusion in patients with chronic liver disease and thrombocytopenia. Gastroenterology. 2018;155(3):705–18.
32. Manzullo E, Sahai S. Preoperative evaluation and management of patients with cancer. Up to Date 2017.
33. Littlewood KE. The immunocompromised adult patient and surgery. Best Pract Res Clin Anaesthesiol. 2008;22(3):585–609.
34. Nagrebetsky A, Al-Samkari H, Davis NM, Kuter DJ, Wiener-Kronish JP. Perioperative thrombocytopenia: evidence, evaluation, and emerging therapies. Br J Anaesth [Internet]. 2019;122(1):19–31. https://doi.org/10.1016/j.bja.2018.09.010.
35. Boxer LA. How to approach neutropenia. Hematology Am Soc Hematol Educ Program. 2012;2012:174–82.
36. Nancy BM. Approach to the adult with pancytopenia. UpToDate. 2020.
37. Shimamura A. Clinical approach to marrow failure. Hematol Am Soc Hematol Educ Prog. 2009:329–37.
38. Rodeghiero F, Tosetto A, Abshire T, Arnold DM, Coller B, James P, et al. ISTH/SSC bleeding assessment tool: a standardized questionnaire and a proposal for a new bleeding score for inherited bleeding disorders. J Thromb Haemost. 2010;8(9):2063–5.
39. Vries MJ, van der Meijden PE, Kuiper GJ, Nelemans PJ, Wetzels RJ, van Oerle RG, et al. Preoperative screening for bleeding disorders: a comprehensive laboratory assessment of clinical practice. Res Pract Thromb Haemost. 2018;2(4):767–77.
40. Šrámek A, Eikenboom JCJ, Briët E, Vandenbroucke JP, Rosendaal FR. Usefulness of patient interview in bleeding disorders. Arch Intern Med. 1995;155(13):1409–15.
41. Chee YL, Crawford JC, Watson HG, Greaves M. Guidelines on the assessment of bleeding risk prior to surgery or invasive procedures: British Committee for Standards in Haematology. Br J Haematol. 2008;140(5):496–504.
42. Velanovich V. The value of routine preoperative laboratory testing in predicting postoperative complications: a multivariate analysis. Surgery. 1991;109(3 I):236–43.
43. Wolberg AS, Campbell RA. Thrombin generation, fibrin clot formation and hemostasis. Transfus Apher Sci. 2008;38(1):15–23.
44. Curry NS, Davenport R, Pavord S, Mallett SV, Kitchen D, Klein AA, et al. The use of viscoelastic haemostatic assays in the management of major bleeding: a British Society for Haematology Guideline. Br J Haematol. 2018;182(6):789–806.
45. Sharma AD, Al-Achi A, Seccombe JF, Hummel R, Preston M, Behrend D. Does incorporation of thromboelastography improve bleeding prediction following adult cardiac surgery? Blood Coagul Fibrinolysis. 2014;25(6):561–70.
46. Walsh M, Kwaan H, McCauley R, Marsee M, Speybroeck J, Thomas S, et al. Viscoelastic testing in oncology patients (including for the diagnosis of fibrinolysis): review of existing evidence, technology comparison, and clinical utility. Transfusion. 2020;60(S6):S86–100.
47. Lancé MD. A general review of major global coagulation assays: thrombelastography, thrombin generation test and clot waveform analysis. Thromb J. 2015;13(1).
48. Escobar MA, Brewer A, Caviglia H, Forsyth A, Jimenez-Yuste V, Laudenbach L, et al. Recommendations on multidisciplinary management of elective surgery in people with haemophilia. Haemophilia. 2018;24(5):693–702.
49. Srivastava A, Santagostino E, Dougall A, Kitchen S, Sutherland M, Pipe SW, et al. WFH guidelines for the management of Hemophilia, 3rd edition. Haemophilia. 2020;26:1–158.
50. Metharom P, Falasca M, Berndt MC. The history of armand trousseau and cancer-associated thrombosis. Cancers (Basel). 2019;11(2).
51. Colman RW, Rubin RN. Disseminated intravascular coagulation due to malignancy. Semin Oncol. 1990;17(2):172–86.

52. Thachil J, Falanga A, Levi M, Liebman H, Di Nisio M. Management of cancer-associated disseminated intravascular coagulation: guidance from the SSC of the ISTH. J Thromb Haemost. 2015;13(4):671–5.
53. Sallah S, Wan JY. Inhibitors against factor VIII in patients with cancer: analysis of 41 patients. Cancer. 2001;91(6):1067–74.
54. Napolitano M, Siragusa S, Mancuso S, Kessler CM. Acquired haemophilia in cancer: a systematic and critical literature review. Haemophilia. 2018;24(1):43–56.
55. Mohri H, Motomura S, Kanamori H, Matsuzaki M, Watanabe SI, Maruta A, et al. Clinical significance of inhibitors in acquired von Willebrand syndrome. Blood. 1998;91(10):3623–9.
56. Richard C, Cuadrado MA, Prieto M, Batlle J, Fernández MF, Salazar MLR, et al. Acquired von willebrand disease in multiple myeloma secondary to absorption of von willebrand factor by plasma cells. Am J Hematol. 1990;35(2):114–7.
57. Bracey AW, Wu AHB, Aceves J, Chow T, Carlile S, Hoots WK. Platelet dysfunction associated with Wilms tumor and hyaluronic acid. Am J Hematol. 1987;24(3):247–57.
58. Tiede A, Rand JH, Budde U, Ganser A, Federici AB. How I treat the acquired von Willebrand syndrome. Blood. 2011;117(25):6777–85.
59. Khorana AA, Francis CW, Culakova E, Kuderer NM, Lyman GH. Thromboembolism is a leading cause of death in cancer patients receiving outpatient chemotherapy [10]. J Thromb Haemost. 2007;5(3):632–4.
60. Sørensen HT, Mellemkjær L, Olsen JH, Baron JA. Prognosis of cancers associated with venous thromboembolism. N Engl J Med. 2000;343(25):1846–50.
61. Auer RAC, Scheer AS, McSparron JI, Schulman AR, Tuorto S, Doucette S, et al. Postoperative venous thromboembolism predicts survival in cancer patients. Ann Surg. 2012;255(5):963–70.
62. Levine M. Treatment of thrombotic disorders in cancer patients. Pathophysiol Haemost Thromb. 1997;27(1):38–43.
63. Agnelli G, Bolis G, Capussotti L, Scarpa RM, Tonelli F, Bonizzoni E, et al. A clinical outcome-based prospective study on venous thromboembolism after cancer surgery: the @RISTOS project. Ann Surg. 2006;243(1):89–95.
64. White RH, Zhou H, Romano PS. Incidence of symptomatic venous thromboembolism after different elective or urgent surgical procedures. Thromb Haemost. 2003;90(3):446–55.
65. Shaw JR, Siegal DM. Pharmacological reversal of the direct oral anticoagulants-a comprehensive review of the literature. Res Pract Thromb Haemost. 2018;2(2):251–65.
66. Gould MK, Garcia DA, Wren SM, Karanicolas PJ, Arcelus JI, Heit JA, et al. Prevention of VTE in nonorthopedic surgical patients. Antithrombotic therapy and prevention of thrombosis, 9th ed: American College of Chest Physicians evidence-based clinical practice guidelines. Chest. 2012;141(2 SUPPL):e227S–77S.
67. Obi AT, Pannucci CJ, Nackashi A, Abdullah N, Alvarez R, Bahl V, et al. Validation of the caprini venous thromboembolism risk assessment model in critically ill surgical patients. JAMA Surg. 2015;150(10):941–8.
68. Khorana A, Kuderer NM, Culakova E, Lyman GH, Francis CW. Development and validation of a predictive model for chemotherapy- associated thrombosis. Blood. 2008;111(10):4902–7.
69. Kakkos SK, Caprini JA, Geroulakos G, Nicolaides AN, Stansby G, Reddy DJ, et al. Combined intermittent pneumatic leg compression and pharmacological prophylaxis for prevention of venous thromboembolism. Cochrane Database Syst Rev. 2016;2016(9).
70. Ho KM, Tan JA. Stratified meta-analysis of intermittent pneumatic compression of the lower limbs to prevent venous thromboembolism in hospitalized patients. Circulation. 2013;128(9):1003–20.
71. Sachdeva A, Dalton M, Lees T. Graduated compression stockings for prevention of deep vein thrombosis. Cochrane Database Syst Rev. 2018;2018(11).
72. Zareba P, Wu C, Agzarian J, Rodriguez D, Kearon C. Meta-analysis of randomized trials comparing combined compression and anticoagulation with either modality alone for prevention of venous thromboembolism after surgery. Br J Surg. 2014;101(9):1053–62.
73. Ockelford PA, Patterson J, Johns AS. A double-blind randomized placebo controlled trial of thromboprophylaxis in major elective general surgery using once daily injections of a low molecular weight heparin fragment (Fragmin). Thromb Haemost. 1989;62(4):1046–9.

74. Bergqvist D. Efficacy and safety of enoxaparin versus unfractionated heparin for prevention of deep vein thrombosis in elective cancer surgery: a double- blind randomized multicentre trial with renographic assessment. Br J Surg. 1997;84(8):1099–103.
75. Tokuhara K, Matsushima H, Ueyama Y, Nakatani K, Yoshioka K, Kon M. Efficacy and safety of thromboembolism prophylaxis with fondaparinux in Japanese colorectal cancer patients undergoing laparoscopic surgery: a phase II study. Int J Surg. 2017;42:203–8.
76. Carrier M, Abou-Nassar K, Mallick R, Tagalakis V, Shivakumar S, Schattner A, et al. Apixaban to prevent venous thromboembolism in patients with cancer. N Engl J Med. 2019;380(8):711–9.
77. Key NS, Khorana AA, Kuderer NM, Bohlke K, Lee AYY, Arcelus JI, et al. Venous thromboembolism prophylaxis and treatment in patients with cancer: ASCO clinical practice guideline update. J Clin Oncol. 2020;38(5):496–520.
78. Bergqvist D, Agnelli G, Cohen AT, Eldor A, Nilsson PE, Le Moigne-Amrani A, et al. Duration of prophylaxis against venous thromboembolism with enoxaparin after surgery for cancer. N Engl J Med. 2002;346(13):975–80.
79. Rasmussen MS, Jorgensen LN, Wille-Jørgensen P, Nielsen JD, Horn A, Mohn AC, et al. Prolonged prophylaxis with dalteparin to prevent late thromboembolic complications in patients undergoing major abdominal surgery: a multicenter randomized open-label study. J Thromb Haemost. 2006;4(11):2384–90.
80. Baglin TP, Brush J, Streiff M. Guidelines on use of vena cava filters. Br J Haematol. 2006;134(6):590–5.
81. Decousus H, Leizorovicz A, Parent F, Page Y, Tardy B, Girard P, et al. A clinical trial of vena caval filters in the prevention of pulmonary embolism in patients with proximal deep-vein thrombosis. N Engl J Med. 1998;338(7):409–16.
82. Douketis JD, Foster GA, Crowther MA, Prins MH, Ginsberg JS. Clinical risk factors and timing of recurrent venous thromboembolism during the initial 3 months of anticoagulant therapy. Arch Intern Med. 2000;160(22):3431–6.
83. Baglin T, Keeling D. Management of venous thromboembolism. Postgrad Haematol Seventh Ed. 2015:830–7.
84. Douketis JD, Spyropoulos AC, Kaatz S, Becker RC, Caprini JA, Dunn AS, et al. Perioperative bridging anticoagulation in patients with atrial fibrillation. N Engl J Med. 2015;373(9):823–33.
85. Balabhadra S, Kuban JD, Lee S, Yevich S, Metwalli Z, McCarthy CJ, et al. Association of inferior vena cava filter placement with rates of pulmonary embolism in patients with cancer and acute lower extremity deep venous thrombosis. JAMA Netw Open. 2020;3(7):e2011079.
86. Franchini M, Marano G, Veropalumbo E, Masiello F, Pati I, Candura F, et al. Patient blood management: a revolutionary approach to transfusion medicine. Blood Transfus. 2019;17(3):191–5.
87. Keding V, Zacharowski K, Bechstein WO, Meybohm P, Schnitzbauer AA. Patient blood management improves outcome in oncologic surgery. World J Surg Oncol. 2018;16(1).
88. Isbister JP, Shander A, Spahn DR, Erhard J, Farmer SL, Hofmann A. Adverse blood transfusion outcomes: establishing causation. Transfus Med Rev. 2011;25(2):89–101.
89. Murphy GJ, Reeves BC, Rogers CA, Rizvi SIA, Culliford L, Angelini GD. Increased mortality, postoperative morbidity, and cost after red blood cell transfusion in patients having cardiac surgery. Circulation. 2007;116(22):2544–52.
90. Isbister JP. The three-pillar matrix of patient blood management-an overview. Best Pract Res Clin Anaesthesiol. 2013;27(1):69–84.
91. Khorana AA, Francis CW, Blumberg N, Culakova E, Refaai MA, Lyman GH. Blood transfusions, thrombosis, and mortality in hospitalized patients with cancer. Arch Intern Med. 2008;168(21):2377–81.
92. Editorial: Blood salvage and cancer surgery: Should we do it? Transfusion. 2009;49(10):2016–8.
93. Gross I, Trentino KM, Andreescu A, Pierson R, Maietta RA, Farmer S. Impact of a patient blood management program and an outpatient anemia management protocol on red cell transfusions in oncology inpatients and outpatients. Oncologist. 2016;21(3):327–32.

7 Nutritional Prehabilitation in Cancer Surgery: Basis and Basics

Rohit Agrawal and Li Xuanhui Janice

7.1 Introduction

Prehabilitation in cancer patient is defined as, "a process on the continuum of cancer care that occurs between the time of cancer diagnosis and the beginning of acute treatment, includes physical and psychological assessments that establish a baseline functional level, identifies impairments, and provides targeted interventions that improve a person's health to prevent or reduce the incidence and the severity of current and future impairments" [1] (Fig. 7.1). The goal of prehabilitation thus is to prevent or reduce the severity of anticipated treatment-related physical impairments and psychological distress so as to facilitate positive outcomes such as improved functional capacity, maintenance of lean mass, reduced surgical complication and better quality of life [2–5]. It's important to understand that role of prehabilitation is not a replacement of rehabilitation, rather to complement it by preparing patients with physical and psychological resilience. Though it's becoming a part of preoperative optimization therapy for cancer patients, there is still some gap in understanding its overall composition, timing and frequency.

Cancer patients are often faced with nutritional challenges and 50–80% were found to have varying degrees of malnutrition in multiple studies [6]. The degree of malnutrition was found to be proportional not only to stage of cancer but also with certain types of cancer for example, patients with head and neck, oesophageal malignancy and pancreatic malignancy were found to be more cachectic. However, a recently conducted review suggested only in <10% of studies nutrition assessment

R. Agrawal (✉)
Department of Anaesthesia and Critical Care Medicine, National University Health System, Singapore, Singapore
e-mail: rohit_agrawal@nuhs.edu.sg

L. X. Janice
Department of Pharmacy, National University Health System, Singapore, Singapore

A. Chakraborty, A. Balakrishnan (eds.), *Prehabilitation for Cancer Surgery*,
https://doi.org/10.1007/978-981-16-6494-6_7

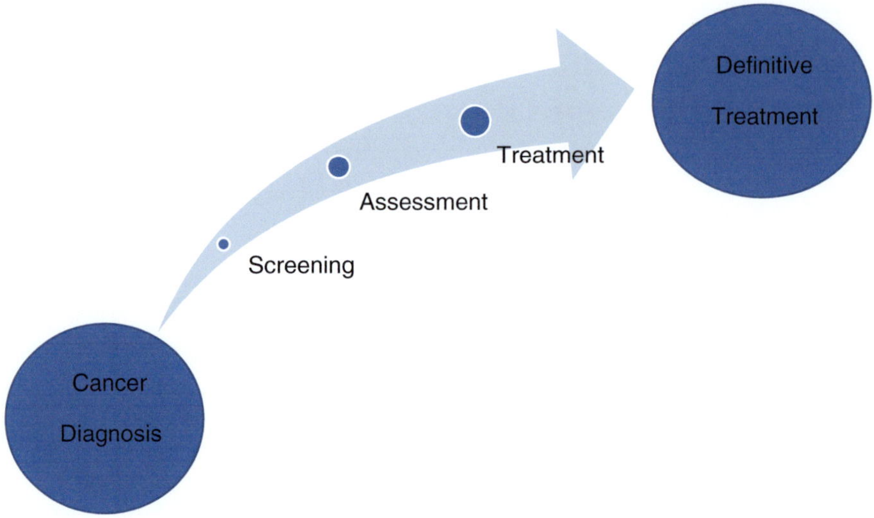

Fig. 7.1 Timing of cancer prehabilitation

was conducted and, in most studies, nutrition assesement tools applied were not validated and <34% of studies discussed nutritional therapy [7]. Thus, creating a need for further studies with more directed nutritional assessment, individually tailored therapy and measurable outcomes which can be used to compare results across studies.

7.2 Definition

7.2.1 Cancer-Associated Malnutrition

Malnutrition can be defined as "a state resulting from lack of intake or uptake of nutrition that leads to altered body composition (decreased fat-free mass) and body cell mass leading to diminished physical and mental function and impaired clinical outcome from disease." However, malnutrition in cancer patients differs significantly from starvation-related malnutrition. Cancer-related malnutrition falls under the category of "chronic disease related malnutrition (DRM)" whereby malnutrition is associated with chronic inflammation. The combination of reduced food intake and metabolic alterations in cancer means that conventional nutrition support may not fully reverse the effects of malnutrition, unlike that seen in starvation-related malnutrition.

The reported prevalence of malnutrition in cancer patients ranges from 20% to up to 80% [8]. Although the prevalence of malnutrition may vary depending on type and stage of cancer, age as well as associated anticancer therapies, differences in definitions and assessments may possibly account for the wide variations seen in studies. The consensus statement by ASPEN or ESPEN can be used for the diagnosis of malnutrition (Tables 7.1 and 7.2).

Table 7.1 Clinical characteristics of malnutrition

Insufficient energy intake (<75% of requirement)
Weight loss (>5% in 3 months)
Loss of skeletal muscle mass
Loss of subcutaneous fat
Localized or generalized oedema
Diminished grip strength

Table 7.2 Diagnosis of malnutrition

ASPEN	ESPEN
The presence of 2 or more indicates malnutrition 1. Insufficient energy intake 2. Weight loss 3. Loss of muscle mass 4. Loss of subcutaneous fat 5. Localized or generalized oedema 6. Diminished functional status as measured by handgrip strength	The presence of either indicates malnutrition 1. BMI <18.5 2. Unintentional weight loss of >10% indefinitely or >5% over the last 3 months + a) BMI <20 (age < 70 years) or <22 (age > 70 years) or + b) Low fat-free mass (<15 kg/m^2 in females and <17 kg/m^2 in males)

7.2.2 Sarcopenia

Sarcopenia is characterized by loss of muscle mass and strength, often associated with loss of physical function. This loss of muscle mass with or without the loss of fat in cancer patients has been shown to be predictive of the risk of post-operative complications and mortality [9, 10]. Severe depletion of muscle is generally classified as an absolute muscularity below the fifth percentile (Table 7.3).

7.2.2.1 Sarcopenic Obesity

It is recognized that sarcopenia can occur in the presence of obesity and traditional approaches of diagnosing malnutrition based on body weight or weight loss may fail to identify such patients at risk. The presence of excess fat and extracellular water may often mask the loss of muscle mass.

As it is increasingly being recognized how sarcopenia influences treatment outcomes in cancer patients, it is important to have sensitive and precise measurements of muscle mass in patients identified to be at risk of malnutrition. The SARC-F may be used as a screening tool to identify patients at risk of sarcopenia in whom further assessments of muscle mass should be done. The SARC-F is a self-reported scoring system which comprises questions assessing different aspects of physical function associated with loss of muscle mass [11].

According to the international consensus on cancer cachexia, CT or MRI is preferred for muscle mass assessments. Besides measurements of muscle mass, assessment of muscle or physical function should also be included as part of the comprehensive nutritional assessment. Several tests like the handgrip strength measured by a hand-held dynamometer or chair rise tests are simple assessments that

Table 7.3 Classification of severe muscle depletion by different methods

	Males	Females
Anthropometry (mid upper arm muscle area)	<32 cm^2	<18 cm^2
Dual energy X-ray absorptiometry (appendicular skeletal muscle index)	<7.26 kg/m^2	<5.45 kg/m^2
CT (lumbar skeletal muscle index)	<55 cm^2/m^2	<39 cm^2/m^2
Bioelectrical impedance (fat-free mass index)	<14.6 kg/m^2	<11.4 kg/m^2

Table 7.4 Sarcopenia assessment

Muscle mass	Muscle strength	Physical performance
Anthropometry Dual energy X-ray absorptiometry CT imaging Bioelectrical impedance	Handgrip test Chair rise test	Timed up and go (TUG) Short physical performance battery (SPPB) Gait speed tests

Table 7.5 Cancer cachexia

Pre-cachexia	Cachexia	Refractory cachexia
Low grade weight loss <5% of total body weight	>5% weight loss or BMI <20 kg/m^2 with >2% wt loss or Sarcopenia with >2% wt loss	Catabolic state from extensive weight loss Disease not responsive to treatments with expected survival <3 months

can be a surrogate for muscle strength and may serve as additional indicators of efficacy of nutrition support (Table 7.4). Other more comprehensive tests like the Timed Up and Go (TUG) and Short Physical Performance Battery (SPPB) tests may also be used.

7.2.3 Cancer Cachexia

Cancer cachexia is a complex multifactorial wasting syndrome characterized by involuntary weight loss and skeletal muscle loss, usually accompanied with progressive functional decline. Cancer cachexia represents a continuum that begins with anorexia and progresses to pre-cachexia, cachexia and then to sarcopenia and refractory cachexia (Table 7.5). It has been estimated that cancer cachexia may be responsible for up to 20% of deaths [12].

Anorexia is often one of the early signs of pre-cachexia. Coupled with the early metabolic changes induced by tumours like impaired glucose tolerance, this may result in some involuntary weight loss. The progression to cachexia is dependent on factors like cancer type and stage, extent of systemic inflammation, anticancer therapies and response.

The Cachexia Score (CASCO) is a comprehensive assessment tool that has been validated for use in cancer patients [13]. It was developed to further classify patients based on the severity of their cachexia, comprising 4 groups, mild, moderate, severe and terminal. This tool consists of 5 main components, weight loss/body composition, inflammation/immunosuppression/metabolic alterations, physical performance, anorexia and quality of life.

7.3 Pathophysiology of Malnutrition in Cancer

The total energy expenditure (TEE) for individuals is the sum total of the resting energy expenditure (REE) and energy expended from physical activity with REE making up the largest component of TEE. However, for cancer patients, several factors may influence REE. These include the energy burden of the tumour, associated metastases, body composition and anatomical alterations that occur in cancer as well as the inflammatory state induced by tumours [14].

It is often thought that cancer patients have higher resting energy expenditures (REE) due to the hypermetabolic state induced by the systemic inflammatory syndrome arising from tumours as well as the energy burden of these tumours. This may vary with types and stages of tumours. In addition, the effects of anticancer therapies may also affect REE. Although REE may be increased in certain subgroups of patients with cancers, it is also noteworthy that when TEE is considered, these may be lower or equivalent to healthy individuals due to the lower activity level of these patients. TEE for individuals with cancers can be variable; however, current ESPEN guidelines suggest it is assumed to be similar to healthy individuals [15] (Fig. 7.2).

7.3.1 Systemic Inflammation Syndrome

A state of inflammation is often activated in patients with cancers. "This is due to" interaction between pro-inflammatory cytokines released by the tumour and an upregulated immune response. Such a state results in several alterations in the metabolic pathways affecting nutrition (Table 7.6) [16–20]. All these result in loss of muscle mass with or without fat loss.

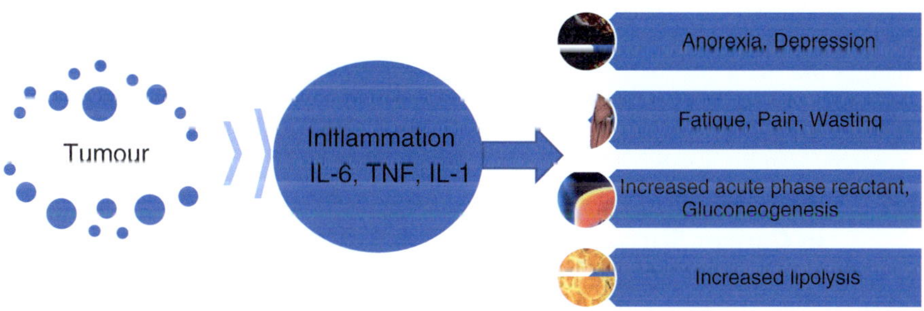

Fig. 7.2 Effect of cancer on nutrition

Table 7.6 Cytokine-mediated effect on protein, carbohydrate and fat metabolism

	Protein	Carbohydrate	Fat
TNF	Increased muscle proteolysis and oxidation Increased hepatic protein synthesis	Increased glycogenolysis, gluconeogenesis, glucose clearance, lactate production Decreased glycogen synthesis	Decreases lipogenesis
IL-1	Increased hepatic protein synthesis	Increased gluconeogenesis, glucose clearance	Increased lipolysis, fatty acid synthesis, decreased LPL synthesis
IL-6	Increased hepatic protein synthesis		Increased lipolysis, fatty acid synthesis
IFN-GAMMA			Decreased lipogenesis and LPL activity, increased lipolysis

1. Protein metabolism: increased muscle catabolism, increase liver synthesis of proteins, decreased muscle protein synthesis.
2. Carbohydrate metabolism: insulin resistance and impaired glucose tolerance, increased gluconeogenesis from amino acid, lactate, etc.
3. Lipid metabolism: increased lipolysis, increased glycerol and fatty acid turnover, similar or increased capacity for lipid oxidation.

7.3.2 Inadequate Nutritional Intake

Either due to primary anorexia caused by cytokines released from tumours disrupting appetite signals from the central nervous system, resulting in reduced appetite and thus reduced intake. This reduced intake is further exacerbated by reversible secondary causes like xerostomia, intestinal obstruction, malabsorption, chemosensory alteration, uncontrolled pain or side-effects of anticancer therapies [18–22].

7.3.2.1 Hypoxic Stress in Tumour Microenvironment

As tumour grows rapidly it may exceed blood supply, resulting in regions of relative hypoxia which in turn triggers a complex (mal-)adaptive mechanism. Tumour metabolism is altered to rely more on glycolysis and less on oxidative phosphorylation, and protection against harmful reactive oxygen species is reduced. These changes are associated with enhanced tumour growth, malignant progression and even resistance to anticancer therapy [23].

7.4 Pathophysiology of Perioperative Stress in Cancer Surgery

In cancer patients, further surgical trauma induces hormonal, haematological, metabolic and immunologic changes which is to counteract the state of surgical stress that challenges metabolic and physiologic equilibrium and thus can further impact

Table 7.7 Impact of surgical resection on nutrition

Organ	Consequences
Tongue or pharynx	Dysphagia
Oesophagus	Dysphagia, gastric stasis/reflux, early satiety, loss of appetite, dumping syndrome, malabsorption of fats
Stomach	Dumping syndrome, anaemia, malabsorption of fats, early satiety, diarrhoea, gastric stasis
Jejunum	Malabsorption of macronutrients and micronutrients
Ileum	Malabsorption of biliary salts, fats, b12
Small intestine	Malabsorption of macronutrients, diarrhoea
Colon	Water and electrolyte loss
Pancreas	Insulin and glucose disorders, malabsorption of macronutrients

nutritional status. This inflammatory state due to surgical stress and tissue injury lead to change in metabolism of glycogen, protein and free fatty acids, leading to diversion of protein for tissue and wound healing, resulting in further loss of lean muscle mass. In patients who are having impaired nutrition due to other factors either diagnosed or undiagnosed, interactions of these surgical factors together with underlying factors determine the overall outcome of patients (Fig. 7.3). Also, cancer surgery which results in radical resection of organs involved in the maintenance of nutritional intake often results in higher risks of malnutrition post-operatively (Table 7.7). It is important to ensure that these patients are optimized preoperatively from a nutritional standpoint and build up reserves if possible. All patients undergoing cancer surgery should be managed within an ERAS pathway.

7.5 Multimodal Prehabilitation

Patients arriving at the doorstep of major elective surgery are likely to be particularly amenable to interventions; however, most surgical pathways are designed with different aims in mind and there are time constraints between the time surgery is first contemplated and the actual surgical date. This may offer a particular "teachable moment" as there is possibility of long-term behavioural change and health benefits by radical shift in ethos and re-design of the "surgical pathway" so that perioperative physicians interact with patients earlier in the perioperative journey. This led to the advent of "Surgery Schools," which gives us the opportunity to share such knowledge with our patients and thereby guide them toward healthier behaviours. Surgery schools also offer the opportunity to manage expectations in relation to the in-hospital surgical journey, improve buy-in to enhanced recovery pathways, and improve psychological preparation for surgery.

Recently, emphasis had been placed on multimodal patient-centred prehabilitation approach. It is basically application of two or more interventions having synergistic effect specifically curated according to patient needs so as to achieve desired health outcomes (Table 7.8). Multimodal prehabilitation interventions comprised of a combination of recommendations by expert consensus which are supported by

Table 7.8 Multimodal prehabilitation

Prehabilitation interventions	Healthcare professionals	Target
Aerobic and resistance training	Physiotherapist, occupational therapist, kinesiologist	To attenuate cardiorespiratory and musculoskeletal deconditioning
Dietary interventions	Dietician and nutritionist	To counteract disease and/or treatment-related malnutrition and to support anabolism and the metabolic cost of exercise
Psychological interventions	Psychologist, psychotherapist and social worker	To reduce stress and associated morbidity To encourage cessation of adverse health behaviours To support intervention initiation and adherence in the pre-treatment setting and establish self-management skills for long-term health behaviour maintenance
Medical optimization	Physician, geriatrician, pharmacist	For assessing/treating anaemia, ect and medication corrections

recent qualitative findings from patient interviews as well as previous research which suggests that comprehensive prehabilitation support via complementary modalities was especially important and well received by people undergoing surgery for lung and colorectal cancer [3–5, 24, 25].

7.6 Nutritional Counselling

All patients should be screened for malnutrition at diagnosis and at routine follow-ups. Patients who are identified to be at malnutrition risk should have a full nutritional assessment done and appropriate interventions depending on their level of malnutrition (Table 7.9). A formal nutritional assessment should also be performed at the time when surgery is decided as part of the preoperative assessment. For patients who are identified to be at risk of malnutrition or identified as malnourished, a multimodal prehabilitation regimen incorporating nutrition support and exercise should be implemented.

Nutritional counselling is one of the interventions utilized for the management of malnourished patients with cancer and a functioning gastrointestinal tract [15]. A dietitian-nutritionist can provide individualized advice to achieve energy and nutrient balance based on the patient's estimated REE, lifestyle, disease state, current intake and food preferences. Counselling needs to address the presence and severity of symptoms such as anorexia, nausea, dysphagia, abdominal bloating or cramping, diarrhoea and constipation. Critical components of nutrition counselling are to: (1) convey to the patient the reasons and goals for nutritional recommendations and (2) motivate the patient to adapt to altered nutritional demand of their disease.

Table 7.9 Elements to be included in a full nutritional assessment

Component	Assessment
Energy and protein intake	Food intake
Barriers to food intake	1. GI function 2. Nutrition impact symptoms (anorexia, dysphagia, nausea etc.) 3. Pain 4. Emotional health
Weight loss and body composition	History of unintentional weight loss, fat-free mass
Muscle mass and function	Anthropometric measures, DEXA, bioelectrical impedance analysis, CT, handgrip strength
Physical function	ECOG score
Systemic inflammation	CRP, albumin, modified Glasgow prognostic score

7.7 Nutritional Screening and Assessment

The American Society for Parenteral and Enteral Nutrition (A.S.P.E.N.) defines nutrition screening as "a process to identify an individual who is malnourished or who is at risk for malnutrition to determine if a detailed nutrition assessment is indicated." Identification of patients with cancer who are at risk for malnutrition based on low body weight (or BMI) and a history of weight loss has become increasingly ineffective due to the global obesity epidemic and the metabolic alterations that occur prior to any measurable change in body weight. Anorexia is recognized as an early risk indicator for malnutrition, and appetite change can occur regardless of a patient's initial weight. Inadequate nutritional intake is confirmed if patients cannot eat for a week or if their energy intake is <60% of estimated requirements for 1–2 weeks [26].

Several screening and assessment tools are available to identify malnutrition risk (Table 7.10). However, including this and other total of 32 nutritional risk assessment tools, identified in 83 studies after a systematic review of the literature, is not an optimal screening tool to be used in the preoperative "at risk" surgical patient population [16]. Nutrition screening and malnutrition risk assessment ideally should be done at cancer diagnosis, though this is not always the case as revealed by a recent review which showed only 1 in 5 US hospitals utilize the formal screening process and only 20% of US GI/oncologic surgical patients received any form nutritional support [27]. Recently, an alternative scoring system, PONS (Preoperative Nutrition Screening) was proposed (Fig. 7.4). The PONS is easy to use and is integrated with a preoperative nutrition care pathway which directs the patient with high risk of malnutrition for further assessment and intervention soon after plan for surgery is confirmed [28].

7.7.1 Laboratory Markers

Laboratory markers like albumin and prealbumin are used in some screening and assessment tools. The production of these proteins is affected by nutritional intake, liver function as well as inflammatory status. Other laboratory markers that have

Table 7.10 Comparison of commonly used nutrition screening tools

Tool	Diet-related	Anthropometry	Weight loss	Severity of illness	Others	Scoring
Malnutrition universal screening tool (MUST)	Nil	BMI	Amount of weight loss >5% weight loss in the past 3–6 months	Presence of acute illness resulting in no nutritional intake >5 days		0–1—No risk of malnutrition 2–5—Risk of malnutrition
Malnutrition screening tool (MST)	Presence of reduced intake from decreased appetite	Nil	Amount of weight loss in the last 6 months	Nil		0—Low risk of malnutrition 1—Medium risk of malnutrition 2—High risk of malnutrition
Nutritional Risk Screening (NRS 2002)	Presence and quantification of reduced food intake in the past week	BMI	Amount of weight loss >5% in the past 1–3 months	Stratified according to severity of illness		3 or more points—Initiate a nutrition care plan
Short nutrition assessment questionnaire (SNAQ)	Presence of decreased appetite over the last month	Nil	Amount of weight loss in the past 1–6 months	Nil	Use of supplemental drinks or tube feeding over the last month	2—Moderate malnutrition 3 or more—Severe malnutrition
Mini nutritional assessment (MNA-SF)	Intake over the past 3 months	BMI Calf circumference	Weight loss during the last 3 months	Presence of acute stress in the past 3 months	Mobility Psychological well-being	12–14 Normal 8–11 at nutritional risk 0–7 malnutrition
PG-subjective global assessment	– Usual vs current intake (patient input) – Presence of nutrition impact symptoms (patient input)	Muscle status – Fat stores – Fluid status	– Weight history (patient input) – Weight loss over last 1 month (scored)	Disease and its relation to nutritional requirements – Metabolic demand	– Usual vs current activities (patient input)	1 no intervention required 2–3 requires nutritional education 4–8 requires nutritional intervention >8 critical need for intervention

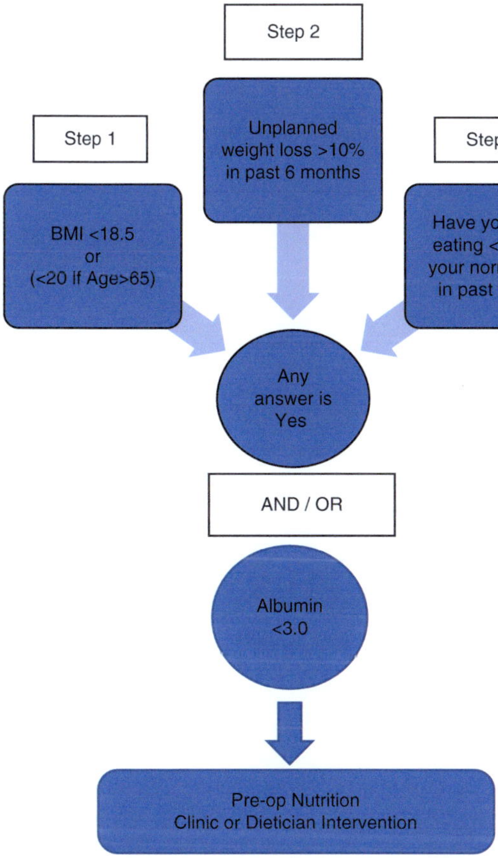

Fig. 7.3 Interaction of tumour and surgical stress on patient outcome

been used include total cholesterol, lymphocyte count and CRP. Most of these suffer from lack of specificity as they may be influenced by the severity of the underlying cancer as well. The Glasgow Prognostic Score (GPS), which is based on CRP and albumin as markers of inflammation, however is highly predictive of inflammation in cancer patients and is widely validated to predict prognosis and mortality [29].

Albumin is one of the most abundant proteins in the serum. It is synthesized in the liver and has a long half-life of approximately 20 days. It is also one of the acute-phase proteins, thus its concentrations are significantly affected by acute stress and inflammation. Systemic inflammation leads to a reduced production of these proteins as well as increasing transcapillary leakage of these proteins, leading to lower concentrations [30]. Other conditions that may lower its concentrations include losses in nephropathies like nephrotic syndrome as well as certain types of enteropathies. Although it has been traditionally used as a marker of malnutrition, it fares poorly in malnutrition not associated with inflammation. Studies have shown that in starvation-related malnutrition in otherwise healthy individuals where malnutrition

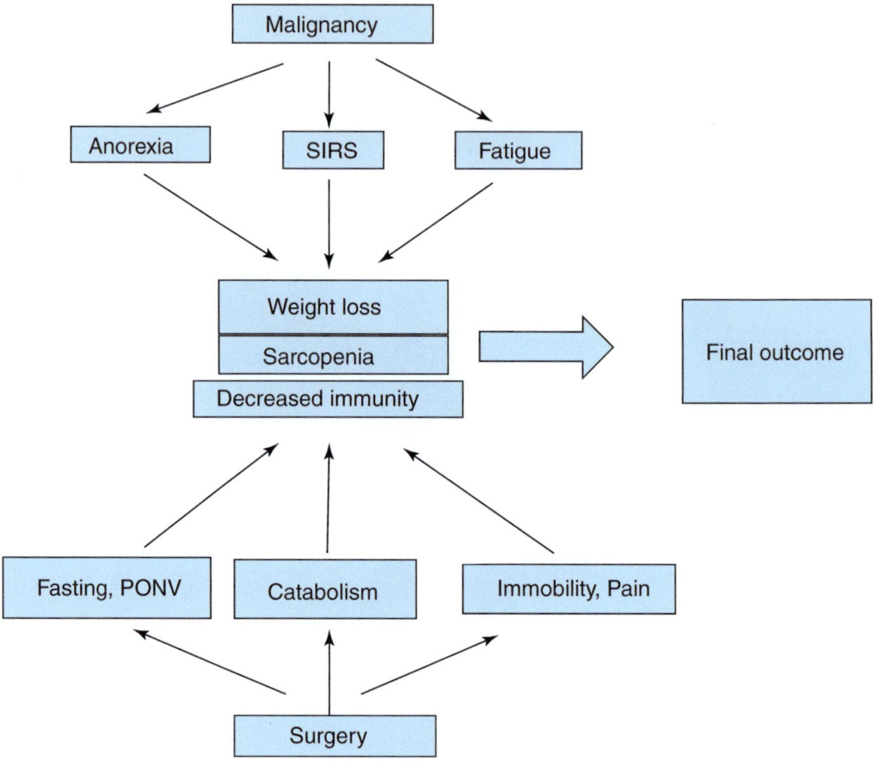

Fig. 7.4 PONS [23]

arises from poor nutritional intake, serum albumin may remain normal despite weight loss till extreme states of starvation are reached [31]. The lack of sensitivity and specificity of albumin has thus led to the move away from these biomarkers in the assessment of nutritional status [32–34]. Albumin, however, has been shown to be a good marker for outcomes in surgical patients [35, 36]. Although it should not be used as a nutritional indicator, it is still recommended to measure these as part of the nutritional assessment as these may help to indicate the inflammatory status of the patient [15]. The Glasgow Prognostic Score (GPS) or modified GPS, a simple scoring system based on concentrations of CRP and albumin, has been shown to be useful in predicting the risk of adverse outcomes in cancer patients [37].

Prealbumin is also a negative acute-phase protein synthesized by the liver. Thus, it suffers the same shortcomings as albumin in its role as a biomarker for nutritional status. However, prealbumin has a shorter half-life of approximately 2–3 days, which makes it a more useful marker of acute changes in nutritional state, in the absence of inflammatory states. Similar to albumin, prealbumin has little role in establishing the diagnosis of malnutrition in cancer patients, although it may be useful as an indicator of response to nutritional therapy when assessed together with other markers of inflammation [37].

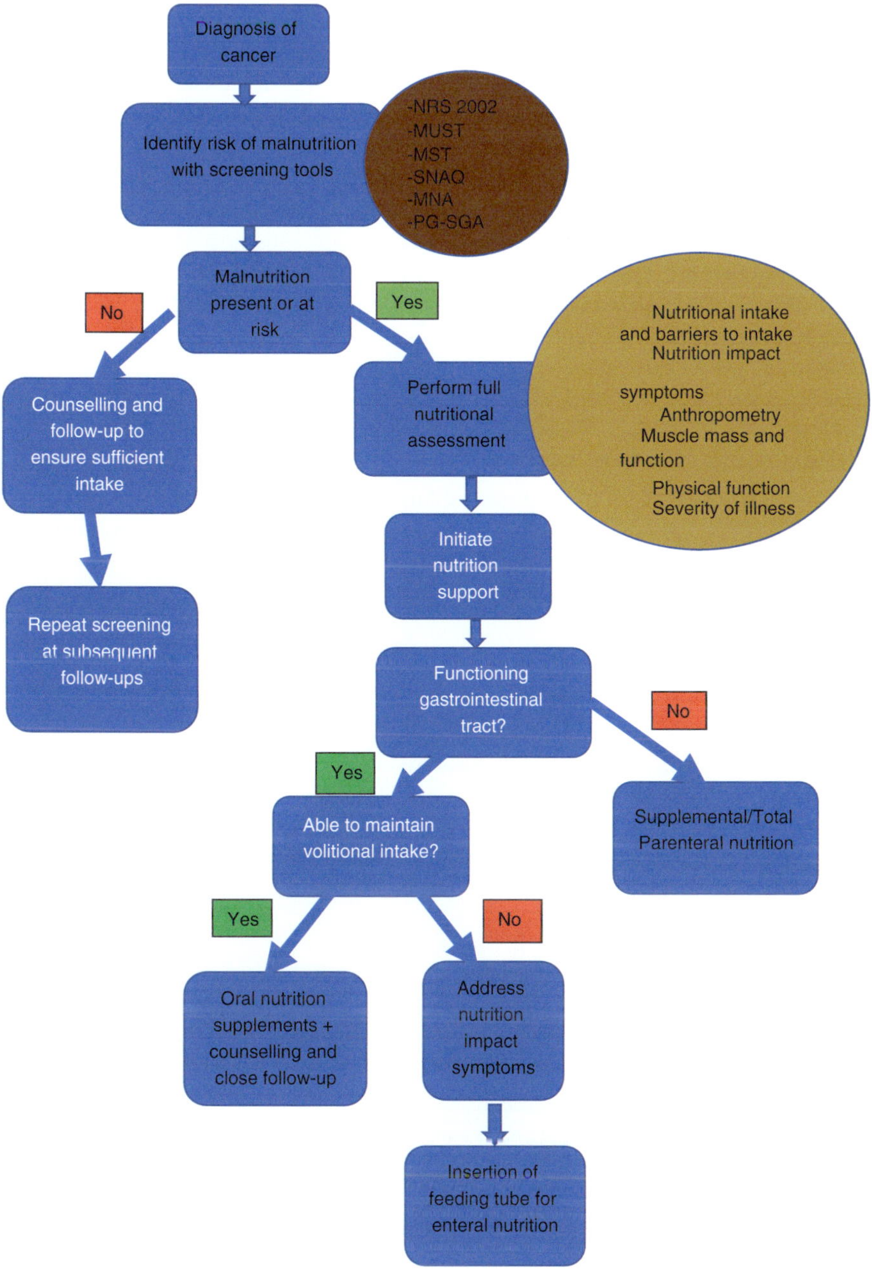

Fig. 7.5 Perioperative nutritional prehabilitation

7.7.2 Imaging Techniques

There is increasing recognition that conventional measures of anthropometry like BMI and weight fail to identify patients who may be at risk of poor outcomes in oncology. This has led to a recent focus on morphometrics, the study of body shape and form, in the area of oncology research [38, 39]. Current studies involving morphometrics have shown negative associations between low muscle mass and cancer-related outcomes like survival and treatment toxicity. Ongoing prospective studies are looking into the utility of such metrics and the ability of interventions to modify these metrics and in turn influence clinical outcomes like survival and reduction of treatment-toxicities.

Dual energy X-ray absorptiometry (DXA), computed tomography (CT) and magnetic resonance imaging (MRI) are all able to quantify adipose and muscle mass and have been regarded as gold standards in the area of morphometric evaluation (Table 7.11). Imaging like CT or MRI are often routinely used in oncology practice to characterize the primary tumour as well as response to treatment. Thus, they may represent a practical option in terms of serial follow-up for changes in body composition. For CT, a single-slice abdominal cross-sectional image, taken at the third lumbar (L3) vertebrae, can be incorporated into algorithms to describe whole body

Table 7.11 Imaging techniques for nutritional screening and assessment

Modality	Measures	Pros	Cons
Anthropometry	Weight, BMI, waist and hip circumference, skinfold	Simple Inexpensive	Insensitive Equations not validated in cancer population Loss in skeletal muscle mass may be masked in obesity or with concurrent gain in adiposity
DXA	Fat mass, FFM and bone mineral	Gold standard High precision and accuracy Reproducible Small radiation exposure	Not widely available Requires trained technicians
CT	Single-slice CT images to estimate muscle mass and fat mass	High precision Differentiation between FFM and fat mass	Radiation exposure Costly Requires interpretation by radiologist
MRI		High precision Differentiation between FFM and fat mass	Costly Not accessible to all Can't be used in presence of metal work Requires interpretation by radiologist
Ultrasound	Muscle thickness Muscle quality	Safe No radiation exposure Easily accessible Portable	Operator-dependent Limited use in obese patients

muscle and adipose volume. However, some of the disadvantages of this modality include the radiation exposure and cost, which would be prohibitive for the sole purpose of body composition assessment, limiting its utility to opportunistic rather than routine for serial follow-up of nutritional interventions. In addition, some cancer cohorts (e.g. breast cancer or prostate cancer) may not require CT images taken in the abdominal area as part of routine care. MRI may be even more cost-prohibitive to be used as a screening and assessment modality for nutritional interventions.

Ultrasound is another non-invasive, low- cost and portable method that is valid for quantifying various muscle dimensions and may be explored in the area of oncological nutrition assessment. Ultrasound measures of muscle have been shown to correlate well with lean body mass assessed with DXA in older adults [40]. Predictive equations have been developed using ultrasound muscle thickness that may be used to estimate appendicular lean soft tissue mass as measured by the gold standard DXA [41]. Studies have also demonstrated the reliability and accuracy of using ultrasound for muscle measurements across various populations and different muscles, although not specifically in the cancer population. There is currently no definitive agreement on which muscle group should be measured and no established criteria for low muscle mass according to ultrasound. There is also a lack of agreement on which muscle group correlates best for functional outcomes. One study has shown that forearm muscle thickness correlates strongly with handgrip strength [41], others have shown that muscle thickness and echo intensity measures in lower limb muscles are associated with functional capacity in older adults [42]. There has also been use of the adductor pollicis muscle thickness as a marker of nutritional status in various populations [43] as well as a prognostic indicator in the oncological setting [44].

It has also been suggested that ultrasound may be used to assess muscle quality as well, which may account for physical performance beyond muscle size. Ultrasound echogenicity has been described to measure muscle quality. The higher the echogenicity, the higher the proportion of slow-twitch muscle fibre and intramuscular adipose tissue, corresponding to lower muscle quality and grip strength [45, 46]. Although this has not been validated in large studies, the plausibility of an association is present. This may thus represent another aspect of muscle analysis but ultrasound can complement current measurements.

The variety of methods currently used in ultrasound muscle measurements and lack of standardized definitions limit its widespread adoption in current clinical practice. However, given its low cost and accessibility, it has huge feasibility to be used as a tool in routine nutritional screening. Further work should be done to validate its use in this setting.

7.8 Nutritional Prehabilitation

Though there is enough evidence to suggest malnutrition, cancer cachexia and sarcopenia is associated with poor outcome but findings of systematic review on prehabilitation therapy are inconsistent in demonstrating effectiveness in reducing post-operative outcome [7]. This could be due to heterogeneity in the study population with patients being combination of different malignancies and at various stages of malnutrition, design not using proper assessment tool, intervention being unimodal or even due to factors like unavailability of nutritional counselling hampering the application of intervention [40]. In different studies conducted in the USA and Europe, it was found that upto 50% of hospitalized patients were malnourished and 40% of those identified as malnourished did not receive any nutritional support. The goal of nutritional prehabilitation is to optimize metabolic status and augment physiologic reserves preoperatively to prevent further worsening of nutritional status which has adverse impacts on post-operative outcomes (Table 7.12).

7.8.1 Components of Nutrition

7.8.1.1 Protein

Positive net muscle protein balance is essential for maintenance or gain of muscle mass. Nutrition in general acts as a potent anabolic stimulus and high postprandial circulating amino acids can stimulate muscle protein synthesis.

Even though protein acts as a building block for muscles and prescribing it based on body composition is ideal, studies prescribing protein based on body weight has shown positive impact on muscle mass. The optimal protein requirements for prevention or treatment of sarcopenia in cancer patients are not well-defined and vary from patient to patient. It ranges from a minimum of 0.2–2.7 mg/kg/day, depending upon the patient tolerance and renal function. A recent review of cancer cachexia studies suggested intake of up to 2 mg/kg/day in patients with active disease to prevent or maintain muscle mass which is in line with the position paper published by ESPEN guidelines. This has to be reduced to 1 and 1.2 mg/kg/day in patients with acute or chronic kidney disease respectively [15, 47].

7.8.1.2 Branched Chain Amino Acids

The branched chain amino acids (leucine, isoleucine, valine) have gained popularity due to their purported benefits of promoting muscle synthesis. Early studies investigating the use of BCAAs in parenteral nutrition in malnourished patients with intra-abdominal adenocarcinoma have suggested benefits in terms of albumin and protein

Table 7.12 Nutrition targets in cancer patients

Nutritional intake	Amount
Energy	20–30 kcal/kg/day (depending upon ambulatory status of patient)
Protein	1–1.5 mg/kg/day (depending upon renal function)
Carbohydrate	<7 mg/kg/day
Fat	1 g/kg/day (100% soybean oil) or 2 g/kg/day (30% soybean oil, 30% medium chain Triglycerides, 25% olive oil, 15% fish oil)
Micronutrients	Vitamins and minerals as per RDA

synthesis [29, 30]. Another study looking at an oral supplementation enriched with leucine may help to stimulate muscle protein synthesis [31]. However, these studies are small and results have yet to be replicated in large-scale studies. Given the uncertain role of BCAAs both in stimulating muscle anabolism in cancer cachexia as well as tumour proliferation, further studies are recommended [32, 33].

7.8.1.3 Carbohydrates and Fats

It is possible that cancer patients may benefit from an altered carbohydrate to fat feeding ratio. The insulin resistance induced by the inflammatory state in cancer often leads to impaired glucose tolerance and utilization. Also, low appetite associated with reduced gut motility may benefit from an energy dense diet consisting of a higher fat to carbohydrate ratio in such cases. In patients requiring parenteral nutrition, this low carbohydrate diet may have additional benefits like reduced risk of infection and low salt and water retention as demonstrated in multiple studies.

7.8.2 Supplements

7.8.2.1 Beta Hydroxy Beta Methylbutyrate (HBM)

It's a metabolite of BCCA, leucine and found in low levels in natural food. HBM has an inhibitory effect on proteolysis and shown to be beneficial in elderly people and patients with COPD and rheumatoid arthritis. Since proteolysis is the main mechanism by which muscle mass is lost in cancer patients, HBM is studied as a nutritional supplement along with a high protein diet in cancer patients. When used as a supplement in doses from 2000 to 3000 mg/day along with arginine and glutamine, early (<5% weight loss), it has shown to maintain or gain lean body mass as opposed to delayed, suggesting nutritional supplements may not benefit in refractory cachexia.

7.8.2.2 Omega-3 Fatty Acid

The long-chain N-3 fatty acid, eicosapentaenoic acid, commonly found in marine oils, helps to attenuate the inflammatory response by competitive antagonism of N-6 polyunsaturated fatty acid thus causing downregulation of PGE2 production and suppression of inflammatory gene productions. Intramuscular deposit of adipose tissue which is implicated in development of insulin resistance and cachexia in cancer patients is found to be reversed by omega 3 fatty acids in some studies. When used with a high protein diet, it is more likely to maintain body composition and prevent muscle loss as compared to isocaloric intake. It also helps to improve appetite, body weight and quality of life. Doses of at least 2000 mg/day have been recommended in order to achieve nutritional benefits.

7.8.2.3 Vitamins and Minerals

Cancer patients are at risk of micronutrient deficiency either due to ongoing metabolic derangement or due to adverse effects of chemo- and radiotherapy. Though a recent systematic review had failed to show advantage of multivitamin supplementation, it was argued by the fact that the study group had severe cachexia which has different metabolic demands. Studies have shown vitamin D supplementation in recommended daily allowance of 600–800 IU is associated with improved muscle mass and strength, especially in patients >65 years. of age. American Cancer society and ESPEN recommend the use of multivitamin-mineral supplements in doses close to daily recommended doses for cancer patients.

7.8.2.4 Immunonutrition

Immunonutrition broadly refers to nutritional formulas that are meant to modulate the activity of the immune system [48]. Increased understanding of cancer immunology and immunotherapy has led to advancements in cancer treatments utilizing the human immune response. This has led to a growing interest in the area of nutrition that may help to module the acquired immune responses and improve outcomes.

Some of the nutrients employed in immunonutrition are listed below (Table 7.13). Immunonutrition formulas usually contain varying amounts of arginine, glutamine, omega-3-fatty acids, essential amino acids and/or nucleotides. Current recommendations from ESPEN strongly support the use of enteral immunonutrition for upper gastrointestinal cancer patients undergoing surgical resection. A recent meta-analysis evaluating a wide range of cancer surgeries has also suggested that enteral immunonutrition helps to reduce post-operative infectious complications and hospital stay in cancer patients. For gastric cancer patients undergoing surgery, it has been found that the optimal combination for these patients in helping to reduce infectious complications and length of stay may be arginine +nucleotides + omega-3-fatty acids and arginine + glutamine + omega-3-fatty acids [49, 50]. The optimal combination of different immunonutrients and their doses are yet to be well-defined for various other subgroups of cancer patients undergoing surgery.

Table 7.13 Immunonutrients and their roles [1, 3]

Immunonutrients	Function
Omega-3-fatty acids	Anti-inflammatory Inhibit the adhesion of lymphocytes to monocytes and reduce the antigen-stimulated reaction of lymphoid cells
S amino acids	Enhance antioxidant status via glutathione synthesis
Glutamine	Nutrient for immune cells (enterocytes, fibroblasts, lymphocytes and macrophages) Improves gut barrier function Precursor for glutathione
Arginine	Substrate for nitric oxide synthesis, stimulates T-lymphocytes proliferation Enhances actions of macrophages and natural killer cells
Nucleotides	Precursors for DNA and RNA Stimulate lymphocytes Affects immune function of macrophage and natural killer cells

7.8.3 Pharmacological Interventions

As mentioned above, cancer cachexia differs significantly from starvation induced cachexia. The ongoing muscle mass loss due to the metabolic aberrations induced by tumours coupled with the inability of intake to meet nutritional requirements means that nutrition support would only be able to partially reverse the effects of malnutrition.

There are currently no FDA-approved medications to treat cancer cachexia; however, several classes of medications have been trialled, however only two classes of medications (progesterone analogues and corticosteroids) have moderate quality of evidence to support their use in cancer cachexia. It should be noted that although these medications may help to improve appetite and weight gain with some improvements in function, they have not been shown to increase muscle mass nor improve mortality. The benefits of these medications need to be weighed against their risks and goals of care. Symptomatic management of cancer or treatment-related effects that may impair nutritional intake like pain, depression, mucositis, nausea, etc. should not be neglected as well.

7.8.3.1 Progesterone Analogues

Megestrol acetate and medroxyprogesterone acetate are the two most common progesterone analogues that have been used to increase appetite. They have been shown to improve appetite with some results in weight gain and possible improvements in quality of life. However, these benefits need to be weighed against the possible higher risks of thromboembolism, oedema and deaths [20].

7.8.3.2 Corticosteroids

The corticosteroids dexamethasone, methylprednisolone and prednisolone have been used to increase appetite in cancer cachexia and especially useful in patients with short life expectancy where it may help to improve overall well-being. However, their beneficial effects are usually transient and are outweighed when adverse effects like myopathy and immunosuppression appear. It is associated with adverse effects like insulin resistance and osteopenia especially when used for long term.

7.8.4 Route

Enteral route being more physiological is able to maintain functional and structural integration of gut mucosa, is associated with less complications and is cheaper. If a patient is not able to tolerate or receive oral feeding, tube feeding should be given either in the form of nasogastric or nasojejunal feeds. In some patients with gastrointestinal malignancies, percutaneous jejunal tube may be required. In patients with moderate to severe degree of malnutrition and who are not able to tolerate enteral nutrition partially or completely, parenteral route can be used. Parenteral route though routinely is not recommended in well-nourished patients on radiotherapy but patients who develop mucositis or radiation enteritis, it can be used for short term (Table 7.14). Combination of enteral and parenteral route is shown to be more effective in reducing chemotherapy-associated complications.

7.8.4.1 Refeeding Syndrome

Refeeding syndrome is defined as the "potentially fatal shifts in fluids and electrolytes that may occur in severely malnourished patients receiving artificial refeeding either enterally or parenterally." The risk of developing refeeding syndrome is related to the degree of malnutrition as well as the period of starvation. The severely malnourished cancer patient is at risk of developing refeeding syndrome, especially if intake in the preceding weeks has been minimal and nutritional support is being planned in anticipation of surgery. It is important to recognize patients who may be at risk and initiate nutrition support cautiously in these patients. In patients who have had minimal intake in the last 5 days, initiation of feeding should not exceed

Table 7.14 Enteral vs parenteral nutrition

	Enteral	Parenteral
Types	Oral, tube feeding (NG, PEG, feeding J)	Partial or complete, peripheral or central line
Indication	All patient should get trial of enteral nutrition	Bowel obstruction Severe mucositis, enteritis or colitis Short bowel syndrome Severe nausea or vomiting
Advantage	– Simple and cheap – Psychological satisfaction – Preserves intestinal mucosal barrier – Stimulates intestinal blood flow and promotes optimal absorption of nutrients – Reduces muscle metabolism – Reduces gut-associated lymphoid system which in turn can be source of activated cells and pro-inflammatory stimulants	– Simple – Can be started early – Able to deliver target calorie and protein from get go – Less need for interruptions due to patient or procedure factors – When time appropriately in indicated patients, shown to increase ventilator free days and improve muscle mass
Disadvantage	– Takes time to establish goal rate and thus target caloric and protein requirement – Independent risk factor for VAP – Risk of sinusitis (NG) or local wound infection (PEG, feeding J) – Intolerance due to vomiting and diarrhoea – Prone for interruptions due to patient or procedure factors – Metabolic derangements like electrolyte imbalance, hyperglycaemia, refeeding syndrome	– Not physiological and associated with disuse atrophy of gut and inflammatory syndrome – Complications related to line placement like bleeding, infection, pneumothorax, etc. – Metabolic derangements like hyperglycaemia, hypercholesterolaemia, hyperchloremic metabolic acidosis and refeeding syndrome – Increased risk steatosis and acalculous cholecystitis – Loss of bone mass

more than half of the estimated requirements in the first few days with close monitoring of electrolytes and clinical status. Before initiation of feeding, electrolytes like potassium, phosphate and magnesium should be repleted and supplemented as necessary. The supplementation of thiamine in doses of 200–300 mg/day is also recommended in these patients.

7.8.5 Timing, Duration and Approach

Once patients are identified to be malnourished, appropriate nutritional interventions should be instituted, especially if surgery is being contemplated. Although it has been traditionally recommended that malnourished patients receive nutrition support for at least 10–14 days before surgery, the optimal period of conditioning required before surgery is ill-defined.

Our suggested approach involves consideration of the patient's nutritional status and urgency of surgical intervention. Nutritional support should be offered in a stepped-up approach, starting with oral nutritional supplements, tube feeding and progressing to parenteral nutrition in cases where enteral nutrition is insufficient or impossible. In severely malnourished patients, a period of at least 10–14 days of nutrition support is recommended before surgery, with a preference to delay surgery if possible. We favour the approach of stratifying nutritional risk (by either PG-SGA or NRS 2002) combined with markers like albumin or prealbumin. Although albumin and prealbumin are not to be used as markers of malnutrition, they may help to identify patients at risk of poor surgical outcomes and in whom nutrition support might be beneficial (Fig. 7.5).

For patients with mild-moderate malnutrition, oral nutritional supplements should be given to ensure that they are meeting their energy and protein needs. For patients with no apparent nutritional risk, assessment needs to be done to ensure that they continue to consume diets that are meeting their needs in the perioperative period. For these patients, a normocaloric diet with a protein intake of at least 1.2–1.5 g/kg is recommended. Even those who may not be malnourished may benefit from a period of nutritional supplements preoperatively, especially those undergoing upper GI surgery as it has been shown to help maintain nutritional status and reduce the severity of post-operative complications [14].

For all patients undergoing cancer surgery, especially upper GI surgery, consideration should be given to provide immune-modulating enteral nutrition for 5–7 days pre-op [15, 29]. Although the optimal components of such "immunonutrition" has not been clearly defined, they are usually enteral formula enriched with omega-3 fatty acids, arginine and ribonucleotides

7.9 Summary

Nutritional prehabilitation in cancer patients should begin at the time of diagnosis. A comprehensive therapeutic plan for the management of the cancer should include nutritional needs and nutritional screening should be performed at time of diagnosis, even if the patient does not appear "malnourished" using conventional definitions of weight and BMI. All patients should undergo a comprehensive nutrition assessment at time of their diagnosis to help identify their risk of developing malnutrition as they progress through their course of treatment. These should not only be limited anthropometric measures and nutritional intake, but expanded to include body composition analysis, functional assessments and identifying potential barriers to nutritional intake and physical activity once cancer treatment is initiated. These measures should be repeated at regular follow-ups (Fig. 7.5). A multimodal approach to nutritional prehabilitation that involves physical exercise and interventions targeting optimal caloric intake should be adopted.

The inflammatory state in cancer leads to altered metabolism in these patients, often resulting in a catabolic state. The additional metabolic stress from surgery further compounds the problem. Thus cancer patients undergoing surgery should be monitored even more closely with regard to their nutritional status. The negative associations between malnutrition and outcomes in cancer patients are well-established and current research has been focusing on the role of nutrition in modifying outcomes like survival and treatment-related toxicities. An adequate intake of calories and protein should be ensured right at the time of diagnosis, with the consideration of immunonutrition in the perioperative period. Nutritional prehabilitation does not stop at the time of surgery, but should be continued into the post-operative period.

References

1. Silver JK, Baima J. Cancer prehabilitation. Am J Phys Med Rehabil. 2013;92(8):715–27. https://doi.org/10.1097/PHM.0b013e31829b4afe.
2. Minnella EM, Bousquet-Dion G, Awasthi R, Scheede-Bergdahl C, Carli F. Multimodal prehabilitation improves functional capacity before and after colorectal surgery for cancer: a five-year research experience. Acta Oncol (Madr). 2017;56(2):295–300. https://doi.org/10.1080/0284186X.2016.1268268.
3. Santa MD, Brahmbhatt P, Lopez C, Baima J, Gillis C, Trachtenberg L, et al. The case for prehabilitation prior to breast cancer treatment. Phys Med Rehabil. 2017;9(9):S305–16. https://doi.org/10.1016/j.pmrj.2017.08.402.
4. Carli F, Silver JK, Feldman LS, McKee A, Gilman S, Gillis C, et al. Surgical prehabilitation in patients with cancer. Phys Med Rehabil Clin N Am. 2017;28(1):49–64. https://doi.org/10.1016/j.pmr.2016.09.002.
5. Halliday L, Wynter-Blyth V, Osborn H, King A, Moorthy K. Adherence to prehabilitation in oesophago-gastric cancer patients. Clin Nutr ESPEN. 2017;19:90. https://doi.org/10.1016/j.clnesp.2017.04.056.
6. von Haehling S, Anker SD. Prevalence, incidence and clinical impact of cachexia: facts and numbers—update 2014. J Cachexia Sarcopenia Muscle. 2014;5(4):261–3.
7. Gillis C, Davies SJ, Carli F, Wischmeyer PE, Wootton SA, Jackson AA, Riedel B, Marino LV, Levett DZH, West MA. Current landscape of nutrition within prehabilitation oncology research: a scoping review. Front Nutr. 2021;8:644723. https://doi.org/10.3389/fnut.2021.644723.
8. White JV, Guenter P, Jensen G, Malone A, Schofield M. Consensus Statement of the Academy of Nutrition and Dietetics/American Society for Parenteral and Enteral Nutrition: characteristics recommended for the identification and documentation of adult malnutrition (undernutrition). J Acad Nutr Diet. 2012;112(5):730–8.

9. White JV, Guenter P, Jensen G, Malone A, Schofield M. Consensus statement: academy of nutrition and dietetics and American Society for Parenteral and Enteral Nutrition. J Parenter Enter Nutr. 2012;36(3):275–83. https://doi.org/10.1177/0148607112440285.
10. Walsh D, Szafranski M, Aktas A, Kadakia KC. Malnutrition in cancer care: time to address the elephant in the room. J Oncol Pract. 2019;15(7):357–9.
11. Erstad BL, Campbell DJ, Rollins CJ, Rappaport WD. Albumin and prealbumin concentrations in patients receiving postoperative parenteral nutrition. Pharmacotherapy. 1994;14(4):458–62.
12. Gibbs J, Cull W, Henderson W, Daley J, Hur K, Khuri SF. Preoperative serum albumin level as a predictor of operative mortality and morbidity: results from the national VA surgical risk study. Arch Surg. 1999;134(1):36–42. https://pubmed.ncbi.nlm.nih.gov/9927128/
13. Kudsk KA, Tolley EA, DeWitt RC, Janu PG, Blackwell AP, Yeary S, et al. Preoperative albumin and surgical site identify surgical risk for major postoperative complications. J Parenter Enter Nutr. 2003;27(1):1–9. https://pubmed.ncbi.nlm.nih.gov/12549591/
14. Purcell SA, Elliott SA, Baracos VE, QSC C, Prado CM. Key determinants of energy expenditure in cancer and implications for clinical practice. Eur J Clin Nutr. 2016;70:1230–8. https://pubmed.ncbi.nlm.nih.gov/27273068/
15. Arends J, Bachmann P, Baracos V, Barthelemy N, Bertz H, Bozzetti F, et al. ESPEN guidelines on nutrition in cancer patients. Clin Nutr. 2017;36(1):11–48. https://pubmed.ncbi.nlm.nih.gov/27637832/
16. Tsoli M, Moore M, Burg D, Painter A, Taylor R, Lockie SH, et al. Activation of thermogenesis in brown adipose tissue and dysregulated lipid metabolism associated with cancer cachexia in mice. Cancer Res. 2012;72(17):4372e82.
17. Argiles JM, Busquets S, Stemmler B, Lopez-Soriano FJ. Cancer cachexia: understanding the molecular basis. Nat Rev Cancer. 2014;14(11):754e62.
18. Fukawa T, Yan Jiang BC, Min-Wen JC, Jun-Hao ET, Huang D, Qian CN, et al. Excessive fatty acid oxidation induces muscle atrophy in cancer cachexia. Nat Med. 2016;22(6):666e71.
19. Martinez-Outschoorn UE, Peiris-Pages M, Pestell RG, Sotgia F, Lisanti MP. Cancer metabolism: a therapeutic perspective. Nat Rev Clin Oncol. 2017;14(1):11e31.
20. Tsoli M, Robertson G. Cancer cachexia: malignant inflammation, tumorkines, and metabolic mayhem. Trends Endocrinol Metab. 2013;24(4):174e83.
21. McAllister SS, Weinberg RA. The tumour-induced systemic environment as a critical regulator of cancer progression and metastasis. Nat Cell Biol. 2014;16(8):717e27.
22. Patel HJ, Patel BM. TNF-alpha and cancer cachexia: molecular insights and clinical implications. Life Sci. 2017;170:56e63.
23. Vaupel P, Hockel M, Mayer A. Detection and characterization of tumor hyp- € oxia using pO2 histography. Antioxid Redox Signal. 2007;9:1221e35.
24. Brahmbhatt P, Sabiston CM, Lopez C, Chang E, Goodman J, Jones J, et al. Feasibility of prehabilitation prior to breast cancer surgery: a mixed methods study. Front Oncol. 2020;10:1–13. https://doi.org/10.3389/fonc.2020.571091.
25. Ferreira V, Agnihotram RV, Bergdahl A, van Rooijen SJ, Awasthi R, Carli F, et al. Maximizing patient adherence to prehabilitation: what do the patients say? Support Care Cancer. 2018;26(8):2717–23. https://doi.org/10.1007/s00520-018-4109-1.
26. van Bokhorst-de van der Schueren MAE, Guaitoli PR, Jansma EP, de HCW V. Nutrition screening tools: does one size fit all? A systematic review of screening tools for the hospital setting. Clin Nutr. 2014;33(1):39–58.
27. Williams JD, Wischmeyer PE. Assessment of perioperative nutrition practices and attitudes—a national survey of colorectal and GI surgical oncology programs. Am J Surg. 2017;213(6):1010–8.
28. McMillan DC. The systemic inflammation based Glasgow prognostic score: a decade of experience in patients with cancer. Cancer Treat Rev. 2013;39(5):534e40.
29. West MA, Wischmeyer PE, Grocott MPW. Prehabilitation and nutritional support to improve perioperative outcomes. Curr Anesthesiol Rep. 2017;7:340–9. https://doi.org/10.1007/s40140-017-0245-2.

30. Hunter DC, Weintraub M, Blackburn GL, Bistrian BR. Branched chain amino acids as the protein component of parenteral nutrition in cancer cachexia. Br J Surg. 1989;76(2):149–53. https://doi.org/10.1002/bjs.1800760215.
31. Deutz NEP, Safar A, Schutzler S, Memelink R, Ferrando A, Spencer H, et al. Muscle protein synthesis in cancer patients can be stimulated with a specially formulated medical food. Clin Nutr. 2011;30(6):759–68.
32. O'Connell T. The complex role of branched chain amino acids in diabetes and cancer. Meta. 2013;3(4):931–45. https://pubmed.ncbi.nlm.nih.gov/24958258/
33. Ericksen RE, Lim SL, McDonnell E, Shuen WH, Vadiveloo M, White PJ, et al. Loss of BCAA catabolism during carcinogenesis enhances mTORC1 activity and promotes tumor development and progression. Cell Metab. 2019;29(5):1151–1165.e6. https://doi.org/10.1016/j.cmet.2018.12.020.
34. Keller U. Nutritional laboratory markers in malnutrition. J Clin Med. 2019;8(6):775. https://doi.org/10.3390/jcm8060775.
35. Lee JL, Oh ES, Lee RW, Finucane TE. Serum albumin and prealbumin in calorically restricted, nondiseased individuals: a systematic review. Am J Med. 2015;128(9):1023.e1–1023.e22. https://pubmed.ncbi.nlm.nih.gov/25912205/
36. Mueller C, Compher C, Ellen DM. A.S.P.E.N. clinical guidelines: nutrition screening, assessment, and intervention in adults. J Parenter Enter Nutr. 2011;35(1):16–24. https://pubmed.ncbi.nlm.nih.gov/21224430/
37. Thomas G, Tahir MR, Bongers BC, Kallen VL, Slooter GD, van Meeteren NL. Prehabilitation before major intra-abdominal cancer surgery: a systematic review of randomised controlled trials. Eur J Anaesthesiol. 2019;36:933–45. https://doi.org/10.1097/EJA.0000000000001030.
38. Gibson DJ, Burden ST, Strauss BJ, Todd C, Lal S. The role of computed tomography in evaluating body composition and the influence of reduced muscle mass on clinical outcome in abdominal malignancy: a systematic review. Eur J Clin Nutr. 2015;69:1079–86. https://doi.org/10.1038/ejcn.2015.32.
39. Dunne RF, Mustian KM, Garcia JM, Dale W, Hayward R, Roussel B, et al. Research priorities in cancer cachexia: The University of Rochester Cancer Center NCI Community Oncology Research Program Research Base Symposium on Cancer Cachexia and Sarcopenia. Curr Opin Support Palliat Care. 2017;11:278–86. https://doi.org/10.1097/SPC.0000000000000301.
40. Nijholt W, Scafoglieri A, Jager-Wittenaar H, Hobbelen JSM, van der Schans CP. The reliability and validity of ultrasound to quantify muscles in older adults: a systematic review. J Cachexia Sarcopenia and Muscle. 2017;8:702–12. https://doi.org/10.1002/jcsm.12210.
41. Abe T, Thiebaud RS, Loenneke JP, Young KC. Prediction and validation of DXA-derived appendicular lean soft tissue mass by ultrasound in older adults. Age (Omaha). 2015;37(6):1–10. https://doi.org/10.1007/s11357-015-9853-2.
42. Mateos-Angulo A, GalÁN-Mercant A, Cuesta-Vargas AI. Ultrasound muscle assessment and nutritional status in institutionalized older adults: a pilot study. Nutrients. 2019;11(6):1247. https://doi.org/10.3390/nu11061247.
43. Pereira PMDL, Neves FS, Bastos MG, Cândido APC. Adductor Pollicis muscle thickness for nutritional assessment: a systematic review. Rev Bras Enferm, Rev Bras Enferm. 2018;71:3093–102. https://pubmed.ncbi.nlm.nih.gov/30517416/
44. Soares BGF d S, Vicentini AP. Use of adductor pollicis muscle thickness in hospitalized or ambulatory patients: a systematic review. Rev Latino-Am Enferm. 2018;26:2960. https://doi.org/10.1590/1518-8345.2045.2960.
45. Stringer HJ, Wilson D. The role of ultrasound as a diagnostic tool for sarcopenia. J Frailty Aging. 2018;7:258–61. https://doi.org/10.14283/jfa.2018.24.
46. Bozzetti F. Basics in Clinical nutrition: nutritional support in cancer. e-SPEN. 2010;5:e148–52. http://clinicalnutritionespen.com/article/S1751499109000651/fulltext
47. Kabata P, Jastrzębski T, Kąkol M, Król K, Bobowicz M, Kosowska A, et al. Preoperative nutritional support in cancer patients with no clinical signs of malnutrition—prospective randomized controlled trial. Support Care Cancer. 2015;23(2):365–70. https://pubmed.ncbi.nlm.nih.gov/25091056/

48. Adiamah A, Skořepa P, Weimann A, Lobo DN. The impact of preoperative immune modulating nutrition on outcomes in patients undergoing surgery for gastrointestinal cancer. Ann Surg. 2019;270(2):247–56. https://journals.lww.com/00000658-201908000-00011
49. Prieto I, Montemuiño S, Luna J, de Torres MV, Amaya E. The role of immunonutritional support in cancer treatment: current evidence. Clin Nutr. 2017;36:1457–64.
50. Buzquurz F, Bojesen RD, Grube C, Madsen MT, Gögenur I. Impact of oral preoperative and perioperative immunonutrition on postoperative infection and mortality in patients undergoing cancer surgery: systematic review and meta-analysis with trial sequential analysis. BJS Open. 2020;4:764–75. https://doi.org/10.1002/bjs5.50314.

Physiotherapy Pre-Habilitation

8

Loy Yijun, Chia Huey Yen, and Chong Cheu Shan Sylvia

8.1 Physiotherapy General Consideration

The concept of "exercise is medicine" has gained significant recognition and trajectory as a form of recommended intervention ([1]). Exercise prescription is commonly done by physiotherapists as well as other healthcare professions such as rehabilitation and sports physicians, exercise therapists as well as sports trainers. The increased recognition of exercise as an integral component and determinant of health status has generated much interest in the advancement of exercise as a form of preventative, restorative as well as interventional therapy ([2]).

This chapter aims to introduce:

- Role of exercise therapy in pre-habilitation.
- Assessments and functional tests commonly used in pre-habilitation.
- Exercise prescription for pre-habilitation.
- Recommendations and considerations for programme set-up.

8.2 Role of Exercise in Pre-Habilitation

The main considerations during the planning of physical rehabilitation prior to the intervention can be classified as:

L. Yijun · C. H. Yen (✉) · C. C. S. Sylvia
Department of Rehabilitation, National University Health System, Singapore, Singapore, Singapore
e-mail: huey_yen_chia@nuhs.edu.sg

A. Chakraborty, A. Balakrishnan (eds.), *Prehabilitation for Cancer Surgery*,
https://doi.org/10.1007/978-981-16-6494-6_8

8.2.1 Patient's Status

This includes:

1. Medical considerations: diagnosis and disease trajectory, comorbidities.
2. Planned interventions: this includes neoadjuvant therapy, curative therapy, as well as adjuvant therapy.
3. Physical function: such as strength, balance, mobility status and endurance.
4. Psychosocial function and needs: includes social support, home environment and long-term care plans and needs.
5. Patient's goals: includes physical roles, responsibilities as well as patient's expectations and readiness for change.

8.2.2 Medical Considerations

The disease process and therapeutic interventions (chemotherapy, hormonal/immunotherapy, radiotherapy/surgery) may cause a toll on both physical and mental health. While pre-habilitation promotes the optimisation of both physical functioning, symptom management and prepares for the stresses induced by surgery or medical therapies, it poses a unique challenge as the parameters of exercise prescription vary greatly between individuals and the time point of their medical journey.

It is advised that while exercise is recommended, the dosage, timing and type of exercise need to be appropriate and titrated to meet the needs and tolerance of the patient. Thoughtful monitoring of a patient's response and tolerance to exercise, their evolving symptoms and needs, will assist in modifications and progression of the exercise prescription. This is especially so for patients who may have complex health or behavioural issues, or medical conditions that may affect their response to exercise.

Regardless of the type or stage of cancer, exercise or physical activity has been found to improve quality of life for cancer patients including reducing and preventing future health complications and disability [3]. There is also strong evidence that exercise helps to cope with debilitating symptoms such as cancer-related fatigue, pain, anxiety and depression [4].

Surgery remains as one of the key interventions both as a diagnostic and therapeutic tool. Pre-habilitation is a proactive form of managing and reducing the medical and functional risk profile of a patient, and the associated potential complications and effects of surgery [5].

Evidence suggests that the effectiveness of exercise interventions may be dependent on the type of surgery as well as the intent of the intervention. For example, post-operative lung complications may be amenable to inspiratory muscle

Table 8.1 Precautions and contraindications for exercise and exercise testing

• Cardiovascular conditions which are suspected, acute, uncontrolled or severe, such as: Cardiac ischaemia, coronary heart disease, cardiac arrhythmias, atrioventricular block, coronary or valve stenosis, heart failure
• Presence of any severe systemic illness, for example, uncontrolled hypertension or diabetes
• Neuromuscular or musculoskeletal problems which may require further investigation, or may be aggravated by exercise
• Acute or severe infections such as pneumonia or thrombophlebitis
• Acute illness or conditions that affect haemodynamic stability or responses to exercise such as anaemia, pulmonary embolism and myocarditis
• Any subjective symptoms which may be aggravated by exercise such as pain/fatigue/nausea/dyspnoea
• Patient's consent: – Risk assessments need to be done in order to ensure suitability and safety of patients for exercise or exercise testing. Appropriate referrals and investigations should be done prior to start or in the presence of any concerns.

Adapted from [3, 15–18]

strengthening prior to cardiac, thoracic or abdominal surgeries [6, 7]. Likewise, specific strengthening exercises prior to orthopaedic surgeries, such as total hip and total knee replacements, may improve post-operative outcomes such as functional recovery and reduced length of stay [8, 9]. Finally, the pre-habilitation of patients who are at the highest risk of having poor outcomes due to poor physical function and reserves, especially in vulnerable groups such as the elderly and the frail population has been shown to be feasible and safe [10–12].

Neoadjuvant chemoradiotherapy has been shown to impact physical fitness and potentially transition a patient from lower to higher surgical risk. Short preoperative time frames available for behavioural and positive lifestyle changes may compound this problem. However, research has shown that fitness improvements and gains can be made in as little as 2 weeks [13, 14]. It is also important to recognise the conditions that might preclude mobilisation, exercise testing or exercise (Table 8.1).

8.3 Physiotherapy Assessment for Pre-Habilitation in Cancer Surgery

A thorough assessment helps to identify potential safety issues and establish a patient's baseline physical, psychological and functional status. This allows customisation of interventions aiming to better prepare and optimise patient's health before starting acute treatments and potentially improve cancer treatment survival outcomes.

8.3.1 Initial Assessment

A good assessment begins with asking the right questions. Detailed but meaningful assessments will offer information which will guide the initial exercise and functional testing, suitable exercise prescription as well as the level of supervision required and triage other suitable services and support. A well-designed programme will then lead to better compliance and effectiveness of the programme.

First and foremost, the physiotherapist should collect a comprehensive yet relevant medical history, investigations such as baseline imaging, laboratory, medication regimens, as well as lifestyle and mobility history such as falls and smoking history. All the information is important to identify existing comorbidities and to understand both the disease and treatment trajectory. In addition, understanding a patient's current functional level, physical fitness, social and emotional status, are essential information which will guide towards a holistic multi-faceted approach to pre-habilitation. Finally, it is important to take into consideration the patient's social history, home or community set-up and support available. These factors have significant implications on a patient's receptiveness, compliance and adherence to rehabilitation programmes.

8.3.2 Physical Assessment

Physical assessment is a wonderful opportunity to gain a general understanding of a patient's current functional status. It is also important to collaborate the subjective and physical findings to obtain an accurate picture of the patient's function. Disease or condition specific assessment tools could also be used and the tools used should be measurable, validated and reliable.

Common physical assessments may include:

- Screening of patient's sensory function: vision/hearing/speech.
- Basic cognition level and processing speed assessment: to assess ability to follow commands. Recommended testing tool: MMSE (mini mental state examination).
- Respiratory assessment: auscultation and cough strength assessment.
- Joint range of motion assessment.
- Muscle strength assessment using manual muscle testing (MMT).
- Neurological assessment: sensation and proprioception.
- Gait and mobility assessment.
- Activity tolerance.

Table 8.2 is an example of how the subjective and physical assessments could be conducted in a systematic way in order to determine the needs of a patient and design a holistic treatment plan.

Table 8.2 Initial Physiotherapy Assessment form

Initial Physiotherapy Assessment Form			
Type of referral	Pre-habilitation/rehabilitation		
Date & time			
Physiotherapist			
Pre-treatment counselling	Done/ not done		
Background			
Diagnosis	Primary medical condition:		
	Type of cancer and stage:		
	Surgery:		
	Chemotherapy:		
	Radiation therapy:		
Past medical history			
Social history	Lives with:; Carer: Yes/no (details)		
	Lift landing: Yes/no, with ____ steps/ stairs		
	Occupation/responsibilities:		
Premorbid status (independent/ level of assistance required)	Premorbid mobility (and type of gait aid):		
	Activities of daily living:		
Falls history	No. of falls within past 1 year:		
Smoking history	Yes/no		
	No. of pack years:		
Frailty assessment results (if any)	Non-frail/pre-frail/frail		
Assessment tool used:			
Relevant investigations (if any)			
Lifestyle	Stage: Precontemplation/contemplation/ preparation/action/maintenance		
	Details:		
Exercise habits	Stage: Precontemplation/contemplation/ preparation/action/maintenance		
	Details:		
	Type of exercise:		
	Frequency/week:		
	Number of min/sessions:		
	Intensity: Low/moderate/high intensity		
Assessment			
Subjective history			
Fatigue assessment	Score: /10 details:		
Pain assessment	Score: /10 details:		
	Location:		
Respiratory assessment	Auscultation:		
	Chest expansion:		
	Cough:		
MMT (score out of 5)		Right	Left
	Upper limb		
	Lower limb		

(continued)

Table 8.2 (continued)

Range of motion	
Sensory function	Speech: Intact/impaired
	Hearing: Intact/impaired
	Vision: Intact/impaired
Sensation	
Proprioception	
Balance assessment	
Cognitive assessment	
Other relevant assessments	
Functional assessment	
Gait assessment	Gait aid:
	Gait:
6 minute walk test result	Distance:
	Max HR:
	Max RPE:
5 times sit to stand test	
10 m gait speed (with 1 m pre and post = 12 m)	
Functional assessment tool:	
e.g.: Functional Independence measure (score out of 7)	Transfers:
	Locomotion (walking):
Stairs:	
Other relevant assessments (if any):	

8.3.3 Exercise and Functional Tests

Exercise and functional tests provide a more in-depth understanding of patient's physical fitness. It guides the prescription and progression of exercise regime appropriately and safely. It can also be used to assess the effectiveness of intervention. Below are some of the commonly used assessments in pre-habilitation:

8.3.3.1 6 min Walk Test (6MWT)

The 6MWT was developed by the American Thoracic Society in 2002. It is a submaximal exercise test used to assess aerobic capacity and endurance. The 6MWT is a self-paced test of walking capacity. Patients are asked to walk as far as possible in 6 min along a flat course. Walking distance is the primary outcome and is recorded in metres or feet. Standardised instructions and encouragement are commonly given during the test. Figure 8.1 below is an example of the 6MWT protocol [19].

Based on Steffen et al. 2002 [20], Table 8.3 below summarises the normative data for community-dwelling elderly with independent functions who were non-smokers with no history of dizziness and did not use assistive devices.

Currently, there has been limited research on minimal clinically important difference (MCID) for 6MWT in cancer population. A MCID of 17.8 m has been established in moderately frail older Asian adults [21] while a MCID between 22 and 32 m has been established for lung cancer patients [22].

6 min walk Test Protocol

Equipment: Blood pressure set, pulse oximeter, a stopwatch, measuring tape, tape to mark start and end points of a 30m corridor, and at least every 3m mark. a cone/ marker to indicate the turnabout point

Set-Up Instructions: Measure a 30-meter distance and mark the start and end points on the floor. Be sure the walkway is straight, clear of any obstacles or changes in surface material.

30m length, marked every 3m

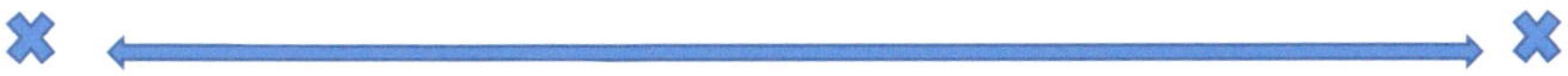

Cones placed at the turnabout points at each end

Assessment Instructions:

Verbal Instructions to Patient [adapted from (19)]:

Instruct the patient as follows:

"The object of this test is to walk as far as possible for 6 minutes. You will walk back and forth in this hallway. You are permitted to slow down, to stop, and to rest as necessary. You may lean against the wall while resting, but resume walking as soon as you are able. You will be walking back and forth around the cones. Remember that the object is to walk AS FAR AS POSSIBLE for 6 minutes, but don't run or jog. Start now, or whenever you are ready."

- After the first minute, tell the patient the following (in even tones): "You are doing well. You have 5 minutes to go.
- When the timer shows 4 minutes remaining, tell the patient the following: "Keep up the good work. You have 4 minutes to go."
- When the timer shows 3 minutes remaining, tell the patient the following: "You are doing well. You are halfway done."
- When the timer shows 2 minutes remaining, tell the patient the following: "Keep up the good work. You have only 2 minutes left."
- When the timer shows only 1 minute remaining, tell the patient: "You are doing well. You have only 1 minute to go."
- Do not use other words of encouragement (or body language to speed up)

Fig. 8.1 Six Minute walk test protocol

Table 8.3 Mean distance in metres by age & gender

Age (Years)	Male	Female
60–69	572 m	538 m
70–79	527 m	471 m
80–89	417 m	392 m

Adapted from [20]

8.3.3.2 Ten Metre Gait Speed (10MGS)

Gait speed is contingent on the smooth integration of multiple organ systems including the musculoskeletal system, cardiopulmonary system and nervous system. Besides being used in the detection of frailty, it is also a strong predictor of future disability, cognitive decline, falls, hospitalisation, institutionalisation and mortality [23].

In 10MGS, gait speed will be assessed using a straight unobstructed course. The test can commence from both static start and rolling start. For a static start, the patient stands at the start of the marked 10 m course. Timing commences from the moment the patient starts walking along the marked 10 m path, and ends when it crosses the 10 m mark. For rolling start, a minimum 1 m acceleration and deceleration zones is recommended [24]. To allow for acceleration and deceleration, the walk will be performed with a 1 metre rolling start, where the patient is already walking when they enter the measuring area. Timing will be started when the toes of the leading foot cross the 1 metre mark and it will be stopped when the toes of the leading foot cross the 11-metre mark. The 10MGS protocol is summarised in Fig. 8.2.

To assess, one should have an idea about the normal mean gait speed (Table 8.4) found in healthy community-dwelling men and women [25].

Studies show [26–30] that gait speed is predictive of higher level function, fall risks, future disability and institutionalisation. A lower gait speed increases the risks (Table 8.5).

8.3.3.3 Five Times Sit to Stand (5xSTS)

The 5xSTS measures lower limb strength, evaluates balance and assesses the risk for falls [31]. For this test, patients will be asked to stand from a chair once without using their arms (arms folded across the chest). For those who are unable to perform the test without using their arms, they can place their hands on their thighs to assist standing. It has been established that adopting this arm position does not confound the test results. All participants who can successfully complete this movement (either with arms folded across the chest or hands placed on their thighs) will then be asked to stand and sit as fast as they can for 5 times. Timing will commence on the command to start and end when the participant sits down after the fifth repetition. Patients should perform the test using the same arm position throughout, using the same chair. Chair heights are generally between 43 and 46 cm. The 5xSTS protocol can be found below:

Five Times Sit to Stand Test Protocol [31]:

Equipment: A stopwatch, a straight back chair with height 45–46 cm and back rest (Fig. 8.3).

Set-Up Instructions:

Assessment Instructions:

Subject began by crossing their arms on their chest and sitting with their back against the chair.

The investigator instructed the subject to stand up fully between repetitions of the test.

10m Gait Speed Test Protocol

Equipment: A stopwatch, measuring tape, tape to mark start and end points

Set-Up Instructions: Measure a 10-meter distance and mark the start and end points on the floor. Be sure the walkway is clear of any obstacles or changes in surface material. An additional 1m acceleration and 1m deceleration is marked at both ends of the 10m distance (total marked distance 12m between cones)

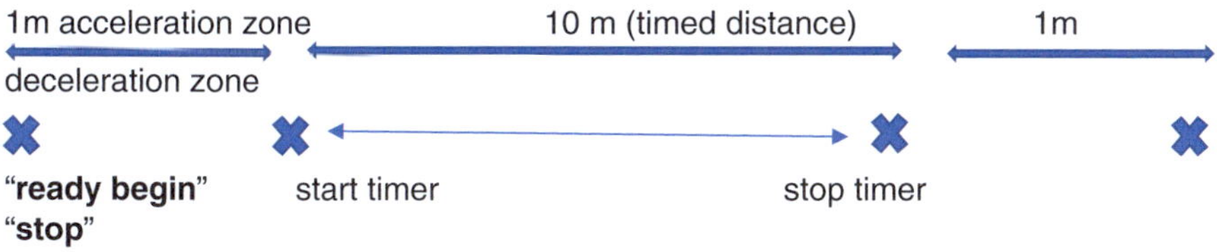

Assessment Instructions:

Have the patient stand at the start point i.e. the start point in the acceleration zone. Patients are encouraged to use their usual gait aid for the test.

Standardized Verbal Instructions to Patient:

- After I say "begin", please walk at your usual comfortable walking pace to the end marker until I tell you that you may stop. Do not talk or stop until you reach the other end.
- Say **"Ready, begin"** and begin timing on the stopwatch when the patient their first foot crosses the 1m mark of the track (after acceleration zone).
- Stop timing on the stopwatch when the patient reaches/crosses the 10 meter mark at the end.
- Say "**Stop**" after the patient has crossed the end point.
- Walk with the patient along the path while he or she is walking for safety. Complete the walking trial two times.
- For each of the two trials, record the time (to the nearest tenth of a second, 0.0 sec) that it took the patient to walk 10 meters.

Record the patient's gait speed (in meters/second) as the average of the two trials:

Trial 1: Gait speed: 10 meters / (time to walk four meters ____ seconds) = ______m/s

Trial 2: Gait speed: 10 meters / (time to walk four meters _____ seconds) = ______m/s

AVERAGE GAIT SPEED: _____m/s

Fig. 8.2 Ten Metre Gait Speed Protocol [24]

Table 8.4 Normal gait speeds for healthy community-dwelling men and women

Normal gait speeds for healthy community-dwelling men and women [6]		
Age (years)	Gender	Average gait speed (m/s)
50–59	Men	1.43
	Women	1.31
60–69	Men	1.34
	Women	1.24
70–79	Men	1.26
	Women	1.13
80–89	Men	0.97
	Women	0.94

Adapted from [25]

Table 8.5 Gait Speed and Implications [26–30]

Gait Speed	
>1 m/s	• >1.1 m/s predictive of completing yard work • > 1.3 m/s climb flights of stairs [26]
<1 m/s	• Will benefit from fall prevention [27] • >0.67 m/s to complete self-care • >0.89 m/s for household activities
<0.6 m/s	• Predicts future risk of falls and hospitalisation • Tend to require assistance for ADL and IADL16 • ≥0.49 to cross street [28]
<0.4 m/s	• Longer length of stay in acute care • Likely to discharge to skilled nursing, inpatient rehab, or nursing home or home health services [26, 29]

Standardised Verbal Instructions to Patient:

- I want you to stand up and sit down 5 times as quickly as you can when I say 'Go'.
- Say **"Go"** and begin timing on the stopwatch.
- Stop timing when the subject's buttocks touched the chair on the fifth repetition.
- For each of the two trials, record the time (to the nearest tenth of a second, 0.0 s) that it took the patient to complete the test.

Record the patient's speed as the average of the two trials:
Trial 1: ______s Trial 2: ______s
AVERAGE timing for five times sit to stand: _______s.

Table 8.6 below is a summary of the normative values for the 5xSTS in the elderly population.

For community-dwelling elderly, a timing of ≥12 s has been established to identify the need for further assessment for fall risk [33].

8.3.3.4 Hand Grip Strength (HGS)

Hand grip strength (HGS) is reflective of overall muscle function and a predictor of cognitive decline, functional limitations, disability, prolonged hospital stays and

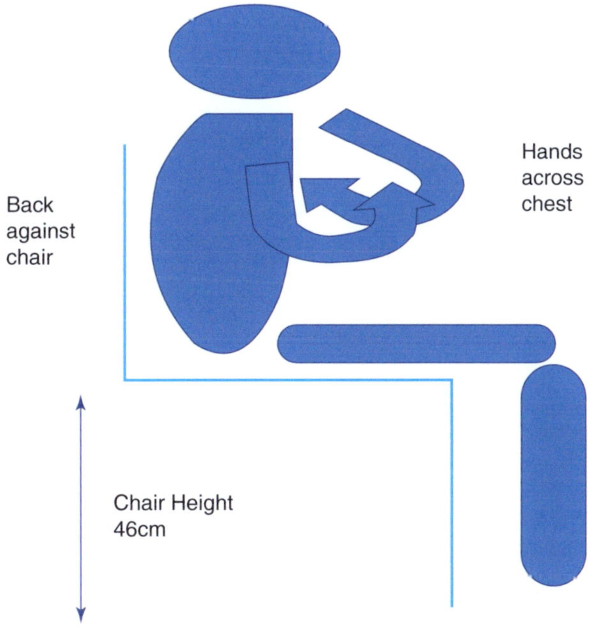

Fig. 8.3 Five times sit to stand set-up

Table 8.6 Mean Normal 5xSTS Performance

Age (Years)	Time (s)
60–69	11.4
70–79	12.6
80–89	14.8

Adapted from [32]

mortality. In addition, its measurement has been well validated and it is easily performed at the bedside [34]. Figure 8.4 below is a summary of the hand grip strength test protocol.

The mean normative values for the hand grip strength, assessed using the Jamar or Martin model, for the elderly population, is summarised in Table 8.7.

A change of 6 kg between tests performed during different sessions will be considered a significant meaningful change [38].

8.3.3.5 Functional Status

Functional status is an important outcome variable to assess when evaluating the impact of a physiotherapy intervention. Here are some of the recommended outcome measures to use;

8.3.3.5.1 Functional Independence Measure (FIM)

The FIM is used to assess and grade the functional status of a person based on the level of assistance he or she requires. FIM scores range from 1 to 7. The grading

Handgrip Strength Test Protocol	
Position	**Subject seated in a chair without arm rests, with feet fully resting on the floor, hips as far back in the chair as possible, and the hips and knees positioned at approximately 90 degrees**
Arm position	Shoulder: adducted and neutrally rotated Elbow: flexed to 90 degrees, forearm should be in midprone (neutral) Wrist: between 15 and 30 degrees of extension (dorsiflexion) and 0-15 degrees of ulnar deviation
Trials	Three trials
Dynamometer	Model: Jamar dynamometer
	Handle position: 2nd
	Acquisition time: at least 3s
	Rest time: at least 15s
Instructions	"This test will tell me your maximum grip strength. When I say go, grip as hard as you can until I say stop. Before each trail, I will ask you 'are you ready?' And then tell you 'Go'. Stop immediately if you experience any unusual pain or discomfort at any point during testing. DO you have any questions? Are you ready? Go!". "Harder.. harder…harder.. Relax"
HGS analysis	Mean of 3 trials

Fig. 8.4 Hand Grip Strength Test Protocol [35, 36]

Table 8.7 Normative Data for community-dwelling older adults by age and gender [37]

Mean (Standard deviation)				
Women	Jamar	Jamar	Martin	Martin
Age	Right hand(kg)	Left hand(kg)	Right hand (kPa)	Left hand(kPa)
60–69	25.3(4.8)	23.6(4.7)	53.7(10.2)	52.4(9.9)
70–79	23.7(5.1)	22.0(4.7)	52.3(12.0)	50.1(11.2)
80+	20.0(4.3)	18.5(4.4)	44.1(9.4)	42.7(10.9)
Men	Jamar	Jamar	Martin	Martin
Age	Right hand(kg)	Left hand(kg)	Right hand (kPa)	Left hand(kPa)
60–69	45.6(8.6)	43.6(8.7)	89.4(16.7)	88.1(17.2)
70–79	42.4(9.1)	40.5(8.5)	83.0(18.2)	79.6(16.2)
80+	34.5(7.2)	32.1(7.0)	64.6(14.5)	64.3(14.7)

categories range from "total assistance with helper = 1" to "complete independence with no helper=7". Scores falling below 6 require another person for supervision or assistance. The higher the score, the more independent the person is.

Tasks that are evaluated using the FIM include bowel and bladder control, transfers, locomotion, communication, social cognition as well as the following six self-care activities:

- Feeding.
- Grooming.
- Bathing.
- Upper Body Dressing.
- Lower Body Dressing.
- Toileting.

The MCID for stroke patients are as below [39]:

- FIM total score: 22 points.
- FIM subscale motor: 17 points.
- FIM subscale cognitive: 3 points.

8.3.3.5.2 Katz Activities of Daily Living

The score for the Katz Activities of Daily Living can range from 0 to 6 and the higher the score, the more independent the person is. Table 8.8 is an example of the Katz Index of Independence in Activities of Daily Living assessment form.

8.3.3.5.3 The Lawton Brody Instrumental Activities of Daily Living

The score ranges from 0 to 8 for women and 0 to 5 for men, to avoid potential gender bias, and again, the higher the score, the more independent the person is. An example of the Lawton Brody Instrumental Activities of Daily Living assessment form is in Table 8.9.

The MCID for both Katz Activities of Daily Living and The Lawton Brody Instrumental Activities of Daily Living for community-dwelling older adults is around 0.5 points [42].

8.3.3.6 Others

Below are some of the other recommended assessments to include while treating cancer patients.

8.3.3.6.1 Fatigue

Fatigue is one of the most frequent complaints of cancer patients and is strongly associated with loss of independence and decreased physical activity and functional decline.

FACIT-Fatigue

The Functional Assessment of Chronic Illness Therapy – Fatigue Scale (FACIT-Fatigue) is a 13-item measure that assesses self-reported fatigue and its impact upon daily activities and function. The MCID for FACIT fatigue has been established to be 3 regardless of direction [43].

Table 8.8 Katz Index of Independence in Activities of Daily Living [40]

Activities Points (1 or 0)	**Independence** (1 Point) **NO** supervision, direction or personal assistance.	**Dependence** (0 Points) **WITH** supervision, direction, personal assistance or total care.
BATHING Points: _________	**(1 POINT)** bathes self completely or needs help in bathing only a single part of the body such as the back, genital area or disabled extremity.	**(0 POINTS)** need help with bathing more than one part of the body, getting in or out of the tub or shower. Requires total bathing
DRESSING Points: _________	**(1 POINT)** get clothes from closets and drawers and put on clothes and outer garments complete with fasteners. May have help tying shoes.	**(0 POINTS)** needs help with dressing self or needs to be completely dressed.
TOILETING Points: _________	**(1 POINT)** goes to toilet, gets on and off, arranges clothes, cleans genital area without help.	**(0 POINTS)** needs help in transferring to the toilet, cleaning self or uses bedpan or commode.
TRANSFERRING Points: _________	**(1 POINT)** moves in and out of bed or chair unassisted. Mechanical transfer aids are acceptable	**(0 POINTS)** needs help in moving from bed to chair or requires a complete transfer.
CONTINENCE Points: _________	**(1 POINT)** exercises complete self-control over urination and defecation.	**(0 POINTS)** is partially or totally incontinent of bowel or bladder
FEEDING Points: _________	**(1 POINT)** gets food from plate into mouth without help. Preparation of food may be done by another person.	**(0 POINTS)** needs partial or total help with feeding or requires parenteral feeding.
TOTAL POINTS: ________ **SCORING:** 6 = high (*patient independent*) 0 = low (*patient very dependent*)		

8.3.3.6.2 Pain

Pain is another common symptom in cancer patients. Pain can be caused by cancer, cancer treatment, or a combination of factors. Therefore, it is important to perform pain assessment. Pain assessment can be done by using the acronym SOCRATES [44]. Table 8.10 summarises the SOCRATES assessment for pain and the example questions.

8.3.3.6.3 Commonly Used Pain Scales

- **Numerical Pain Rating Scale (NPRS):** point scale of (0–10). Figure 8.5 is an example of the NPRS, which is commonly used for assessment of pain.
- **Visual Analogue scale (VAS)** with pain faces scale. Refer to Fig. 8.6 for an example of VAS assessment of pain.
- **Categorical score** (mild, moderate, severe).

8.3.3.6.4 Quality of Life (QOL)

Quality of life (QOL) means different things to different individuals, groups and cultures. The WHO [48] has defined QOL as:

Table 8.9 Lawton Brody Instrumental Activities of Daily Living [41]

Scoring: For each category, circle the item description that most closely resembles the client's highest functional level (either 0 or 1).			
A. Ability to Use Telephone		**E. Laundry**	
1. Operates telephone on own initiative—Looks up and dials numbers, etc. 2. Dials a few well-known numbers. 3. Answers telephone but does not dial. 4. Does not use telephone at all.	1 1 1 0	1. Does personal laundry completely. 2. Launders small items—Rinses stockings, etc. 3. All laundry must be done by others.	1 1 0
B. Shopping		**F. Mode of transportation**	
1. Takes care of all shopping needs independently. 2. Shops independently for small purchases. 3. Needs to be accompanied on any shopping trip. 4. Completely unable to shop.	1 0 0 0	1. Travels independently on public transportation or drives own car. 2. Arranges own travel via taxi, but does not otherwise use public transportation. 3. Travels on public transportation when accompanied by another. 4. Travel limited to taxi or automobile with assistance of another. 5. Does not travel at all.	1 1 1 0 0
C. Food preparation		**G. Responsibility for own medications**	
1. Plans, prepares and serves adequate meals independently. 2. Prepares adequate meals if supplied with ingredients. 3. Heats, serves and prepares meals, or prepares meals, or prepares meals but does not maintain adequate diet. 4. Needs to have meals prepared and served.	1 0 0 0	1. Is responsible for taking medication in correct dosages at correct time. 2. Takes responsibility if medication is prepared in advance in separate dosage. 3. Is not capable of dispensing own medication.	1 0 0
D. Housekeeping		**H. Ability to handle finances**	
1. Maintains house alone or with occasional assistance (e.g. "heavy work domestic help"). 2. Performs light daily tasks such as dishwashing, bed making. 3. Performs light daily tasks but cannot maintain acceptable level of cleanliness. 4. Needs help with all home maintenance tasks. 5. Does not participate in any housekeeping tasks.	1 1 1 1 0	1. Manages financial matters independently (budgets, writes checks, pays rent, bills, goes to bank), collects and keeps track of income. 2. Manages day-to-day purchases, but needs help with banking, major purchases, etc. 3. Incapable of handling money.	1 1 0
Score		**Score**	
Total score__________________ A summary score ranges from 0 (low function, dependent) to 8 (high function, independent) for women and 0 through 5 for men to avoid potential gender bias			

"... an individual's perception of their position in life in the context of the culture and value systems in which they live and in relation to their goals, expectations, standards and concerns. It is a broad ranging concept affected in a complex way by

Table 8.10 Pain Assessment—SOCRATES [45]

Letter	Aspect	Example Questions
S	Site	Where is the pain? Location of the pain
O	Onset	When did the pain start? Sudden or gradual? Progressive or regressive?
C	Character	What is the pain like? (sharp, dull)
R	Radiation	Does the pain radiate anywhere?
A	Associations	Any other signs or symptoms associated with the pain?
T	Time course	Does the pain follow any pattern?
E	Exacerbating/relieving factors	Does anything change the pain?
S	Severity	How bad is the pain? (using pain scale)

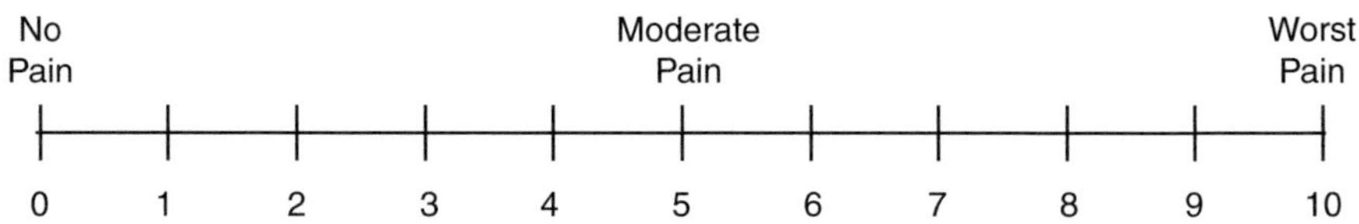

Fig. 8.5 Numerical Pain Rating Scale [46]

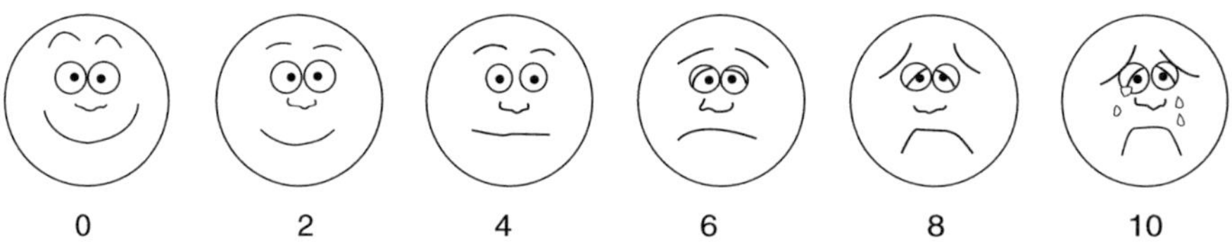

Fig. 8.6 Visual Analogue Scale [47]

the person's physical health, psychological state, personal beliefs, social relationships and their relationship to salient features of their environment".

Using QOL measures can guide clinicians towards a more patient-centred and meaningful care.

European Organization for Research and Treatment in Cancer Quality of Life Questionnaire 30item (EORTC QLQ-C30)

The EORTC QLQ-C30 is a questionnaire developed to assess quality of life in cancer patients. It has high reliability and validity in different groups of cancer patients and the test–retest reliability is optimal. The EORTC QLQ-C30 comprises 30 items, 24 of which are aggregated into 9 multi-item scales: 5 functioning scales (physical, role, cognitive, emotional and social); 3 symptom scales (fatigue, pain, and nausea and/or vomiting) and 1 global health-status scale. The remaining six single items assess symptoms of dyspnea, appetite loss (AP), sleep disturbance, constipation, diarrhoea and financial impact.

Based on a study by King [49], mean differences no less than 10 points are widely regarded as clinically meaningful for the QLQ-C30 in randomised clinical trials.

Table 8.11 SMART Goals [52]

S	Specific	Goals are direct, detailed and meaningful.
M	Measurable	Goals are quantifiable and can be tracked to monitor progress or success.
A	Attainable	Goals are realistic and achievable based on patient's condition
R	Relevant	Goals are in line with patient's needs and expectation
T	Time-bound	Goals have a definite time frame and a completion date.

The MCIDs varied by QLQ-C30 scale, direction (improvement vs deterioration) and anchor. The MIDs for within-group change ranged from 5 to 14 points (improvement) and − 14 to −4 points (deterioration), and MIDs for between-group change over time ranged from 4 to 11 points and from −18 to −4 points. Correlation-weighted MIDs for most QLQ-C30 scales ranged from 4 to 10 points in absolute values [50].

8.3.3.7 Patient Goals and Expectation

Lastly, the fundamental part of pre-habilitation or rehabilitation is identifying patient goals and expectation. Goal setting is "the formal process whereby a rehabilitation professional or a multidisciplinary team, together with the patient and/or their family, negotiate goals" [51]. One common method of goal setting has been derived from the acronym: SMART, which is demonstrated in Table 8.11 below.

Goal setting is used to direct interventions towards a specific outcome and can result in greater patient satisfaction and improved recovery [51]. Goals can also be used to evaluate the success of physiotherapy interventions.

8.4 Physiotherapy Exercise Prescription

Despite a lack of consensus over the dosage, duration and type of exercises for rehabilitation, general recommendations agree that most patients may benefit from some form of pre-habilitation activity. This may range from inspiratory muscle training for patients with respiratory conditions, to range of motion or stretching exercises to address stiffness of joints or tight muscles, to strengthening exercises of certain major muscle groups. Interventions may also include more dynamic activity such as balance retraining, aerobic or endurance training, or more specialised exercise programmes to meet the needs of patients.

Exercise is generally safe and effective for patients with cancer [53]. The optimal prescription of exercise for patients with cancer starts with a comprehensive history and physical examination of cardiac, pulmonary, neurological, and musculoskeletal signs and symptoms [53]. Following the assessments, a better understanding of the patient's impairment, functional limitations as well as disabilities, both current and anticipated issues, could be better addressed from the start.

As patients with cancer can present with different patho-physiology, medical management, prognosis and health behaviours, it is vital for therapists to be cognizant of the challenges in prescribing an exercise programme. It is also important to be mindful of the changes that can occur throughout the programme and to modify the prescription accordingly. Nonetheless, ascertainment and discussion of the following may aid in effective individualised exercise prescription:

- Current exercise behaviour of the patient.
- Motivation level to exercise.
- Patient's understanding of exercise and the significance.
- The needs and goals of the patient.

8.4.1 Monitoring before/during/Post Exercise

Patients participating in an exercise class managed under an institution should ideally have their vitals measured and assessed prior to, during and post exercises. The extent and frequency of monitoring is dependent upon the patient's condition, tolerance and response to exercise, as well as the type of exercises prescribed. It is important that records be kept as it would help to track the progress and tolerance of the patient, as well as to use the parameters to guide the subsequent exercise prescriptions. It is also strongly encouraged that patients be educated on the implications of these parameters and learn to self-monitor the parameters (if indicated) when they are exercising on their own.

Common parameters measured:

- **Blood pressure (BP)**: The BP response to exercise should be monitored prior to and after the exercise session. Patients with volatile or BP range bordering on the lower or higher limits should be checked in between exercises to ensure exercise safety. Patients who have had their BP medications must notify their therapists prior to the exercise session.
- **Heart Rate (HR)**: It is recommended that the resting HR, HR during exercise and post-exercise HR be measured. Targeted HR during exercise should be calculated prior to the exercise programme, and patients are taught to monitor their own HR and corresponding rate of perceived exertion prior, during and after the exercises. Heart Rate Recovery (HRR) has been demonstrated to be an invaluable resource in predicting cardiovascular response to exercise (HRR).
- **Peripheral capillary oxygen saturation (SpO2)**: The SpO2 should be monitored prior to, during and after the end of an aerobic exercise. The monitoring of SpO2 response to exercise is important for patients with lung and/or heart conditions or other medical conditions affecting oxygenation. For selected populations who present with desaturations during exercise, such as patients with pulmonary conditions or cardiac conditions such as heart failure, ambulatory oxygen may be used as a supplementary aid to improve exercise endurance. Oxygen therapy during exercise might reduce dyspnoea and improve saturations, therefore increasing tolerance towards higher level and duration of exercise to attain higher exercise gains [54].

- **Fatigue**: Physical activity has demonstrated to be effective in the treatment for cancer-related fatigue [55–57]. The numerical fatigue rating scale can be used for the assessment of fatigue before and following the end of exercise session.
- **Pain**: The numerical rating scale (NRS) for pain can be used to assess pain score. The presentation of a new pain, changes in intensity, site or nature of pain, warrants appropriate assessment or investigations prior to the commencement of exercise. This is especially important for patients with cancer who are at risk of metastatic conditions, or in the elderly inactive population who are at higher risk of developing musculoskeletal injuries.
- **Weight**: Tracking of weight is important for certain populations such as patients who are at risk of fluid retention, or experiencing involuntary muscle loss such as patients with cancer. Trending their weight will allow the physiotherapists to refer them on to appropriate services such as the dietician or managing physicians.
- **Self-reported symptoms**: It is important that patients are educated on signs and symptoms which may preclude, modify or require a termination of exercise. It is important that patients understand the implications of the symptoms and action plan in the event they experience them. It is recommended that all education materials include the common languages supplemented with pictorial examples to facilitate patient's education and understanding. Figure 8.7 includes written and pictorial descriptions of these signs and symptoms.
- **Ratings of perceived exertion (RPE)**: The Borg RPE is used to rate the breathlessness and exertion during an activity [58]. The RPE can be used to guide the modification and prescription of exercises based on the patient's tolerance and reported exertion (Fig. 8.8). It is also of particular importance in rating and measuring intensity in patients whose exercise response cannot be based on heart rate changes, for example patients who have irregular heart rate, on beta blocker medications or have pacemakers. A BORG scale might assist in a patient's ability to rate their exertion and encourage self-monitoring.

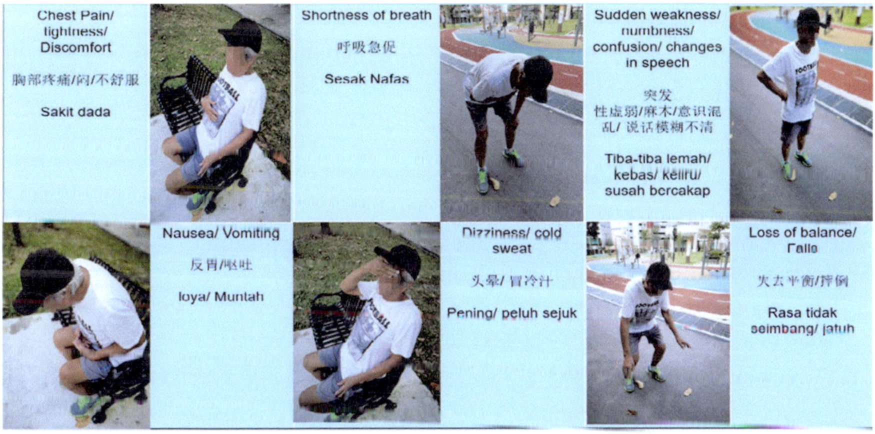

Fig. 8.7 Signs and symptoms that precludes exercise

Rating	Perceived Exertion	Feels Like
0	At rest	Effortless
1	Very light	
2	Somewhat light	Easy to breathe/ able to speak normally comfortable
3	Moderate	
4	Somewhat hard	
5	Hard	Breathing heavily/ Can speak in sentences
6		
7	Very Hard	Short of breath/ Able to say a few words/ a phrase
8		
9	Very, Very Hard	Hard to catch a breath/ Barely say a few words
10	Maximum Exertion	Out of breath. Unable to talk.

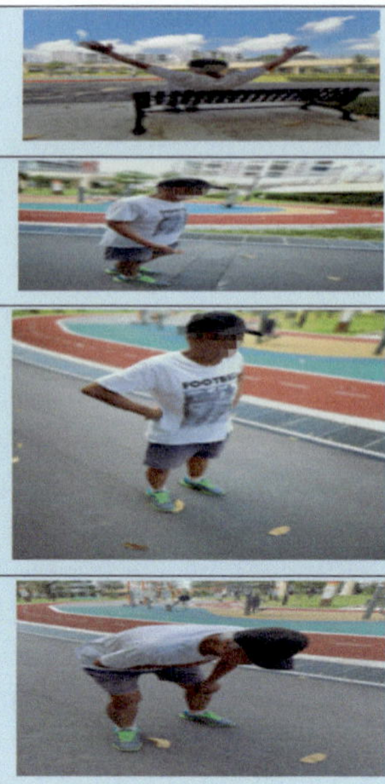

Fig. 8.8 An example of a BORG scale [58]

- **Heart rate (HR) monitoring**: The heart rate responses from the 6MWT can be adopted; the heart rate reserve (HRR) is calculated using the Karvonen formula (Fig. 8.10). The ACSM recommends moderate intensity between 40 and 60% of HRR.

Fig. 8.10 Formulas used to calculate the intensity of aerobic exercise. Abbreviations: HRmax, maximal heart rate; HRR, heart rate reserve; RHR, resting heart rate. Adapted from [4]

Example of suggested assessments.

Table 8.12 presents a summary of possible parameters and when they can be measured during an exercise programme.

8.4.2 The FITT Principle

The FITT principle is widely used for exercise prescription:

- Frequency (F): The number of sessions per week.
- Intensity (I): How hard per session.
- Time (T): The duration for each session.
- Type (T): Exercise modality.

Exercise programme can be prescribed tailored to an individual's needs and ability (Fig. 8.9) [59].

Table 8.12 Summary of parameters monitoring

Pre Programme	Pre and post session	After each exercise item
Resting blood pressure	Pre/post-exercise BP	Heart rate
Resting heart rate	Pre/post-exercise HR	RPE scale
Height: Cm; weight (kg)		
Blood glucose level (if applicable)	Pre/post blood glucose level (if applicable)	
Fatigue level in last 24 h/ last week	Pre/post fatigue score (rate 1–10)	
Presence of pain/score/location		
Sensation changes since last visit		
Any falls after last visit	HOW DID you feel about the session today? Rate 1–10	HOW DID you feel about this exercise today? Rate 1–10
Other relevant information (if any)		

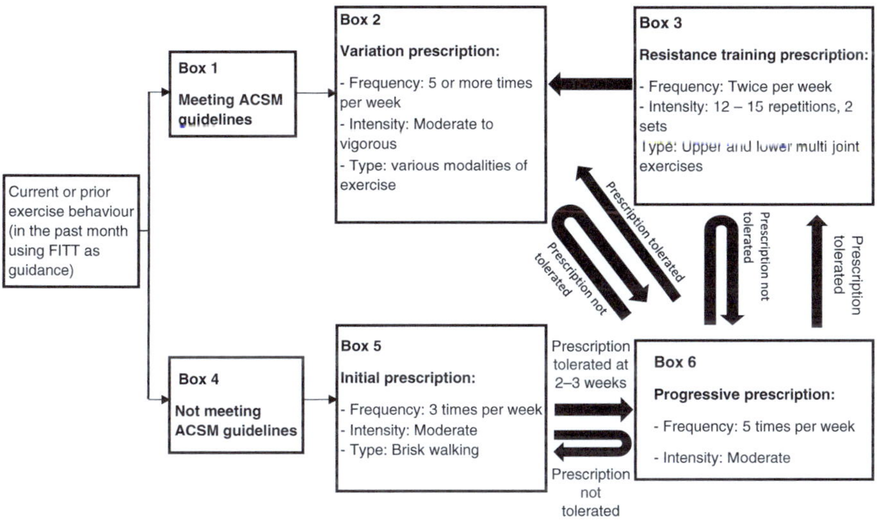

Fig. 8.9 Individualised exercise programme prescription

8.4.3 Types of Exercises

8.4.3.1 Aerobic Exercise

For most patients with cancer, walking is typically preferred, even though stationary cycling is more suitable for frail elderly patients and patients with gait or coordination difficulties.

According to the American College of Sports Medicine (ACSM) guidelines, patients are encouraged to aim for ≥150 min per week of moderate or ≥75 min per week of vigorous aerobic exercise per week. Subsequently, exercise levels can be progressed by varying the frequency, intensity, type and time of exercise every

2–3 weeks (Fig. 8.9: Box 1 and Box 2). For patients who do not meet the ACSM guidelines (Fig. 8.9: Box 4), a lower intensity introductory prescription is recommended (Fig. 8.8: Box 5).

Once exercise is well-tolerated, the frequency and duration of exercise can be increased until the recommendation of ≥150 min per week of moderate intensity is achieved (Fig. 8.9: Box 6).

The intensity of the aerobic exercise can be explained using the following measures:

- **Talk-test**: Moderate exercise is defined as an activity when one can speak comfortably in sentences, and vigorous exercise is an activity when one is unable to converse.
- **Ratings of perceived exertion (RPE)**: The Borg RPE is used to rate the breathlessness and exertion during an activity [58].
- **Heart rate (HR) monitoring**: The heart rate responses from the 6MWT can be adopted; the heart rate reserve (HRR) is calculated using the Karvonen formula. The ACSM recommends moderate intensity between 40 and 60% of HRR. Fig. 8.10 summarises the formulas that are used to calculate the intensity of aerobic exercise.

8.4.3.2 Resistance Exercise

Resistance exercises are important in increasing muscle mass and preventing deterioration for all patients with cancer [53]. For patients with cachexia and those who aerobic exercise is contraindicated, resistance exercises should be the key focus. The recommended frequency for resistance exercise is 2–3 days per week (with 48-hour recovery), and the intensity set between 40 and 60% of 1-repetition maximum (1RM) for 1–3 sets of 8–12 repetitions (up to a maximum of 15 repetitions) [60].

Resistance training for the major muscle groups is commonly performed using:

- Elastic bands.
- Free weights.
- Resistance machines.
- Own body weight.

Age-predicted maximum heart rate

HRmax = 220 – age

Karvonen formula:

% HRR = ([HRmax – RHR] x % intensity) + RHR

Fig. 8.10 Common formulae for prediction of heart rate. Abbreviations: HRmax, maximal heart rate; HRR, heart rate reserve; RHR, resting heart rate

8.4.3.3 Flexibility Training

Flexibility training is recommended for 2–7 days per week, with a slow and static stretch for 10–30 s up to 4 repetitions [60]. It is suggested that general stretches for major muscle groups should be performed, with particular attention given to muscles which may be limited by preoperative treatment.

Table 8.13 below shows an example of a home exercise programme prescribed for a patient who does not meet the recommended ACSM guideline.

8.4.3.4 Balance Exercises

Balance training is an important part of exercise programme especially in the population most at risk of having balance impairments such as the elderly, the patients with neurological diseases and the population with impaired sensory, proprioceptive, or vestibular systems [61]. For patients who may have drug-induced peripheral neuropathy due to their neoadjuvant chemotherapy, it is imperative to educate them on appropriate falls risk management and prevention.

Training strategies for both static and dynamic balance [61] include:

- Varying base of support (from wide base to narrow base).
- Varying the stability of the dependent surfaces they are sitting/standing/moving on
- Variation of input from the functioning sensory systems (e.g. changing visual/proprioceptive/vestibular inputs) to rehabilitate or challenge the impaired system.
- Increasing task complexity or concurrent multitasking, e.g. counting in multiples of 3 while trying to balance on a foam platform.
- Varying from self-generated inner perturbation to external perturbations.
- Increasing the intensity or frequency or duration of perturbation.

Table 8.13 An example of home exercise programme for a patient who does not meet the ACSM criteria

Aerobic exercise	Resistance exercise	Flexibility training
15 min of brisk walking for 3–4 days/week at moderate intensity Progressing to 20–25 min in the next week	A resistance band can be used to train the major muscle groups: • Shoulder press. • Shoulder abductions. • Triceps. • Biceps. • Hip flexors. • Hip abductors. • Quadriceps. 12–15 repetitions for 2 sets, done over 2–3 days/week	A slow, static stretch of 10–30 s can be performed for the major muscle groups: • Upper trapezius. • Levator scapulae. • Shoulder posterior capsule. • Wrist flexors and extensors. • Trunk side flexors. • Quadriceps. • Hamstrings. • Calf muscles.
Additional 15 min of stationary cycling at moderate intensity for 1–2 days/week in the next week	Additional set can be performed in the next week if exercises are well-tolerated	Stretches can be done prior to and after aerobic and resistance exercises

8.4.4 Education

Patient education is essential in empowering patients, which can improve the motivation level. Moreover, patients may experience lesser anxiety and experience better post-op outcomes. The pre-habilitation patient education should include:

- The importance of exercise prior to surgery.
- The FITT principles of exercise.
- Comprehensive education on the post-op recovery journey.
- Home exercise programme (HEP) prescription and monitoring.

8.4.5 Special Considerations

- **Fatigue**: Severe fatigue (ε 7/10) is contraindicated for exercise. Patients with mild or moderate levels of fatigue should start from a low intensity and be monitored for the response to exercise.
- **Bone metastasis or osteoporosis**: Patients with bone metastasis or osteoporosis should avoid high impact or contact activities.
- **Malnutrition**: Patients with altered water and/or food intake may present with electrolyte imbalance. Monitor heart rate and rhythm closely during exercise.

8.5 Starting a Pre-Habilitation Programme (PHP)

A pre-habilitation programme that supports the physical, functional and psychosocial needs of patients will go a long way in optimising their health prior to the commencement of medical or surgical therapies.

Preparation for a pre-habilitation programme (PHP) includes:

1. Programme set-up.
2. Physiotherapist requirement and manpower planning.
3. Delivery Model.

8.5.1 Programme Set-up and Equipment Planning

8.5.1.1 Preparation Prior to Start of a Programme

1. **Programme recruitment and exclusion criteria**: This is dependent on both the programme set-up and the skills set of the physiotherapists and other healthcare members involved in the care [3].
2. **Exercise assessment and training guidelines**: The guidelines should include the type of assessments to be conducted, time points of reassessments, exercise prescription based on assessment outcomes, as well as progression and adaptation of exercise regime based on patient's changing needs [18].

Table 8.14 Commonly used equipment

Aerobic	Weight bearing modalities such as treadmills, elliptical
	Non-weight bearing modalities such as recumbent bikes, upper limb ergometers
Resistance training	Free weights/dumb bells
	Exercise resistance band
	Weight machines
Balance	Foam mats, gym balls, parallel bars

3. **Emergency protocols**: It is crucial that facility emergency protocols and equipment are in place prior to the start of the programme, to manage any potential adverse events that might occur during the exercise programme [18].
4. All protocols should ideally be reviewed on an annual basis to ensure that the information is updated and relevant.

8.5.1.2 Equipment Set-up

The planning of equipment for the facility is ultimately dependent on the type of patients anticipated to be utilising the service. A set-up with a thoughtful range of equipment should be ideally available to address the varying physical limitations such as poor balance, poor tolerance or physical strength. A summarised list of equipment that are commonly used for different types of exercises is illustrated in Table 8.14.

In a predominantly elderly adult patient population, it is recommended that equipment which can be used by a greater cohort of patients might serve to encourage participation and optimise usage and space.

For example:

(a) A bicycle with recline back support might be appropriate for both frailer and fitter patients versus an upright bike which might be difficult for a frailer patient to manage.
(b) Patients who are predominantly wheelchair bound might benefit from a wheelchair assessment upper limb arm ergometer, or wheelchair compatible reclining bike for aerobic exercises.
(c) Equipment with assisted mode might be appropriate for patients who are too weak to initiate or sustain exercise for a reasonable amount of time.

8.5.1.3 Programme Costs

Evaluating the cost-effectiveness of the programme is important for sustainability and accountability towards the stakeholders investing in the programme. From the patient's perspective, the out of pockets costs have been a significant factor in compliance and participation.

For insured or subsidised patient, it is also important to acknowledge that aside from the direct costs of the programme, transportation costs and income costs are also potential barriers to participation [62].

8.5.2 Physiotherapist Requirement

8.5.2.1 Physiotherapist Competency

Physiotherapists delivering the PHP should be minimally trained in basic cardiac life support (BCLS) and have experience or expertise in exercise prescription for their target populations [3]. Framework from associations such as the American College of Sports Medicine Clinical Exercise Specialist course is an example of training which qualifies the participant with skills in exercise assessment, monitoring and reassessment, development of intervention plan and implementation of programme.

For example, expertise required for conducting a programme for patients with orthopaedic conditions would vary greatly from the expertise required for patients with oncological conditions. Physiotherapists should be able to demonstrate core competence in the following areas:

8.5.2.1.1 Knowledge

1. Demonstrate clinical knowledge and evidence based information specific to the population they are working with.
2. Identify precautions and contraindications to exercise and assessments.
3. Understand the implications of assessments and clinical reasons for implementation.

8.5.2.1.2 Clinical Skills

1. Conduct appropriate screening, assessments and functional tests.
2. Demonstrate implementation of appropriate exercise programmes, including but not limited to: monitoring of parameters and patient response.
3. Demonstrates the set-up and use of exercise equipment, as well as patient handling skills.
4. Ability to engage, understand and communicate with the patient, including effective patient education.
5. Ability to take into consideration the evolving needs, expectations and goals of the patient involved during the sessions and modify the sessions accordingly.

Physiotherapists who are managing the programme would be encouraged to develop training guidelines and protocols based on their programme's needs and to standardise quality of care within their institution [18].

Suggested competencies for programme lead include:

1. Overall team management involved in the PH programme.
2. Establishing, maintaining and evaluation of measurable goals of PH programme.
3. Development of framework and implementation of programme.
4. Development of training guidelines and competency assessments for staff training.
5. Facility set-up and maintenance.

8.5.3 Manpower Considerations for Exercise Programme

8.5.3.1 Group Class Ratio

The recommended ratios may range from 1:3 to 1:12. This may be dependent on:

1. The type of patients they manage (e.g. stability of medical conditions, patients cognition status, exercise response),
2. The level of expertise, training and the availability of supervising physiotherapists and supporting assistants,
3. The preferences of patients.

Patients who may be better suited for individual/small group exercise sessions include:

- Those who require higher level of assistance for mobility, exercise or at high falls risk.
- Those who have more complex medical issue/need which necessitate closer supervision and monitoring.

Patients who may be better suited for larger group exercise sessions:

- Those who are medically stable and functionally more independent.
- Those who may benefit from the social support and dynamics of a group set-up.

Figure 8.11 below is a summary of factors which may guide a physiotherapist in deciding the location, the level of supervision and the size of class suitable for a patient.

8.5.4 Delivery Models Considerations

8.5.4.1 Hospital-Based Inpatient Services

Patients who are reviewed while being admitted within the institution have the benefit of accessing onsite medical and rehabilitative services. However, patients tend to be sicker with confounding acute conditions which necessitates thoughtful exercise prescription, appropriate for their functional and overall health status.

Patients who are undergoing investigations or supportive therapies need to have their exercise programme paced and titrated to their condition for that day. For example, patients who may be undergoing electrolyte or blood product replacements might be better reviewed after their infusion.

Patients who are admitted during their pre-habilitation period also have the advantage of multiple supervised sessions within a day. There is strong evidence to support additive effects of exercise sessions, e.g. 2 sessions of 20 min exercise sessions versus 1 session of 40 min, for patients who are physically weaker or medically less stable. ACSM recommends a minimum of 10 min per exercise session.

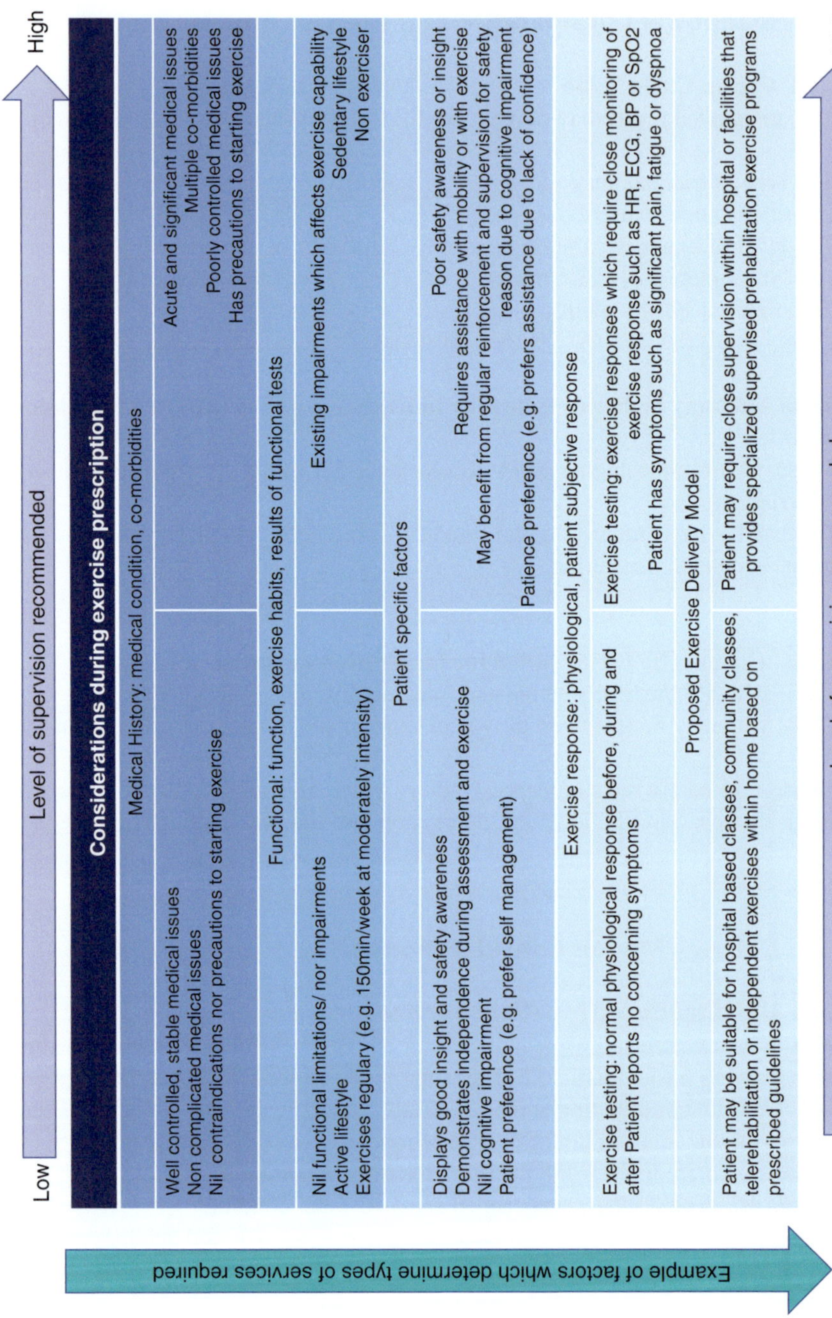

Level of supervision recommended
Low
High
Considerations during exercise prescription
Medical History: medical condition, co-morbidities
Well controlled, stable medical issues
Non complicated medical issues
Nil contraindications nor precautions to starting exercise
Acute and significant medical issues
Multiple co-morbidities
Poorly controlled medical issues
Has precautions to starting exercise
Functional: function, exercise habits, results of functional tests
Nil functional limitations/ nor impairments
Active lifestyle
Exercises regulary (e.g. 150min/week at moderately intensity)
Existing impairments which affects exercise capability
Sedentary lifestyle
Non exerciser
Patient specific factors
Displays good insight and safety awareness
Demonstrates independence during assessment and exercise
Nil cognitive impairment
Patient preference (e.g. prefer self management)
Poor safety awareness or insight
Requires assistance with mobility or with exercise
May benefit from regular reinforcement and supervision for safety reason due to cognitive impairment
Patience preference (e.g. prefers assistance due to lack of confidence)
Exercise response: physiological, patient subjective response
Exercise testing: normal physiological response before, during and after Patient reports no concerning symptoms
Exercise testing: exercise responses which require close monitoring of exercise response such as HR, ECG, BP or SpO2
Patient has symptoms such as significant pain, fatigue or dyspnoa
Proposed Exercise Delivery Model
Patient may be suitable for hospital based classes, community classes, telerehabilitation or independent exercises within home based on prescribed guidelines
Patient may require close supervision within hospital or facilities that provides specialized supervised prehabilitation exercise programs
Level of supervision recommended
Low
High
Example of factors which determine types of services required

Fig. 8.11 Recommended level of supervision

8.5.4.2 Hospital-Based Outpatient Services

Location of facility can be a boon to encourage participation and compliance for patients [63]. Accessibility of facilities has been reported to be a significant cause of participation barrier for participants [62]. Commuting time which may be affected by proximity and availability of public transport, parking spaces as well as distance to travel to the facility for patients with mobility issues, are factors influencing patient participation [64].

8.5.4.2.1 Within the Facility

It is recommended that accessibility within the facility is optimised for inclusiveness, mobility and safety. This includes compliance with wheelchair manoeuvrability guidelines and recommended space allowances.

The elimination of curbs and steps as far as possible within the facility will serve to improve ease of wheelchair access as well as risk of falls secondary to tripping.

This is also a teaching opportunity for patients to have a good idea of what a safe space set-up might look like to encourage safe mobility (e.g. placement of rails within common toilets, decluttered spaces within the exercise gym, slip proof surfaces or mats on exercise areas).

8.5.4.2.2 Availability of Services

Availability of PHP sessions such as availability of programmes suited for the patient, timing of sessions and number of sessions available prior to therapy commencement date, are known factors in determining the programme uptake and compliance. It is recommended that the programmes are offered to patients who might benefit most from the PHP in the event of resource limitations [3].

8.5.4.3 Community and Home Based Programmes

Community programmes are also an excellent centre-based resource for patients who do not require specialised supervision or services during pre-habilitation. Enrolment in community programmes is also a good alternative for patients who are unable to travel to the acute healthcare facility.

Home based exercise programmes have been shown to be just as beneficial for patients compared to centre-based supervised programmes. It is particularly prudent to be intentional in establishing safe and effective home based programmes as it allows patients with transport limitations to have the access to exercise programmes that they are able to perform on their own.

It is recommended that emphasis be placed on educating patients on the exercises which they are able to perform within their own home or within community programmes, and encourage participation and improve self-efficacy during these sessions. For example, a prescription of a 10-min walk on the treadmill is translatable into a 10-min walk within their own neighbourhood. Patients can be taught to use water filled bottles as weights, as well as other home equipment as exercise props.

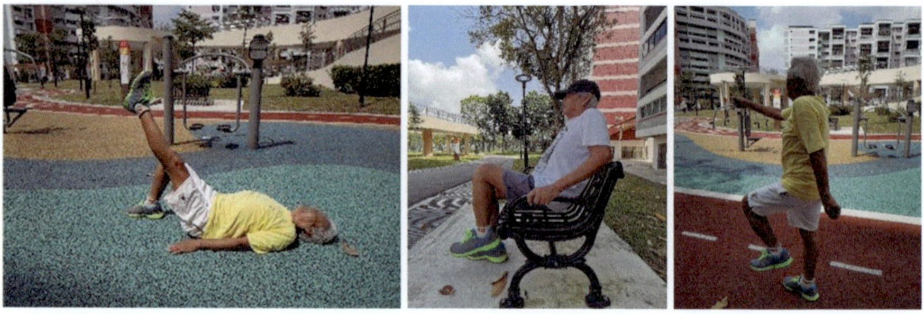

Fig. 8.12 Alternative positioning: Lying versus seated versus standing exercise

8.5.4.3.1 Level of Supervision

Based on the subjective and objective assessments conducted, the level of supervision might vary depending on patient condition as well as the type of exercise prescribed. It is also important to assess the risk factors for varying exercises implemented within the patients' homes. For example, a high level balance exercise might require the presence of a caregiver to negate the potential falls risk, or a variation of a standing exercise could be performed in a stable seated position instead.

For example, alternative starting positions for a similar task (Fig. 8.12) can be performed either in a lying, sitting or standing position. Depending on the patient's level of requirement of supervision, an alternative position can be chosen to mitigate risk of fall.

8.5.4.4 Telerehabilitation

The increasing availability and efficiency of telehealth resources has been a great tool for extending resources and contact into satellite locations such as patients homes and facilities without onsite specialised services. Capacity of monitoring and feedback from patients to their therapists, communication and delivery of information and resources has been shown to improve out of hospital-based outcomes for exercise interventions.

Development of responsive programmes which are adaptive to different needs of patients, e.g. audio feedback and visual aids such as videos and images, tracking of vitals and self-reporting tools, video-conferencing are valuable resources and tools for patients and caregivers. Use of telerehabilitation has been demonstrated to be as least as effective as centre-based programmes in modifying risk factors and improving functional capacities. Combined with the cost-effectiveness of telerehabilitation, this seems to be a viable option as a delivery model [65].

References

1. Schmitz KH, Campbell AM, Stuiver MM, Pinto BM, Schwartz AL, Morris GS, et al. Exercise is medicine in oncology: engaging clinicians to help patients move through cancer. CA Cancer J Clin. 2019;69(6):468–84.

2. Pate RR, Pratt M, Blair SN, Haskell WL, Macera CA, Bouchard C, et al. Physical activity and public health: a recommendation from the Centers for Disease Control and Prevention and the American College of Sports Medicine. JAMA. 1995;273(5):402–7.
3. Tew GA, Ayyash R, Durrand J, Danjoux GR. Clinical guideline and recommendations on pre-operative exercise training in patients awaiting major non-cardiac surgery. Anaesthesia. 2018;73(6):750–68.
4. Campbell KL, Winters-Stone KM, Patel AV, Gerber LH, Matthews CE, May AM, et al. An executive summary of reports from an international multidisciplinary roundtable on exercise and cancer: evidence, guidelines, and implementation. Rehabil Oncol. 2019;37(4):144–52.
5. Banugo P. Amoako D. Bja Educ: Prehabilitation; 2017.
6. Mans CM, Reeve JC, Elkins MR. Postoperative outcomes following preoperative inspiratory muscle training in patients undergoing cardiothoracic or upper abdominal surgery: a systematic review and meta analysis. Clin Rehabil. 2015;29(5):426–38.
7. Katsura M, Kuriyama A, Takeshima T, Fukuhara S, Furukawa TA. Preoperative inspiratory muscle training for postoperative pulmonary complications in adults undergoing cardiac and major abdominal surgery. Cochrane Database Syst Rev. 2015;10
8. Moyer R, Ikert K, Long K, Marsh J. The value of preoperative exercise and education for patients undergoing total hip and knee arthroplasty: a systematic review and meta-analysis. JBJS Rev. 2017;5(12):e2.
9. Wang L, Lee M, Zhang Z, Moodie J, Cheng D, Martin J. Does preoperative rehabilitation for patients planning to undergo joint replacement surgery improve outcomes? A systematic review and meta-analysis of randomised controlled trials. BMJ Open. 2016;6(2).
10. Milder DA, Pillinger NL, Kam PCA. The role of prehabilitation in frail surgical patients: a systematic review. Acta Anaesthesiol Scand. 2018;62(10):1356–66.
11. Dronkers JJ, Lamberts H, Reutelingsperger I, Naber RH, Dronkers-Landman CM, Veldman A, et al. Preoperative therapeutic programme for elderly patients scheduled for elective abdominal oncological surgery: a randomized controlled pilot study. Clin Rehabil. 2010;24(7):614–22.
12. Bruns ERJ, van den Heuvel B, Buskens CJ, Van Duijvendijk P, Festen S, Wassenaar EB, et al. The effects of physical prehabilitation in elderly patients undergoing colorectal surgery: a systematic review. Color Dis. 2016;18(8):O267–77.
13. Durrand J, Hackett R, Yates D, Danjoux G. Prehabilitation. In: Perioperative Medicine–Current Controversies. Springer; 2019. p. 15–47.
14. Faithfull S, Turner L, Poole K, Joy M, Manders R, Weprin J, et al. Prehabilitation for adults diagnosed with cancer: a systematic review of long-term physical function, nutrition and patient-reported outcomes. Eur J Cancer Care (Engl). 2019;28(4):e13023.
15. NICE NI for H and CE. Routine preoperative tests for elective surgery. Vol. 121, BJU International. 2018.
16. ACSM AC of SM. ACSM's Guidelines for Exercise Testing and Prescription. 2010.
17. Wolin KY, Schwartz AL, Matthews CE, Courneya KS, Schmitz KH. Implementing the exercise guidelines for cancer survivors. J Support Oncol. 2012;10(5):171.
18. Balady GJ, Chaitman B, Driscoll D, Foster C, Froelicher E, Gordon N, et al. Recommendations for cardiovascular screening, staffing, and emergency policies at health/fitness facilities. Circulation. 1998;97(22):2283–93.
19. ATS A. ATS statement, guidelines for the six-minute walk test. Am J Respir Crit Care Med 2002;166:111–117.
20. Steffen TM, Hacker TA, Mollinger L. Age-and gender-related test performance in community-dwelling elderly people: six-minute walk test, berg balance scale, timed up & go test, and gait speeds. Phys Ther. 2002;82(2):128–37.
21. Kwok BC, Pua YH, Mamun K, Wong WP. The minimal clinically important difference of six-minute walk in Asian older adults. BMC Geriatr. 2013;13(1):1–5.
22. Granger CL, Holland AE, Gordon IR, Denehy L. Minimal important difference of the 6-minute walk distance in lung cancer. Chron Respir Dis. 2015;12(2):146–54.
23. Middleton A, Fritz SL, Lusardi M. Walking speed: the functional vital sign. J Aging Phys Act. 2015;23(2):314–22.

24. Graham JE, Ostir GV, Fisher SR, Ottenbacher KJ. Assessing walking speed in clinical research: a systematic review. J Eval Clin Pract. 2008;14(4):552–62.
25. Lusardi MM, Pellecchia GL, Schulman M. Functional performance in community living older adults. J Geriatr Phys Ther. 2003;26(3):14.
26. Ostir GV, Berges I, Kuo Y-F, Goodwin JS, Ottenbacher KJ, Guralnik JM. Assessing gait speed in acutely ill older patients admitted to an acute care for elders hospital unit. Arch Intern Med. 2012;172(4):353–8.
27. Kennedy DM, Stratford PW, Riddle DL, Hanna SE, Gollish JD. Assessing recovery and establishing prognosis following total knee arthroplasty. Phys Ther. 2008;88(1):22–32.
28. Studenski S, Perera S, Wallace D, Chandler JM, Duncan PW, Rooney E, et al. Physical performance measures in the clinical setting. J Am Geriatr Soc. 2003;51(3):314–22.
29. Rabadi MH, Blau A. Admission ambulation velocity predicts length of stay and discharge disposition following stroke in an acute rehabilitation hospital. Neurorehabil Neural Repair. 2005;19(1):20–6.
30. Bohannon R, Andrews AW. Comfortable walking speed: Norms for adults derived using meta-analysis. In: NIH Toolbox Conference: Bethesda, MD. 2008.
31. Buatois S, Perret-Guillaume C, Gueguen R, Miget P, Vançon G, Perrin P, et al. A simple clinical scale to stratify risk of recurrent falls in community-dwelling adults aged 65 years and older. Phys Ther. 2010;90(4):550–60.
32. Bohannon RW. Reference values for the five-repetition sit-to-stand test: a descriptive meta-analysis of data from elders. Percept Mot Skills. 2006;103(1):215–22.
33. Tiedemann A, Shimada H, Sherrington C, Murray S, Lord S. The comparative ability of eight functional mobility tests for predicting falls in community-dwelling older people. Age Ageing. 2008;37(4):430–5.
34. Bohannon RW. Grip strength: an indispensable biomarker for older adults. Clin Interv Aging. 2019;14:1681.
35. Sousa-Santos AR, Amaral TF. Differences in handgrip strength protocols to identify sarcopenia and frailty-a systematic review. BMC Geriatr. 2017;17(1):1–21.
36. MacDermid J, Solomon G, Valdes K. Clinical assessment recommendations. American Society of Hand Therapists; 2015.
37. Desrosiers J, Bravo G, Hebert R, Dutil E. Normative data for grip strength of elderly men and women. Am J Occup Ther. 1995;49(7):637–44.
38. Nitschke JE, McMeeken JM, Burry HC, Matyas TA. When is a change a genuine change?: a clinically meaningful interpretation of grip strength measurements in healthy and disabled women. J Hand Ther. 1999;12(1):25–30.
39. Beninato M, Gill-Body KM, Salles S, Stark PC, Black-Schaffer RM, Stein J. Determination of the minimal clinically important difference in the FIM instrument in patients with stroke. Arch Phys Med Rehabil. 2006;87(1):32–9.
40. Wallace M, Shelkey M. Katz index of independence in activities of daily living (ADL). Urol Nurs. 2007;27(1):93–4.
41. Lawton MP, Brody EM, Médecin U. Instrumental activities of daily living (IADL). Gerontologist. 1969;9:179–86.
42. Suijker JJ, van Rijn M, ter Riet G, van Charante EPM, de Rooij SE, Buurman BM. Minimal important change and minimal detectable change in activities of daily living in community-living older people. J Nutr Health Aging. 2017;21(2):165–72.
43. Cella D, Eton DT, Lai J-S, Peterman AH, Merkel DE. Combining anchor and distribution-based methods to derive minimal clinically important differences on the functional assessment of cancer therapy (FACT) anemia and fatigue scales. J Pain Symptom Manag. 2002;24(6):547–61.
44. Swift A. The importance of assessing pain in adults. Nurs Times. 2015;111(41):12–4.
45. Gregory J. Use of pain scales and observational pain assessment tools in hospital settings. Nurs Stand. 2019;34
46. Williamson A, Hoggart B. Pain: a review of three commonly used pain rating scales. J Clin Nurs. 2005;14(7):798–804.

47. Wong DL, Baker CM. Pain in children: comparison of assessment scales. Pediatr Nurs. 1988;14(1):9–17.
48. WHO W. The World Health Organization quality of life assessment (WHOQOL): position paper from the World Health Organization. Soc Sci Med 1995;41(10):1403–1409.
49. King MT. The interpretation of scores from the EORTC quality of life questionnaire QLQ-C30. Qual Life Res. 1996;5(6):555–67.
50. Musoro JZ, Coens C, Fiteni F, Katarzyna P, Cardoso F, Russell NS, et al. Minimally important differences for interpreting EORTC QLQ-C30 scores in patients with advanced breast cancer. JNCI Cancer Spectr. 2019;3(3):pkz037.
51. Wade DT. Goal setting in rehabilitation: an overview of what, why and how. Clin Rehabil. 2009;23(4):291–5.
52. Doran GT. There'sa SMART way to write management's goals and objectives. Manag Rev. 1981;70(11):35–6.
53. Jones LW, Eves ND, Peppercorn J. Pre-exercise screening and prescription guidelines for cancer patients. Lancet Oncol. 2010;11(10):914–6.
54. Hardinge M, Annandale J, Bourne S, Cooper B, Evans A, Freeman D, et al. British Thoracic Society guidelines for home oxygen use in adults: accredited by NICE. Thorax. 2015;70(Suppl 1):i1–43.
55. Stricker CT, Drake D, Hoyer K-A, Mock V. Evidence-based practice for fatigue management in adults with cancer: exercise as an intervention. In: Oncology nursing forum. Oncology Nursing Society; 2004. p. 963.
56. Watson T, Mock V. Exercise as an intervention for cancer-related fatigue. Phys Ther. 2004;84(8):736–43.
57. Mitchell SA, Hoffman AJ, Clark JC, DeGennaro RM, Poirier P, Robinson CB, et al. Putting evidence into practice: an update of evidence-based interventions for cancer-related fatigue during and following treatment. Clin J Oncol Nurs. 2007;18:38–58.
58. Williams N. The Borg rating of perceived exertion (RPE) scale. Occup Med (Chic Ill). 2017;67(5):404–5.
59. Metkus TS Jr, Baughman KL, Thompson PD. Exercise prescription and primary prevention of cardiovascular disease. Circulation. 2010;121(23):2601–4.
60. Azevedo MJ, Viamonte S, Castro A. Exercise prescription in oncology patients: general principles. Rehabilitación. 2013;47(3):170–8.
61. Klatt BN, Carender WJ, Lin CC, Alsubaie SF, Kinnaird CR, Sienko KH, et al. A conceptual framework for the progression of balance exercises in persons with balance and vestibular disorders. Phys Med Rehabil Int. 2015;2(4).
62. Chen AW, Koh YT, Leong SW, Ng LW, Lee PS, Koh GC. Post community hospital discharge rehabilitation attendance: self-perceived barriers and participation over time. Ann Acad Med Singap. 2014;43(3):136–44.
63. Clark AM, King-Shier KM, Spaling MA, Duncan AS, Stone JA, Jaglal SB, et al. Factors influencing participation in cardiac rehabilitation programmes after referral and initial attendance: qualitative systematic review and meta-synthesis. Clin Rehabil. 2013;27(10):948–59.
64 Resurrección DM, Moreno-Peral P, Gómez-Herranz M, Rubio-Valera M, Pastor L. Caldas de Almeida JM, et al. factors associated with non-participation in and dropout from cardiac rehabilitation programmes: a systematic review of prospective cohort studies. Eur J Cardiovasc Nurs. 2019;18(1):38–47.
65. Jiang X, Ming W-K, You JHS. The cost-effectiveness of digital health interventions on the management of cardiovascular diseases: systematic review. J Med Internet Res. 2019;21(6):e13166.

Psycho-Social Prehabilitation Before Surgery in Oncology

9

Soumitra Shankar Datta and Arnab Mukherjee

9.1 Introduction: Psycho-Social Aspects of Prehabilitation

Prehabilitation involves optimising and improving the patient's functional capacity before surgery to improve the post-operative outcome [1]. Recent approaches to prehabilitation have encouraged multimodal approaches that encompass psycho-social interventions, addressing nicotine dependence and alcohol dependence side by side optimising physical factors as functional capacity [2]. This is particularly important in oncology. Psychiatric disorders affected more than 1 billion people worldwide according to the global burden of diseases study [3] and patients diagnosed with cancer are at high risk of psychological distress and mental health disorders [4]. One in six patients with cancer suffers from depression at some point during their care [5]. The present chapter will be discussing the various psychological factors relevant to cancer-related prehabilitation. There are separate sections dedicated to treating special groups of patients as children and adolescents and those who are differently abled. We aim to provide an overview for oncology clinicians and mental health professionals, on the topic of psycho-social prehabilitation, so that they can integrate this into their day-to-day clinical practice.

S. S. Datta (✉)
Department of Palliative Care and Psycho-oncology, Tata Medical Centre, Kolkata, West Bengal, India

MRC Clinical Trials Unit, Institute of Clinical Trials & Methodology, University College London, London, UK

A. Mukherjee
Department of Palliative Care and Psycho-oncology, Tata Medical Centre, Kolkata, West Bengal, India

A. Chakraborty, A. Balakrishnan (eds.), *Prehabilitation for Cancer Surgery*,
https://doi.org/10.1007/978-981-16-6494-6_9

9.2 Assessment of Pre-Existing and Newly Diagnosed Psychiatric Morbidities Before Surgery

Cancer patients with anxiety and depression were found to be at great risk of longer hospitalisations and accrued increased healthcare-related costs [6]. A recent review looking at the preoperative psychological factors affecting surgical outcomes across a range of surgeries grouped the existing research into three broad categories, namely a) mood-related factors (anxiety, depression, perceived stress, anger, and others), b) attitudinal factors (self-efficacy, locus of control, and others) and c) personality-related factors as quantified by standardised personality inventories [7]. The rates of psychological morbidity are high in oncology and the specific role of psychological interventions before cancer surgeries have received some attention but there is a paucity of randomised trials on the topic as reported by the authors of this review [8].

One approach is to screen all cancer patients prior for psychological distress and unmet mental health needs at the onset of treatment [4]. However, this approach is resource-intensive and very few studies describe successful implementation strategies for universal distress management [9]. The other approach is to use psychiatric screening for specific high-risk patients as physical multi-morbidities [10] and past psychiatric conditions and those with other risk factors [11].

The pre-surgical assessment should include an assessment to elicit past and present psychiatric morbidities and psychological wellness. Common questions that are likely to help in identifying past or current psychiatric conditions in cancer patients before surgery and make referrals to psycho-oncology teams are suggested in Table 9.1.

Table 9.1 Possible interview questions before surgery

SN	Possible questions to explore emotional health during a pre-surgical period	Purpose
1	Have you ever accessed professional care for an emotional problem? If you have, when was that and what treatment did you receive? How long was the treatment?	Eliciting past psychiatric history
2	How is your sleep?	Exploring sleep problems
3	How would you rate your mood currently?	Exploring the present emotional state
4	Are you worried about your present health condition?	Screening for health related anxities
5	Are you taking any medicines to help your sleep, anxiety, and low mood?	Exploring present psychiatric conditions
6	Have you in the past or currently use any addictive substances?	Screening for past and present substance use
7	Have you ever been a smoker or user of tobacco in any form	Screening for past and present tobacco use
8	Are you worried about the post-operative period?	Screening for anticipatory anxiety
9	Have you ever found it difficult to follow health advice given to you by any healthcare professionals?	Screening for adherence-related problems
10	Do you want to tell us anything else about how you feel?	Open-ended last question

It is possibly best to have the assessment well ahead of the date of the elective surgery, more than 1–2 weeks before the hospital admission. This gives the health care professional an opportunity to address any unmet mental health needs and help the patient to get ready emotionally for the procedure. It may be better to make this a routine procedure such that patients do not feel uneasy. With the increased focus on mental health in the past decade, most patients feel good after this assessment experience [12].

9.3 Understanding the Expectations of the Patient and Having a Realistic Discussion

During prehabilitation, it is not unusual for patients to expect a reassuring stance from the treating team, that following the surgery, their health will be better. It is important to be realistic when such discussions happen so that there is no misunderstanding later in the course of treatment. For complicated surgeries like head and neck cancer surgeries and intra-abdominal/thoracic onco-surgeries, the surgical and anaesthesia team should explain the restrictions that the patient may face in the immediate post-operative period so that patient gets a chance to prepare for this. A good example would be explaining the temporary (or permanent) nature of a tracheostomy that may be needed for a patient undergoing surgery for oral and head and neck cancers. This discussion allows the treating team to understand the expectations of the patient as well. There may be occasions when the patient is very anxious and is misinformed based on the information they encountered on the internet. Clinicians should offer a chance to the patients to discuss their worries. Patients can be directed to credible sources of information on the internet and this will help the patient in his or her realistic appraisal of the situation.

9.4 Common Psychological Concerns before Surgeries and their Impact on Outcome

Over the last few decades, survival related to cancer has improved with better management of the surgical site, more acceptable cosmetic outcomes, and reduced treatment time and hospital visits [13]. Even with such advancements in treatment options, receiving the diagnosis of cancer continues to be very stressful and most patients find it difficult to cope with. During treatment of cancer, may remain preoccupied with body image issues secondary to loss of an organ or adjuvant chemotherapy-related hair loss. Following treatment completion, patient may have longer-term worries related to changes in their bodies as lymphedema following axillary clearance for breast cancer, adapting to sexual intimacy as a survivor, stress caused potential problems related to procreation in men and childbearing in women, and fear of passing the cancer gene to the future generation. There can be significant worries related to fear of recurrence [13–16]. Anticipatory and procedural anxiety may lead to an increase in substance use. People often develop psychiatric morbidities first time after the diagnosis of cancer and data suggest cancer-specific survival is shorter in patients who develop first onset mood, anxiety, substance abuse disorders after the diagnosis of cancer [17]. Psychological prehabilitation thus remains a desired goal to improve the coping skills of the patient to contribute to the recovery following surgery [8, 18–20]. Studies have shown attitudinal factors like self-efficacy and perceived control, personality factors like neuroticism, and the presence or absence of a psychiatric diagnosis like depression influence surgical outcomes [7]. Higher preoperative anxiety, depression, and lower self-efficacy were found to be associated with post-operative pain or impaired recovery [7, 21]. A recent meta-analysis showed psychological prehabilitation among patients undergoing surgery for prostate cancer showed beneficial outcomes on mood and cancer-specific quality of life including cancer worries and sexual function [22]. Similar interventions among breast cancer patients showed reduced psychological distress, anxiety, and depression 3 months post-surgery regarding loss of a breast, after one year of surgical treatment. Psycho-educational interventions help to improve activity level for patients undergoing radiotherapy as well [22].

9.5 Communicating with Patients and Families before Surgery: Finding the Right Balance Between Too Much and Too Little Information

Clinicians often face an ethical and moral dilemma when deciding about the extent of information that is reasonable to be shared with a patient and family before a complicated procedure. Modern clinical care expects clinicians to be open and honest about the expected effects and adverse effects of any treatments that a patient may undergo. However, the depth of this discussion may be related to the technicalities involved in the procedure the patient is about to undergo. Previous research from India has shown that cancer clinicians often individualise the discussion based on their perception of the patient's ability to process the information [23]. Other factors as existing levels of health information campaigns and health information delivery systems are also important mediums that may help in achieving the correct balance [24]. Translation of complicated medical information to simple visual representations has been attempted so that patient education material is friendly yet informative to patients, their caregivers, and the lay members of the public [25]. There is also some evidence supporting that repeating the health information more than once increases the probability of recalling the health recommendation [26]. Having a well-engaged patient is likely to improve patient satisfaction and better symptomatic and disease outcome and hence communication before any complex surgeries is crucial.

9.6 Optimising Psychotropic Medications Before Surgery

While prescribing psychotropic medications, there could be two potential situations that clinicians face. Some patients may be already on psychiatric medications, and other patients may have newly identified psychiatric conditions warranting the need for medication at all.

In the former situation, it is highly recommended to obtain a detailed medication history and the contexts in which the patient has prescribed these medications. In certain situation, minor short-term alterations may be preferred by the anaesthetist and surgical team, e.g. skipping lithium for 2–3 days before surgery so that it does not interfere with cardiac depolarisation. In all other situations, it is often preferred to continue the same chronic medications the patient is on. However, this will need to be reviewed in the post-operative period depending on the physical parameters of the patient on a day-to-day basis.

When the treating physician or surgeons feel the patient has a previously unidentified psychiatric condition needing treatment, before starting on psychotropic medication, it may be worthwhile to get an opinion from a consultant psychiatrist. Occasionally the onset of treatment for a long-standing psychiatric condition may be delayed till the surgery is over. If the symptoms are significantly impacting on the quality of life, interacting with the physical symptoms, or is identified to be posing a risk of treatment non-adherence to the disease for which the patient is seeking treatment, the start of psychiatric treatment may have to be done even before the surgery. This judgement to start psychotropic medications before surgery is to be based on individualised patient care decisions for the person who is accessing treatment, his or her levels of social support, the severity of psychiatric symptoms, and the risk posed to himself and others.

9.7 Multimodal Prehabilitation Over Single Modal Prehabilitation

Research has demonstrated that surgical specialists may find it difficult to inform patients about the prognosis of a disease, break the bad news to patients, discuss the probable length of life after surgery, inform patients about potential negative consequences of surgery such as those on sexual functioning and psychological well-being post-treatment and may end up minimising the patient's distress related to these [14, 27]. The tendency to reserve referral for formal psychiatric assessment only for those patients with severe psychopathology may make the team struggle with managing angry, controlling, demanding patients who may refuse to engage in post-operative care [27].

Although physical prehabilitation may have an impact on psychological well-being and vice versa, there is presently a move towards multimodal prehabilitation. One study exploring prehabilitation in patients undergoing radical prostatectomy showed that patients who received home-based moderate-intensity exercise had improved physical and psychological well-being in the post-operative period, as compared to control group patients, who received treatment as usual [28]. A recent review [29] concluded that single modality preoperative interventions as "nutritional interventions" or only "exercise" did not have any impact on the post-operative outcome as regards the duration of hospitalisation or complications for traditional prostatectomy. On the other hand, multimodal approaches targeting post-operative functional state was found to be effective and safe [29].

The indications for a formal psychiatric assessment before surgery includes: a) pre-existing psychiatric condition, b) pre-existing substance-related problems, c) complex surgeries that may impact the post-operative functioning, e.g. amputations, surgeries for oral cancer, surgeries that may impact fertility, d) patients who are very anxious, e) any other behaviour of the patient that the treating team is unable to explain, f) severe co-existent or co-incidental social stressor as family bereavement, g) poor social support. Other than those mentioned above there may be situations where involving a mental health professional will be useful in preoperative care planning.

9.8 Prehabilitation for Special Groups: Connecting Prehabilitation with Rehabilitation

9.8.1 Children and Adolescents

There has been recent interest in specific models of prehabilitation suited to the needs of adolescents and young adults [30]. Research has explored the feasibility of group-based interventions, delivered remotely on physical aspects of rehabilitation as children aged 8–20 years awaiting below-knee amputation or limb-sparing surgery for lower extremity sarcoma [31]. However, there is a paucity of research on psychological prehabilitation interventions for children and adolescents. The promising trend of using digital and remote interventions that may be acceptable to children and adolescents needs further exploration in the future. A study on the effect of preoperative educational video on the post-operative outcome of daycare surgery of children undergoing dental and ENT (ear, nose, and throat) surgical procedures showed that the intervention was effective in reducing post-operative pain in children as compared to control arm receiving treatment as usual [32].

9.8.2 Differently Abled

A recent review of health information systems for disability-related rehabilitation in low-and-middle-income countries (LMICs) found it to be weak and fragmented in many parts of the world [33]. Even in high-income countries, a study from the USA on war veterans and service members has demonstrated higher rates of rehospitalisation in the first year of treatment, in patients with traumatic brain injury acquired through a military deployment [34]. Managing illnesses in the context of a disability can pose additional challenges to patients and their caregivers. The role of prehabilitation in those with disabilities requires further exploration as this is likely to help patients in their recovery.

9.8.3 Patients with Substance Misuse Problems

A Cochrane review has concluded that intensive perioperative alcohol cessation intervention offered over 4–8 weeks, can result in complete cessation of alcohol use preoperatively and reduced rates of post-operative surgical complications [35]. As regards tobacco dependence, free access to nicotine replacement patches, before elective surgeries, stimulated interests in smokers to attempt quitting as compared to the control group, but the effect of the intervention was often very short-lasting except for a small proportion of patient who managed to quit for a longer time [36]. It is important to note that even short-term cessation is not without its benefits for post-operative outcomes.

9.9 Prehabilitation in the Post-Pandemic Era

As the world recovers from the SARS-CoV-2 pandemic, a discussion on prehabilitation cannot be overemphasised as the world goes through the grief of losing the near and dear ones, recovering from a period of loss of faith in a value system that we had taken for granted. Unique challenges of providing psychological support to hospitalised cancer patients in times of the pandemic have been reported from India [37]. In a multidisciplinary consensus statement by the Association of Anaesthetists, the Centre for Peri-operative Care, the Federation of Surgical Specialty Associations, the Royal College of Anaesthetists, and the Royal College of Surgeons of England empathised the role of multimodal prehabilitation for elective surgeries on patients who are COVID-19 survivors for a better post-operative outcome [38]. The above guideline talks about multidisciplinary patient optimisation.

9.10 Conclusions

Surgical recovery has to happen to a person who has a body as well as a mind. We all have the same organ systems but we may think and act differently and patients with cancer are no exception. Human life is a functional concept at its best. That is what made us human. Thus, not surprisingly, physical healing is often complemented by a balanced psychological state. Psychological prehabilitation before surgery is likely to impact both bodily recovery and emotional well-being of the patient following the surgery.

References

1. Banugo P, Amoako D. Prehabilitation. BJA Educ. 2017;17(12):401–5.
2. Myers J, Niebauer J, Humphrey R. Prehabilitation coming of age: implications for cardiac and pulmonary rehabilitation. J Cardiopulm Rehabil Prev. 2021;25
3. Rehm J, Shield KD. Global burden of disease and the impact of mental and addictive disorders. Curr Psychiatry Rep. 2019;21(2):10.
4. Holland JC, Andersen B, Breitbart WS, Buchmann LO, Compas B, Deshields TL, et al. Distress management. J Natl Compr Cancer Netw JNCCN. 2013;11(2):190–209.
5. Bravery B, Loughman S, Murphy M. Depression treatment research in people with cancer does not reflect cancer prevalence: findings from a systematic review. Evid Based Ment Health 2020;23(4):155–60.

6. Mausbach BT, Decastro G, Schwab RB, Tiamson-Kassab M, Irwin SA. Healthcare use and costs in adult cancer patients with anxiety and depression. Depress Anxiety. 2020;37(9):908–15.
7. Levett DZH, Grimmett C. Psychological factors, prehabilitation and surgical outcomes: evidence and future directions. Anaesthesia. 2019;74(S1):36–42.
8. Tsimopoulou I, Pasquali S, Howard R, Desai A, Gourevitch D, Tolosa I, et al. Psychological Prehabilitation before cancer surgery: a systematic review. Ann Surg Oncol. 2015;22(13):4117–23.
9. McCarter K, Fradgley EA, Britton B, Tait J, Paul C. Not seeing the forest for the trees: a systematic review of comprehensive distress management programs and implementation strategies. Curr Opin Support Palliat Care. 2020;14(3):220–31.
10. Jing Z, Li J, Fu PP, Wang Y, Yuan Y, Zhao D, et al. Physical multimorbidity and lifetime suicidal ideation and plans among rural older adults: the mediating role of psychological distress. BMC Psychiatry. 2021;21(1):78.
11. Castro-Figueroa EM, Torres-Blasco N, Rosal MC, Castro WP, González-Lorenzo ME, Vélez H, et al. Preferences, use of and satisfaction with mental health services among a sample of Puerto Rican cancer patients. PLoS One. 2019;14(7):e0216127.
12. Schofield PE, Butow PN, Thompson JF, Tattersall MHN, Beeney LJ, Dunn SM. Psychological responses of patients receiving a diagnosis of cancer. Ann Oncol. 2003;14(1):48–56.
13. Fallowfield L, Jenkins V. Psychosocial/survivorship issues in breast cancer: are we doing better? J Natl Cancer Inst. 2015;107(1):335.
14. Hermelink K, Berndt U, Haidinger R. Alleviating the breast cancer experience: a plea for psycho-oncology. Breast Care Basel Switz. 2015;10(2):82–3.
15. Weis J. Psychosocial Care for Cancer Patients. Breast Care. 2015;10(2):84–6.
16. Zimmermann T. Intimate relationships affected by breast cancer: interventions for couples. Breast Care. 2015;10(2):102–8.
17. Zhu J, Fang F, Sjölander A, Fall K, Adami HO, Valdimarsdóttir U. First-onset mental disorders after cancer diagnosis and cancer-specific mortality: a nationwide cohort study. Ann Oncol. 2017;28(8):1964–9.
18. Johanning J, Hall D. Successful Prehabilitation: a Noble goal. J Am Geriatr Soc. 2018;66(10):1869.
19. Lehto RH, Cimprich B. Anxiety and directed attention in women awaiting breast cancer surgery. Oncol Nurs Forum. 1999;26(4):767–72.
20. Nosarti C, Roberts JV, Crayford T, McKenzie K, David AS. Early psychological adjustment in breast cancer patients: a prospective study. J Psychosom Res. 2002;53(6):1123–30.
21. Foster C, Haviland J, Winter J, Grimmett C, Chivers Seymour K, Batehup L, et al. Pre-surgery depression and confidence to manage problems predict recovery trajectories of health and wellbeing in the first two years following colorectal cancer: results from the CREW Cohort Study. PLoS ONE [Internet]. 2016 12 [cited 2021 May 12];11(5). https://www.ncbi.nlm.nih.gov/pmc/articles/PMC4865190/
22. Treanor C, Kyaw T, Donnelly M. An international review and meta-analysis of prehabilitation compared to usual care for cancer patients. J Cancer Surviv. 2018;12(1):64–73.
23. Datta SS, Tripathi L, Varghese R, Logan J, Gessler S, Chatterjee S, et al. Pivotal role of families in doctor–patient communication in oncology: a qualitative study of patients, their relatives and cancer clinicians. Eur J Cancer Care (Engl). 2017;26(5):e12543.
24. Kim KL. Predictors of cancer information overload: findings from a national survey [Internet]. Professor T.D. Wilson; [cited 2021 Mar 19]. https://d-scholarship.pitt.edu/25116/2/paper326.html
25. Pimjai Sudsawad S. Center on Knowledge Translation for Disability and Rehabilitation Research (KTDRR) KT Library - Research Quality [Internet]. 2007 [cited 2021 Mar 19]. https://ktdrr.org/ktlibrary/articles_pubs/ktmodels/
26. McDonald J, McDonald P, Hughes C, Albarracín D. Recalling and intending to enact health recommendations: optimal number of prescribed behaviors in multibehavior messages. Clin Psychol Sci. 2017;5(5):858–65.

27. Burton MV, Parker RW. Psychological aspects of cancer surgery: surgeons' attitudes and opinions. Psychooncology. 1997;6(1):47–64.
28. Santa Mina D, Hilton WJ, Matthew AG, Awasthi R, Bousquet-Dion G, Alibhai SMH, et al. Prehabilitation for radical prostatectomy: a multicentre randomized controlled trial. Surg Oncol. 2018;27(2):289–98.
29. Minnella EM, Carli F, Kassouf W. Role of prehabilitation following major uro-oncologic surgery: a narrative review. World J Urol. 2020;31
30. McCann L, McMillan KA, Hewitt C. An e-Prehabilitation System of Care for Teenagers and Young Adults Diagnosed With Cancer: Protocol for a Qualitative Co-Design Study. JMIR Res Protoc [Internet]. 2018 Sep 12 [cited 2021 Mar 19];7(9). Available from: https://www.ncbi.nlm.nih.gov/pmc/articles/PMC6231758/
31. Corr AM, Liu W, Bishop M, Pappo A, Srivastava DK, Neel M, et al. Feasibility and functional outcomes of children and adolescents undergoing preoperative chemotherapy prior to a limb-sparing procedure or amputation. Rehabil Oncol Am Phys Ther Assoc Oncol Sect. 2017 Jan;35(1):38–45.
32. Chartrand J, Tourigny J, MacCormick J. The effect of an educational pre-operative DVD on parents' and children's outcomes after a same-day surgery: a randomized controlled trial. J Adv Nurs. 2017;73(3):599–611.
33. McPherson A, Durham J, Richards N, Gouda H, Rampatige R, Whittaker M. Strengthening health information systems for disability-related rehabilitation in LMICs. Health Policy Plan. 2017;32(3):384–94.
34. Tran J, Hammond F, Dams-O'Connor K, Tang X, Eapen B, McCarthy M, et al. Rehospitalization in the first year following veteran and service member TBI: a VA TBI model systems study. J Head Trauma Rehabil. 2017;32(4):264–70.
35. Egholm JW, Pedersen B, Møller AM, Adami J, Juhl CB, Tønnesen H. Perioperative alcohol cessation intervention for postoperative complications. Cochrane Database Syst Rev. 2018;11:CD008343.
36. Webb AR, Coward L, Soh L, Waugh L, Parsons L, Lynch M, et al. Smoking cessation in elective surgical patients offered free nicotine patches at listing: a pilot study. Anaesthesia. 2020;75(2):171–8.
37. Mukherjee A, Chatterjee M, Chattopadhyay S, Bhowmick C, Basu A, Bhattacharjee S, et al. Psycho-oncology service provisions for hospitalised cancer patients before and during the COVID-19 pandemic in an oncology Centre in eastern India. Ecancermedicalscience. 2021;15(1226):1–15.
38. El-Boghdadly K, Cook TM, Goodacre T, Kua J, Blake L, Denmark S, et al. SARS-CoV-2 infection, COVID-19 and timing of elective surgery: a multidisciplinary consensus statement on behalf of the Association of Anaesthetists, the Centre for Peri-operative Care, the Federation of Surgical Specialty Associations, the Royal College of Anaesthetists and the Royal College of Surgeons of England. Anaesthesia. 2021;18

10 The Role of Pain Management in Cancer Prehabilitation

Sarah Dawson and Kiran K. Koneti

10.1 Introduction and General Considerations

"Controlling pain should be an essential part of cancer treatment… when pain is managed effectively, people can enjoy time with family and friends, rest better and continue many of their daily activities, like work, school and play. No one should live or die in pain."

Dr. Etienne Krug, Director of WHO's Department for the Management of Noncommunicable Diseases.

Pain is a significant burden amongst cancer patients, affecting approximately 53% of patients overall, and 59% of patients undergoing active treatment [1]. Pain is often multi-factorial and multi-faceted; it may be resultant of the disease process itself such as inflammation, compression and ischaemia from the tumour mass, or may result from disease treatment such as chemotherapy, radiotherapy or surgery [2]. The pain experienced by cancer patients is further compounded by psychological factors such as anxiety, depression and grief reactions [3].

Physical aspects of pain cannot be treated effectively in isolation from other aspects of pain such as anxiety and spiritual aspects of suffering, holistic assessment and treatment must encompass all of these aspects [4]. In general pain management should involve treating the cause of the pain wherever possible [5], for instance fixation of pathological fractures and use of antibiotics to treat infection. If the cause

S. Dawson
Specialty Registrar in Anaesthesia, Northern School of Anaesthesia,
Newcastle upon Tyne, UK
e-mail: sarah.dawson48@nhs.net

K. K. Koneti (✉)
Consultant in Anaesthesia and Pain Management, STS NHS Foundation Trust,
Sunderland, UK
e-mail: kiran.koneti@nhs.net

A. Chakraborty, A. Balakrishnan (eds.), *Prehabilitation for Cancer Surgery*,
https://doi.org/10.1007/978-981-16-6494-6_10

cannot be removed entirely, treatment should be directed at the underlying disease process, e.g. palliative radiotherapy or use of bisphosphonates to treat symptomatic hypercalcaemia. Where these treatments are not indicated or fail, optimisation of oral opioids provides the mainstay of treatment in the majority of patients.

10.1.1 Goals of Pain Control

Severe pain can interfere with mobility, fitness, nutrition, sleep and mood. Effective pain control is required to enable patients to maximally benefit from prehabilitation, in addition to enhancing their quality of life. The goal of good pain control is to optimise the patient's comfort and function (see Fig. 10.1) whilst avoiding adverse effects from analgesics. This is best achieved through a multimodal, multidisciplinary and holistic approach tailored to each patient.

10.2 Assessment of Cancer Pain

Making a detailed evaluation of pain, including its causes, severity and effects on the patient's daily life, is an important first step towards designing an effective management plan [3]. Assessment of pain at the earliest opportunity allows an appropriate treatment strategy to be implemented early during the course of prehabilitation prior to surgery.

Pain assessment tools, such as the brief pain inventory [6] (BPI, see Fig. 10.2 below), can play an important role in evaluating pain and monitoring the effectiveness of treatment. The BPI concisely registers the location, character and intensity of the pain, in addition to treatments which have been trialled, and the effect which the pain has on the patient's daily life. The burden of pain may be further increased by psychosocial factors including social and financial difficulties or overall disease prognosis. Assessment and reassessment of pain at regular intervals is key to establishing whether a treatment is efficacious and safe, as well as minimising and addressing side effects. Patients with particularly complex pain issues may benefit from expertise from a pain specialist at an early stage [7].

Goals of good pain control	
Physical	Improve ambulation and levels of activity Enable prehab programs to increase fitness Enable participation in activities important to patient
Social and emotional	Improve motivational status Improve mood Enable sense of control
Prognostic	Opioid minimisation and impact on disease recurrence Reduce chronic pain post-surgery

Fig. 10.1 Goals of good pain control

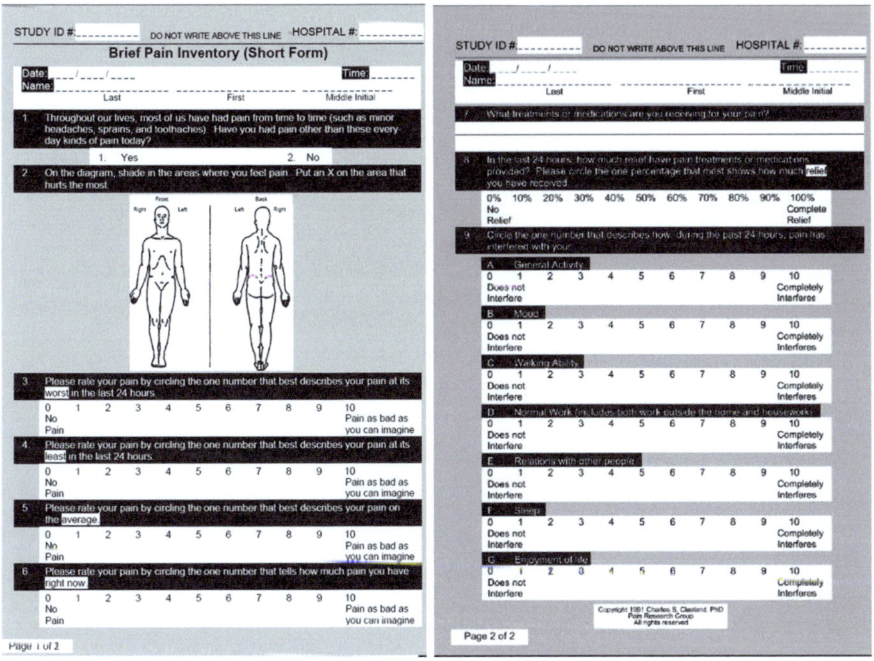

STUDY ID #:__________ DO NOT WRITE ABOVE THIS LINE HOSPITAL #:__________

Brief Pain Inventory (Short Form)

Date: ___/___/___ Time: _______

Name: __________ __________ __________

Last First Middle Initial

1. Throughout our lives, most of us have had pain from time to time (such as minor headaches, sprains, and toothaches). Have you had pain other than these every-day kinds of pain today?

1. Yes 2. No

2. On the diagram, shade in the areas where you feel pain. Put an X on the area that hurts the most.

Front Back Right Left Left Right

3. Please rate your pain by circling the one number that best describes your pain at its worst in the last 24 hours.

0 1 2 3 4 5 6 7 8 9 10
No Pain — Pain as bad as you can imagine

4. Please rate your pain by circling the one number that best describes your pain at its least in the last 24 hours.

0 1 2 3 4 5 6 7 8 9 10
No Pain — Pain as bad as you can imagine

5. Please rate your pain by circling the one number that best describes your pain on the average.

0 1 2 3 4 5 6 7 8 9 10
No Pain — Pain as bad as you can imagine

6. Please rate your pain by circling the one number that tells how much pain you have right now.

0 1 2 3 4 5 6 7 8 9 10
No Pain — Pain as bad as you can imagine

Page 1 of 2

STUDY ID #:__________ DO NOT WRITE ABOVE THIS LINE HOSPITAL #:__________

Date: ___/___/___ Time: _______

Name: __________ __________ __________

Last First Middle Initial

7. What treatments or medications are you receiving for your pain?

8. In the last 24 hours, how much relief have pain treatments or medications provided? Please circle the one percentage that most shows how much relief you have received.

0% 10% 20% 30% 40% 50% 60% 70% 80% 90% 100%
No Relief — Complete Relief

9. Circle the one number that describes how, during the past 24 hours, pain has interfered with your:

A. General Activity
0 1 2 3 4 5 6 7 8 9 10
Does not Interfere — Completely Interferes

B. Mood
0 1 2 3 4 5 6 7 8 9 10
Does not Interfere — Completely Interferes

C. Walking Ability
0 1 2 3 4 5 6 7 8 9 10
Does not Interfere — Completely Interferes

D. Normal Work (includes both work outside the home and housework)
0 1 2 3 4 5 6 7 8 9 10
Does not Interfere — Completely Interferes

E. Relations with other people
0 1 2 3 4 5 6 7 8 9 10
Does not Interfere — Completely Interferes

F. Sleep
0 1 2 3 4 5 6 7 8 9 10
Does not Interfere — Completely Interferes

G. Enjoyment of life
0 1 2 3 4 5 6 7 8 9 10
Does not Interfere — Completely Interferes

Copyright 1991 Charles S. Cleeland, PhD
Pain Research Group
All rights reserved

Page 2 of 2

Fig. 10.2 The *Brief Pain Inventory* C Cleeland, Handbook of Pain Assessment, The Guilford Press, New York (1991), pp. 378–382

10.3 Cancer Pain Pathophysiology

10.3.1 Mechanisms of Pain in Cancer Patients

Understanding the mechanisms that can cause cancer pain is an important part of providing effective treatment. Cancer patients experience pain for a variety of different reasons, the pain may be nociceptive (i.e. arising from somatic tissues or viscera) or neuropathic (arising from a lesion or disease of the somatosensory nervous system). Most commonly there will be an overlap, and patients will present with a mixture of the two. Eighty percent of patients will experience more than one type of pain [2]. Differences between nociceptive and neuropathic pain are outlined below (Fig. 10.3).

10.3.2 Causes of Pain in Cancer Patients

The majority of pain experienced by cancer patients, around 75%, is directly attributable to their cancer [2]. The remainder is evenly split between pain relating to cancer treatment and pain unrelated to cancer, including pre-existing pain conditions such as chronic back pain, fibromyalgia and diabetic neuropathy (see

	Nociceptive		
Pain Type	Somatic	Visceral	Neuropathic
Definition	Pain caused by physiological activation of pain receptors		Pain caused by lesion of dysfunction of the somatosensory nervous system
Mechanism	Natural physiological transduction		Ectopic impulse generation, among others
Arises from	MSK system	Viscera e.g. GI tract, pancreas	Injury to central or peripheral nervous system
Localisation	Well-localised	Diffuse/ poorly localized, referred pain	Can follow a nerve path or be poorly diffuse
Quality of Symptoms	Achy, dull, throbbing, sore	Gnawing, squeezing, cramping	Shooting, burning, tingling, electric-shock
Examples	Pathological fracture	Capsular liver pain, mucositis	Radiation induced neuritis, paraneoplastic phenomena
Hypersensitivity	Uncommon		Present (Allodynia/Hyperalgesia)
Treatment	Good response (conventional analgesics)		Poor-moderate response (anti-depressants, anti-epileptics)

Fig. 10.3 Differences between nociceptive (somatic and visceral) and neuropathic pain

Fig. 10.4). The tumour itself may cause pain by local mass effect, causing compression, obstruction, ischaemia, inflammation and oedema of surrounding neural and non-neural tissues. Depending on the disease process, there may be paraneoplastic phenomena with the production of anti-Hu and Yo antibodies causing peripheral neuropathy or neuritis.

Where tumour deposits are present in bone, activation of osteoclasts via local production of mediators, including interleukin 1 and 6, results in increased bone resorption providing further space for the tumour to expand. This alters the structural integrity of the bone, and may result in pain through abnormal weight distribution or pathological fractures [2]. The increased osteoclastic activity also causes hypercalcaemia, through systemic release of calcium stores from bone, which may result in abdominal, muscle and bone pain. Osteoclasts themselves also contribute to local acidosis and can cause damage to peripheral nerve endings.

Local Mass Effect	Treatment related	Paraneoplastic	Associated conditions
Inflammation Compression Ischemia Oedema Bowel obstruction	Radiation neuritis and cystitis Chemotherapy induced neuropathy Mucositis Surgery	Anti-neuronal antibodies causing peripheral neuropathy	Infection Hypercalcaemia Osteoporosis Prolonged immobility/ pressure ulcers Lymphoedema Constipation

Fig. 10.4 Summary of causes of pain in cancer patients

Treatments for cancer including chemotherapy and radiotherapy frequently result in pain. Chemotherapy-induced peripheral neuropathy affects a high proportion of patients receiving specific neurotoxic drugs such as taxanes, and platinum-based drugs such as cisplatin and oxaliplatin. Radiotherapy causes inflammation and pain in structures through which the radiation beam must pass, e.g. skin (radiation dermatitis), or other nearby structures depending on the location of treatment (radiation cystitis and radiation-induced neuritis).

Oral mucositis can result from radiotherapy (usually due to direct necrotic and inflammatory effects) or chemotherapy (as a result of low white cell count). Mucositis is common but can be severe and result in additional treatment challenges. Patients may have reduced appetite, resulting in malnutrition or be at increased risk of bacterial, viral or fungal infection due to a loss of integrity of the mucous membranes. Although mild mucositis may respond to simple treatments such as ice chips and topical therapies, opioids either as lozenges or administered intravenously may be required to control symptoms in more severe cases.

Surgery itself is another important cause of pain in cancer patients. Cancer patients make up a high proportion of patients undergoing procedures such as thoracotomy, mastectomy and limb amputation which are all recognised to be at high risk for development of persistent pain syndromes. Often these treatments are combined, with patients undergoing adjuvant chemo- or radiotherapy, both of which are risk factors for persistent surgical pain. The perioperative management of surgical pain and its implications are addressed later in this chapter (see Sect. 10.7).

10.4 Pain Pathways

10.4.1 Overview of Ascending and Descending Pain Pathways

The pain pathway is the neuroanatomical tract responsible for the transduction of sensory stimuli to the sensation of pain. Chemical and mechanical stimuli are transduced into electrical signals by specialised nociceptors on the free nerve endings of primary sensory afferent fibres (A™ and c fibres). The action potential generated then passes up the nerve fibre and is transmitted to the cell body in the dorsal root ganglion, before being transmitted to the dorsal horn of the spinal cord, terminating in lamina I, II and V. Here the primary afferents synapse with second-order neurones, which decussate before ascending in the contralateral spinothalamic tract to the ventral posterolateral (VPL) nucleus in the thalamus. Third-order neurones then project from this nucleus in the thalamus to the primary somatosensory cortex (see Fig. 10.5), giving rise to the conscious perception of pain in relation to its anatomical site and character.

The spinoparabrachial tract is responsible for the cognitive-affective component of pain. Like the spinothalamic tract, the spinoparabrachial tract also arises from the dorsal horn where the primary sensory afferents synapse with a second-order neurone. The spinoparabrachial tract ascends and has connections with several higher structures including the ventromedial hypothalamus, amygdala, anterior cingulate and medial pre-frontal cortices. It is the spinoparabrachial tract which is thought to convey emotional aspects of pain which makes pain "unpleasant".

A descending system is responsible for suppressing pain, through modulation and inhibition of ascending signals at the level of the dorsal horn in the spinal cord. The structures involved in this descending system include the limbic system, anterior cingulate cortex, amygdala, the periaqueductal gray and the rostral ventral medulla (see Fig. 10.5, above). If anxiety, fear and sleeplessness feed into the limbic

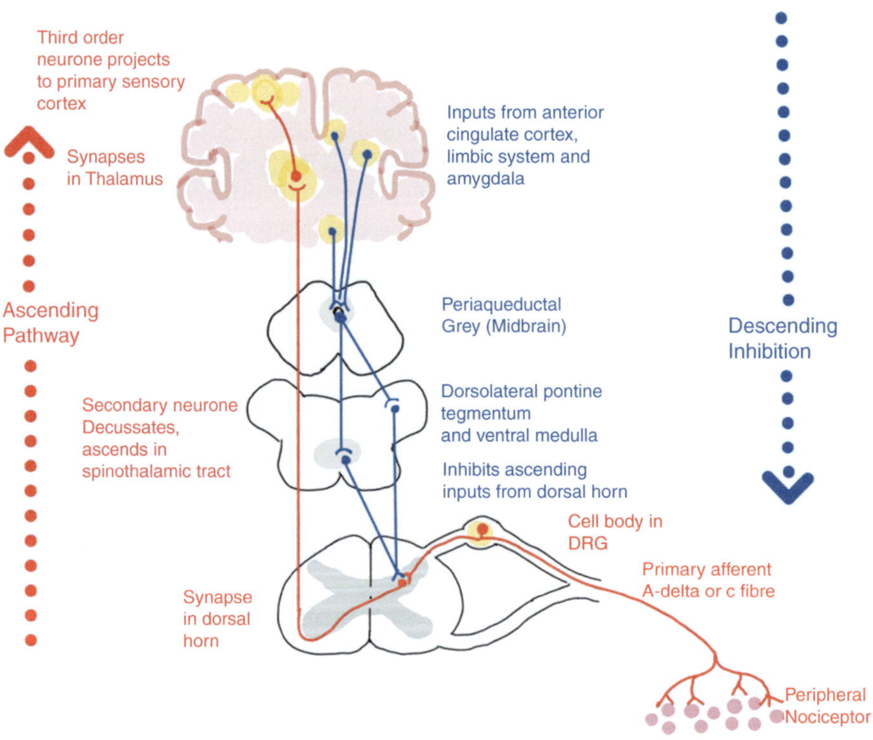

Fig. 10.5 Overview of the pain pathways

system and cortex, descending modulation and inhibition are reduced, and the result is an increase in pain.

10.4.2 Interaction between Cancer Cells and Pain Pathway

Cancer cells are highly metabolically active tissue, when metabolic activity outstrips nutrient and oxygen supply areas of necrosis develop. Cancer cells can actively secrete a range of pro-inflammatory, pain-inducing chemicals into their local environment including tumour necrosis factor-α, interleukins and nerve growth factor. The local inflammatory response recruits lymphocytes and macrophages, which secrete further pro-inflammatory substances into the local interstitium including histamine, interleukins, prostaglandins, leukotrienes, hydrogen ions, potassium ions, bradykinin and adenosine triphosphate [2]. This inflammatory "sensitising soup" results in peripheral sensitisation by lowering the threshold potential at peripheral nociceptors, increasing the likelihood that a stimulus will give rise to an action potential and be perceived as pain. The local tissue oedema resulting further impedes oxygen and nutrient supply, resulting in further necrosis and inflammation.

The tumour itself may cause direct mechanical compression of free nerve endings or axons by mass effect. This either causes direct stimulation of the mechanoreceptors at the free nerve endings, or damages the nerve fibre by compressing its blood supply, the vasa nervorum, both of which lead to neuropathic pain. Damage to nervous tissue can lead to peripheral sensitisation lowering the threshold at which an action potential will be generated. Central sensitisation can also occur at the level of the dorsal horn through NMDA receptor activation, which blocks descending inhibition from inhibitory interneurons and results in an overall gain in afferent signals. When put together this results in a greater number of inputs to higher centres; non-painful stimuli are perceived as painful (allodynia) and painful stimuli are perceived as more painful (hyperalgesia). Put simply, this central and peripheral wind-up of pain pathways caused by pro-inflammatory mediators and direct mass effect results in the cancer patient feeling more pain.

10.5 Treatment of Cancer Pain

Analgesic drugs including the WHO analgesic ladder [8] remain the mainstay of the management of cancer pain. Other treatment strategies such as disease-modifying treatments, anaesthetic interventions, surgery, psychological, physiotherapeutic and spiritual interventions have an important role in some patients [9].

10.5.1 WHO Analgesic Ladder

The WHO analgesic ladder [8] (Fig. 10.6) was developed in 1986 and disseminated worldwide. It remains the cornerstone of management, with the choice of drug

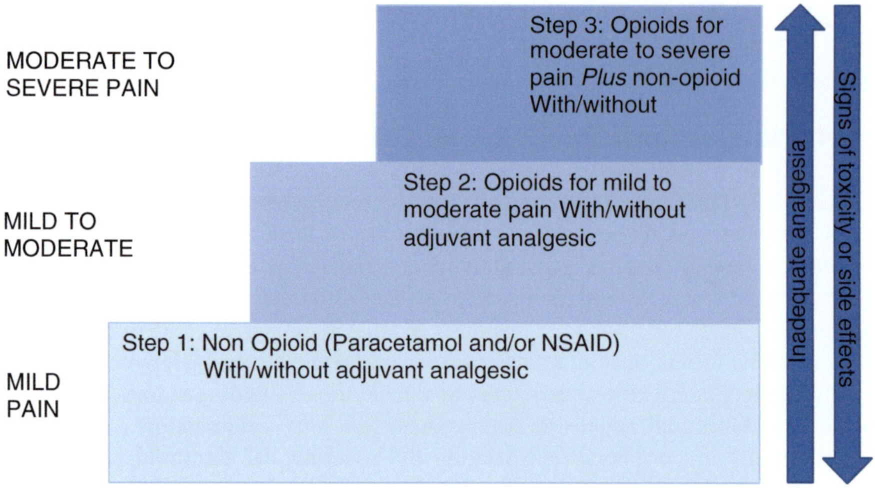

Fig. 10.6 The WHO analgesic ladder for cancer pain. Adapted from *WHO guidelines for the use of analgesics in cancer pain.* V Ventafridda, L Saita et al. Int J Tissue React. 1985;7(1):93–6

being based on the severity of the pain and not the stage of the disease. Drugs should be given in standard doses, at regular intervals. Patients should be started on an analgesic that is appropriate to the type and severity of their pain. In patients presenting with severe pain, it is recommended that patients are started on a combination of paracetamol and/or NSAID with an opioid such as oral morphine (i.e. step 3 below) to try and control symptoms. However, a more cautious approach may be required in patients who are opioid naïve and elderly. A patient who is on maximum dose codeine (240 mg per 24 h) is receiving the equivalent of 24 mg oral morphine per day. A patient requiring this amount of weak opioid will probably be able to tolerate a strong opioid without adverse events, but an opioid naïve elderly patient may have significant side effects even from low doses of strong opioids, so it may be prudent to start with a weaker opioid such as codeine in these cases.

10.5.2 Pharmacological: Opioids

Opioid medications, when titrated appropriately, can provide effective analgesia in approximately 70% of patients with cancer pain [5]. A wide variety of routes of administration may be utilised (see Fig. 10.7), but the oral route is usually preferred unless a patient is unable to tolerate taking tablets. Morphine remains the most commonly prescribed opioid for patients with severe pain, probably due to familiarity, availability and price. Comparative trials for opioids in cancer pain are difficult to perform due to the heterogeneous population and ethical considerations [4], so head-to-head data is very limited. The balance between efficacy and side effects varies amongst opioids due to pharmacokinetics, routes of administration and absorption and genetic variability in responses and drug metabolism [9]. The initial

	Examples	Distinguishing Features	Cautions	Formulation	Suggested initial dose
Weak opioids	Codeine	useful as anti-pertussive/ alleviating SOB	variable metabolism via CYP2D6 constipating	Oral tablets and liquid, injectable	30mg 4-6H (IR) 60mg 12H (CR)
	Tramadol	less constipating, affects neurotransmission at serotonin and noradrenaline	drug interactions with antidepressants : SSRIs and TCAs	Oral tablets/capsules (slow or immediate release), injectable	25-50mg 4-6H (IR) 50-100mg 12H (CR)
Strong opioids	Morphine	Gold standard analgesic for severe cancer pain	Active metabolites accumulate in renal failure	Oral tablets (slow or immediate release) and liquid, injectable	5-10mg 4H (IR) 20-30mg 12H (CR)
	Hydromorphone	Useful for patients requiring high dose opioid Less nausea/vomiting/sedating than morphine	Hydromorphone and metabolites may accumulate in renal failure	Oral tablets and liquid, injectable	1-2mg 4H (IR) 2-4mg 12H (CR)
	Oxycodone	Less CNS effects than morphine Combined formulation with naloxone	Accumulates in renal failure	Oral tablets (slow or immediate release) and liquid	5mg 4H (IR) 10-20mg 12H (CR)
	Fentanyl	May be given parenterally Lozenges have rapid onset for breakthrough pain Safer in renal impairment	Very potent-limits usage in opioid naive patients	Transdermal patch, transmucosal lozenge, injectable	12.5-25mcg/hr 72hr patch
	Methadone	Blocks re-uptake noradrenaline and 5HT useful in neuropathic pain No active metabolites	Very prolonged half life Difficult to convert dosing Multiple drug interactions Long QT	Tablet or liquid, injectable	3-5mg 8H
	Buprenorphine	Partial agonist-antagonist Safer in renal impairment Can be given in patches	Fever may increase absorption	Transdermal patch, transmucosal lozenge, injectable	17.5-35mcg/hr patch every 84-96H

Fig. 10.7 Opioids used in the treatment of cancer pain

choice of opioid should be based on the assessment of the individual, which route of administration is preferred, and the basic pharmacology and properties of the drug. The latter is particularly important for patients with renal impairment, due to accumulation of drug and metabolites. Fentanyl, alfentanil, hydromorphone and buprenorphine are usually the preferred drugs in these patients, but all require careful monitoring.

10.5.2.1 Initiation and Dose Titration

When a strong opioid such as morphine is initiated, the dose must be titrated to effect. One method to achieve this is to prescribe a regular dose of morphine with a rapid onset and short duration of action (such as oramorph). This is taken every four hours, with additional "extra" doses of the same amount given for breakthrough pain as required [4]. After one or two days the total daily dose requirement can be calculated, and the regular dose can be adjusted accordingly until pain relief is satisfactory. The regular four hourly dose required to do this can vary hugely from 5–10 mg to in excess of 200 mg. Prescribing oral morphine 5–10 mg every 4 h in opioid naïve patients without renal impairment is a reasonable starting point.

Once the required dose has been established, it may be more convenient to switch to controlled-release preparation taken every once or twice daily for maintenance, with additional doses of immediate-release preparation (usually 1/6th of the total required daily dose) prescribed as needed for breakthrough pain. Patients with advancing disease usually have escalating pain, and the analgesic dose requirements should be reviewed frequently to make sure pain relief is adequate. Conversely, patients who have a reduced burden of disease following surgery, chemotherapy or radiotherapy may have improved pain, and their dose may need to be reduced to minimise side effects.

10.5.2.2 Routes of Administration

When a patient is unable to take medication by mouth, other routes of administration should be considered. For patients already established on oral morphine, the rectal route may be appropriate, as the rectal bioavailability of morphine is very similar to oral bioavailability [4], so the same dose regime may be continued, and the need to switch to an alternative opioid is avoided. Alternatively, a different opioid that can be administered transdermally such as fentanyl or buprenorphine may be utilised in patients. Oral lozenges (fentanyl, buprenorphine) can be used in this case for breakthrough pain. For some patients, it may be more convenient to convert to parenteral administration via a subcutaneous infusion with a portable syringe driver. Subcutaneous administration is generally preferred over intravenous administration in this context, as it avoids the need for intravenous cannulation, which can be difficult and also painful for the patient. The maintenance dose of oral morphine should be halved to get the equianalgesic dose of subcutaneous morphine required. Conversion factors to oral morphine equivalent for commonly used opioids are outlined in Fig. 10.8, below.

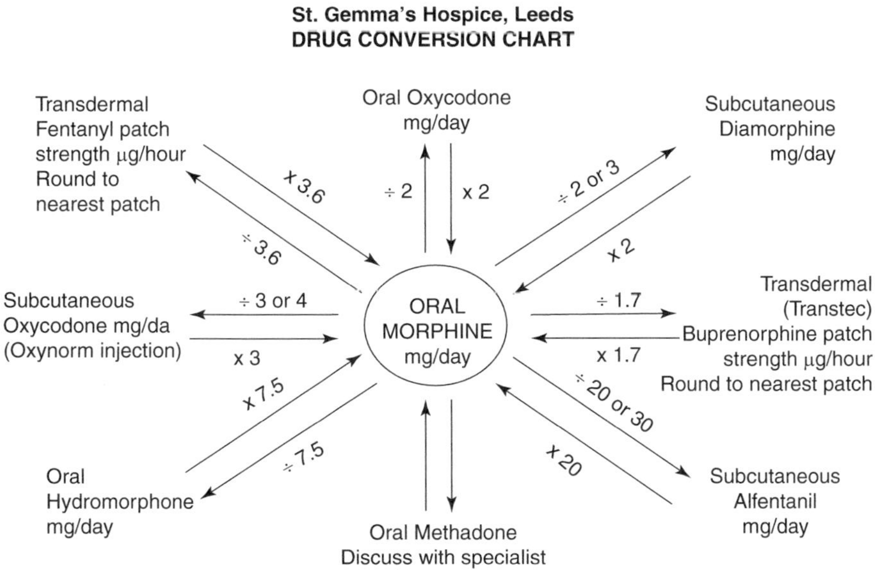

Fig. 10.8 Equivalent analgesic doses, *Pharmacotherapy for cancer pain.* Oxberry SG, Simpson KH. CEACCP 2005; 5(6): 203–206

10.5.2.3 Opioid Rotation

If patients have inadequate pain control or develop adverse side effects prior to effective pain control, opioid rotation is sometimes considered to see if an alternative opioid may be more effective, or better tolerated [9]. Broadly these patients fall into two groups (see Fig. 10.9):

Patients recently initiated on an opioid who fail to achieve adequate analgesia ("morphine non-responders") or have dose-limiting side effects.

Patients who have been established on opioid for some time, but have escalating dose requirements due to disease progression or drug tolerance.

Opioid tolerance describes the reduction in both clinical efficacy and central side effects of a drug. As such patients require progressively higher doses to maintain good control of their pain. If the tolerance to the analgesic action develops disproportionally to the tolerance of side effects, the side effects that result from higher doses needed for effective analgesia, and may limit the dose tolerated. Opioid cross-tolerance is thought to be incomplete, due to different mu-opioid receptor subtypes, and the varying action of each opioid at each of these subtypes. Thus if a patient develops tolerance to one opioid, e.g. morphine, switching to an alternative opioid may have a better analgesic side effect profile based on their different actions at the varying subtypes of mu-opioid receptor.

Trial data in this area is limited, with most data coming from open studies or small case series, however, it has been suggested 50–80% of patients will achieve a clinical improvement after opioid switching [9]. The reasons why some patients will respond to one opioid in preference to another is still not well understood, but

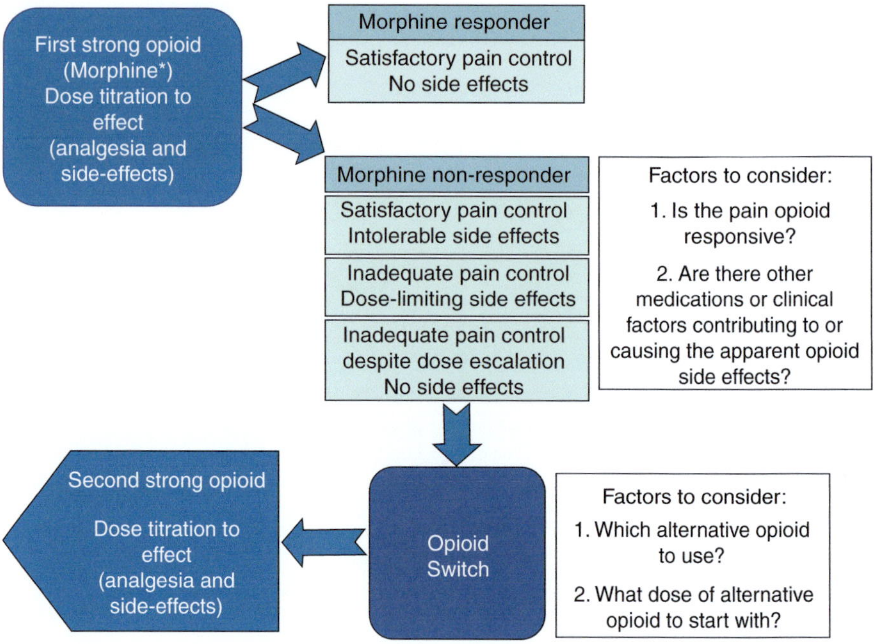

Fig. 10.9 Considerations in opioid rotation, *Differences between opioids: pharmacological, experimental, clinical and economical perspectives*

it is thought likely related to inter-individual genetic differences in pharmacokinetics and pharmacodynamics. One of the potential benefits of opioid switching is it may allow effective analgesia at a lower equivalent dose, for this reason, the equivalent dose is often reduced by 30–50% when switching to a different opioid.

AM Drewes, RD Jensen, et al. Br J Clin Pharmacol. 2013 Jan; 75(1): 60–78.

10.5.2.4 Adverse Effects

The adverse effects of opioids are well recognised. Up to 80% of patients taking opioids for cancer pain will experience unwanted side effects [2]. These side effects include drowsiness, nausea, constipation and dry mouth. Side effects are usually worse during the first few days of therapy and settle over the first week [5]. Drowsiness will often settle, though if sedation remains problematic it should be treated with either dose reduction, opioid rotation, or a stimulant medication such as methylphenidate. Side effects such as nausea and vomiting should be minimised by prophylactic treatment with regular antiemetics such as cyclizine, ondansetron or metoclopramide. Constipation is very often persistent, and patients started on opioids should also be prescribed a regular laxative. Dry mouth can be troublesome to patients, though is often overlooked, but can be successfully treated with simple measures such as frequent cold drinks, ice chips or an artificial saliva spray.

Less common side effects include confusion, hallucinations, itch and ventilatory depression. If side effects continue to be problematic, dose reduction, opioid rotation or co-administration of a specific antagonist such as naloxone may be useful. The combination of confusion, agitation, vivid dreams, and visual and auditory hallucinations should alert healthcare providers to the diagnosis of opioid toxicity [4], which should be managed by dose reduction, low-dose haloperidol to treat agitation, and ensuring adequate hydration status. Problems such as opioid dependency and addiction are thankfully rare in cancer patients, when opioids are prescribed appropriately.

10.5.3 Pharmacological: Non-opioids

Non-opioid medications used in the treatment of cancer pain include paracetamol, non-steroidal anti-inflammatory drugs (NSAIDs), antidepressants, anticonvulsants, ketamine, topical capsaicin, corticosteroids and bisphosphonates (see Fig. 10.10.)

The term "adjuvant analgesic" is used to describe a drug whose primary indication is for something other than pain, but has useful analgesic properties in treating some pain conditions. Rather than simply adopting the WHO approach, which treats "adjuvants" as optional, there is increasing evidence for the benefit of routinely combining opioids with these other pharmacological agents for synergistic effects, reducing opioid requirement and toxicity [10]. In the context of cancer-related pain, these drugs can be further grouped into two broad categories:

- Drugs used to treat neuropathic pain where opioids have been inadequate, e.g. antidepressants, anticonvulsants, ketamine.
- Drugs used to target a specific cancer pain syndrome, e.g. bone pain, pain from an obstructed viscus, capsular pain, muscle spasms.

10.5.3.1 Simple Analgesics: Paracetamol and NSAIDS

Analgesics such as paracetamol and NSAIDs are typically utilised in the early stages of the WHO analgesic ladder, and have been shown to improve pain control when given in combination with an opioid, compared to using opioids alone [11]. Paracetamol is a simple, cheap, and well-tolerated analgesic, which is the first step of the WHO ladder [8]. It is rapidly absorbed following oral administration, though rectal and parenteral routes can be used if the patient is unable to take medications orally. Although it is effective when given alone for mild pain, in cancer pain paracetamol is more often used in combination with weak or strong opioids. The number needed to treat (NNT) for paracetamol is around 3.6 in the acute pain setting, but when co-administered with opioids it increases their analgesic efficacy [11]. Although the mechanism of action is still not fully understood, it is thought to inhibit central prostaglandin synthesis, without affecting peripheral cyclo-oxygenase receptors, so it has fewer side effects than other anti-inflammatory agents.

Non-steroidal anti-inflammatory drugs (NSAIDs) may be used alone or alongside paracetamol as a first step on the WHO ladder for mild pain [8]. Their utilisation alongside a weak or strong opioid had also been shown to increase the efficacy of analgesia in patients with cancer pain in meta-analyses [11]. NSAIDs act

Drug	Example(s)	Indication(s)
Paracetamol	-	Mild to moderate pain, co-administration with opioids
NSAIDs	Ibuprofen, Diclofenac COX-2 inhibitors	Bone pain,Soft tissue infiltration Hepatomegaly
Antidepressants	Amitriptyline Venlafaxine	Nerve compression or infiltration Paraneoplastic neuropathies
Anticonvulsants	Gabapentin, Pregabalin Carbamazepine	Nerve compression or infiltration, Paraneoplastic neuropathies Chemo-induced neuropathy
NMDA receptor antagonists	Ketamine	Opioid reduction in severe refractory pain
Topical therapies	Capsaicin	Post-surgical neuropathic pain
Corticosteroids	Dexamethasone	Liver capsular pain, cerebral metastases
Bisphosphonates	Pamidronate Zoledronic acid	Bone Pain

Fig. 10.10 Non-opioid medications used in the treatment of cancer pain

through inhibition of the cyclo-oxygenase pathway to reduce the production of prostacycline (PGI2) and prostaglandins (such as PGE2), which mediate pain and the pro-inflammatory response through production of cytokines and migration of leukocytes (see Fig. 10.11). However, cyclo-oxygenase enzymes also have important housekeeping functions including protection of the GI tract (via PGE2), kidneys (PGI2 and PGE2) and platelet function (thromboxane A2). Non-specific inhibition of this pathway therefore leads to predictable side effects such as gastric ulceration and renal dysfunction. Patients should be prescribed gastric protection such as a proton pump inhibitor (e.g. omeprazole) prophylactically to reduce the risk of gastric ulcers.

Newer agents such as celecoxib specifically inhibit the COX-2 isoenzyme, which is considered the inducible isoenzyme during painful stimuli. This selectivity spares the inhibition of COX-1, which is thought to be constitutive in the GI tract and required for normal gastrointestinal function, hence these drugs have a more favourable side effect profile. Nevertheless they have still been implicated in causing renal impairment, and one agent, rofecoxib, has been withdrawn because of cardiovascular risks, so caution is needed when using other drugs of the same class.

10.5.3.2 Treatment of Neuropathic Pain

Adjuvant analgesics may be particularly useful in the treatment of neuropathic pain, which may be a result of the disease process or a side effect from cancer treatments. There is an absence of high-quality evidence specific to treating tumour-related neuropathic pain, although decades of experience and efficacy data from antidepressant use in non-cancer neuropathic syndromes suggest a trial of therapy for patients

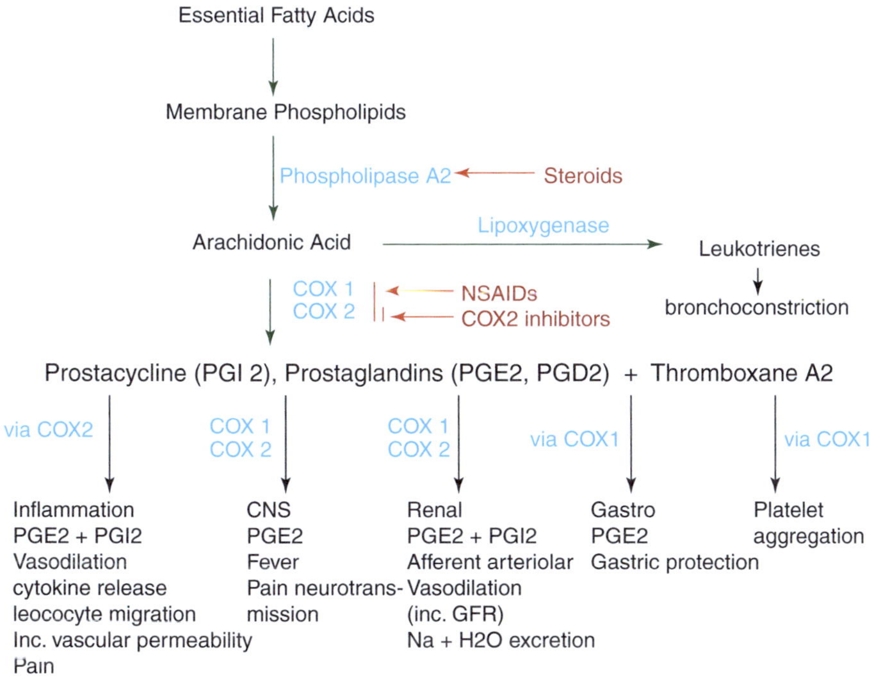

Fig. 10.11 Mechanism of action and side effects of steroids and NSAIDs

with cancer-related neuropathic pain, not adequately controlled by conventional analgesics (i.e. opioids in combination with paracetamol and/or NSAIDs). Two of the most commonly utilised groups of medications which fall into this category are antidepressants and anticonvulsants.

10.5.3.3 Antidepressants

Older, less specific antidepressants such as tricyclics seem more effective in the treatment of neuropathic pain than newer classes of antidepressants [5] such as selective serotonin reuptake inhibitors (SSRIs), which target fewer receptor types. The NNT for 50% reduction of pain compared to placebo for amitriptyline (a tricyclic antidepressant) is 2–3 for most pain conditions compared to 6–7 for SSRIs. Venlafaxine (which inhibits the reuptake of both serotonin and noradrenaline) has less evidence than tricyclics, but can also be useful particularly for patients in whom low mood and neuropathic pain co-exist. The benefit in analgesia with antidepressants seems to occur even without an effect on mood, but as depression and difficulty sleeping often co-exist with poorly controlled pain effects on mood and help with sleep are both useful. The starting dose should be low (e.g. amitriptyline 10 mg) and is usually taken at night. Side effects are common, and often limit the use of tricyclics [4], they include sedation, blurred vision, and dry mouth, but at higher doses, postural hypotension, cardiac arrhythmias, urinary and sexual problems can occur, although this is less common.

10.5.3.4 Anticonvulsants

Like antidepressants, there is no strong evidence to advocate the use of anticonvulsants in the treatment of cancer-related neuropathic pain; however, there is a strong body of evidence that supports their use in non-cancer-related neuropathic pain conditions [5]. Drugs which are frequently used in this context include gabapentin, pregabalin, carbamazepine and sodium valproate [4]. Carbamazepine is the agent of choice in patients with trigeminal neuralgia (for tumours compressing the trigeminal nerve), with NNT of 2–3. Gabapentin and pregabalin both have anti-hyperalgesic and anti-allodynic properties in a variety of neuropathic pain syndromes, and trials have demonstrated up to 30% of patients achieve a 50% reduction in the pain compared to placebo [5]. Like antidepressants, the use of anticonvulsants may be limited by side effects, which are frequent and include dizziness and somnolence. Antidepressants may be used in combination with anticonvulsants to treat neuropathic pain, but given the lack of data regarding their efficacy specific to cancer pain it is good practice to introduce one agent at a time, and discontinue it if there is no improvement in analgesia.

10.5.3.5 Ketamine

Ketamine is an N-methyl-d-aspartate (NMDA) receptor antagonist. NMDA receptors are important in the modulation of ascending pain pathways at the level of the dorsal horn in the spinal cord. Ketamine has been utilised in chronic pain to treat a variety of pain syndromes such as central pain, and pain associated with nerve trauma or spinal cord injury, which are refractory to high-dose opioids. It may be administered by a variety of different routes including orally, intravenously and subcutaneously. Data on the efficacy of ketamine in the treatment of cancer pain is very limited. A Cochrane review from 2017 [12] found insufficient evidence to comment on the benefits and harm in using ketamine as an adjunct to opioids in cancer pain. Nevertheless, ketamine is occasionally used in refractory cancer pain as an adjuvant analgesic for its opioid-sparing benefits [10], particularly in patients who may have opioid-induced hyperalgesia. Limiting its use are significant side effects, which include sedation, delirium and hallucinations, especially at higher doses.

10.5.3.6 Topical Therapies

Capsaicin is the ingredient in chilli peppers which produces its "heat". When applied to the skin, it causes depolarisation of nociceptors and release of substance P. With repeated application stores of substance P within the nociceptors become deleted, leading to decreased pain perception. This is useful in patients with neuropathic pain causing hyperalgesia or allodynia. Trials have shown capsaicin cream is effective in reducing post-surgical neuropathic pain, for instance following mastectomy [10]. Application is required 3–4 times daily of 0.025% or 0.075% cream. It may cause severe burning pain initially (related to the release of substance P from nociceptors), so may be better tolerated if preceded by application of a topical local anaesthetic or oral analgesia.

10.5.3.7 Treatment of Bone Pain

Bone pain is a common problem in palliative care, a population which is likely distinct to that undergoing prehabilitation prior to cancer surgery. Radiotherapy is usually considered when bone pain is focal. Multifocal bone pain may benefit from adjuvant treatment with an NSAID, corticosteroid or bisphosphonates [10]. Bisphosphonates inhibit osteoclast activity, and hence reduce bone resorption in a variety of illnesses. Their analgesic efficacy is well established in a variety of cancers.

10.5.4 Interventional Approaches

Cancer pain management by medicines alone might be challenging and a substantial number of cancer patients do not achieve effective pain control with medication alone. Interventional pain management can complement this. There are various interventions used in managing this pain across the globe. The techniques depend on the site, type and stage of cancer along with limitations with risks, complications, resources and costs involved. The main role of these techniques is to target the neural pathways—either temporarily or making it permanent. The temporary solutions might involve blocks with local anaesthetics, neurolytic substances, etc., whilst the permanent solutions might come in the form of neurodestructive techniques—radiofrequency, thermal coagulation, cryofreezing, cordotomies, surgical destruction, etc. Destructive techniques aim to cause irreversible conduction block by physical disruption of nervous tissue. Non-destructive techniques use pharmacological agents or electrical stimulation to achieve reversible conduction block. However, patient selection with multidisciplinary pain management can offer the best solutions for patients. All interventions designed to relieve cancer pain carry attendant risk, and these must be weighed against potential benefits. Overall, 8% of patients with cancer pain may require nerve blocks, 3% neurolytic blocks and 3% neuraxial techniques.

10.5.4.1 Methods of Nervous Tissue Destruction

10.5.4.1.1 Pharmacological

The agents most commonly used for this purpose are 50–100% alcohol and 3–12% phenol, although ammonium salts and glycerol may occasionally still feature.

Alcohol causes intense pain on injection, and can be mixed with local anaesthetic to mitigate this. It causes dehydration of axons, extraction and precipitation of membrane proteins, cerebrosides, and cholesterol, leading to oedema and sclerosis of the myelin sheath and axonal damage. It is hypobaric when injected intrathecally.

Phenol causes protein precipitation and axonal damage in a similar manner. It is more viscous and diffuses less freely through tissues than alcohol, and has a local anaesthetic effect, causing a sensation of warmth followed by numbness. Like local anaesthetics, overdose may lead to cerebral and cardiovascular toxicity, and doses are generally limited to <1 g for a single procedure. Unlike alcohol, it is believed to have a greater affinity for vascular than neural tissue, and may be made hyperbaric relative to cerebrospinal fluid when prepared in oil.

Ammonium salts cause a non-specific axonopathy but are used less commonly due to doubts about effectiveness. Glycerol can be applied to the gasserian (trigeminal) ganglion to cause axonolysis and demyelination.

10.5.4.1.2 Radiofrequency Current

By passing an alternating current of 50–500 kHz through tissues, resultant molecular oscillation causes a heating effect which can be used to ablate peripheral and central sensory pathways. Current is concentrated at the uninsulated needle tip, causing very localised heating of up to 5 mm around the distal 5–10 mm of the radiofrequency needle. Precision of needle placement is therefore vital. In conventional radiofrequency, the needle tip is heated to 80–90 °C for 60–90 s, with temperature monitored via a thermocouple. In pulsed radiofrequency, the temperature is kept below 43 °C (above this, most mammalian proteins begin to denature and tissue damage occurs) by the use of 2 Hz, 20 ms pulses of alternating current for 3–5 min. This is considered less effective than continuous radiofrequency by many experts, but as no tissue damage occurs, dysaesthesias, motor block and deafferentation pain syndromes are not considered a problem with this technique. Its mode of action is unknown, but appears to disrupt axonal electrical transmission and may have an immunomodulatory effect.

10.5.4.1.3 Surgical

Peripheral and central neural tissues may be divided surgically, but in practice, such procedures are rarely performed. Examples include midline myelotomy (creating a segmental midline incision in the spinal cord to interrupt decussating spinothalamic fibres) for pelvic visceral cancer pain, and dorsal root entry zone lesioning.

10.5.4.1.4 Non-destructive Techniques

Local anaesthetic with or without steroid may be deposited or infused around nerves to cause reversible conduction block and pain relief. Peripheral nerve, peripheral field or spinal cord stimulation may be used in the cancer pain setting to modulate nociceptive traffic.

10.5.4.1.5 Injection into Tissues and Joints

Injections into soft tissue and joints are often performed in the management of common chronic non-cancer pain syndromes, such as myofascial pain or painful arthropathy. A patient with cancer who develops one of these painful conditions should be considered a candidate for the appropriate intervention, as long as they do not have a contraindication (e.g., coagulopathy or leukopenia, pneumothorax), and the decision to proceed or not should be based on a careful assessment of benefits, risks, alternative treatments and the overall goals of care.

10.5.4.1.6 Somatic Blocks

These involve peripheral nerve or plexus blocks in similar manner to temporary peripheral blocks, but with different agents, e.g. brachial, lumbar, paravertebral and nerve root blocks. These could give pain relief for around 3 weeks when phenol is used.

10.5.4.1.7 Visceral Blocks

Most visceral innervation is via the autonomic nervous system, with pain fibres in both sympathetic and parasympathetic nerves. Depending on the area of cancer, various plexus can be targeted, e.g. coeliac, superior hypogastric plexus, etc.

10.5.4.2 Central Blocks

These are usually in the form of use of pharmacological agents as single shot (phenol or alcohol) or infusion of agents via intrathecal/epidural catheters. With use of neurolytic solutions, there is risk of motor block and limit sensory loss in areas unaffected by pain. Especially disruption of motor function to bladder, bowel and lower limb limit the use of these treatments at times. There are also intrathecal drug delivery (ITDD) systems using various agents including opioids, ziconotide (a presynaptic calcium channel blocker). These can be completely external devices or implantable devices—depending on the longevity of life, etc.

10.5.4.3 Percutaneous Cervical Cordotomy

This technique involves creating a precise radiofrequency lesion in the lateral spinothalamic tract at the C1/2 level contralateral to the side of the pain, interrupting decussated second-order pain fibres and selectively abolishing pain and temperature sensation from the affected half of the body. Owing to some second-order spinothalamic fibres decussating several spinal segments above or below their distal synaptic connections, cordotomy may only reliably be used to treat pain below the level of the C4 dermatome (i.e. below the clavicle). It is usually achieved percutaneously using radiofrequency current, but open surgical approaches are possible. It is effective, with 83% of patients undergoing the procedure able to halve their opioids, and 38% to stop them completely [13]. It is used mainly for refractory chest wall pain secondary to mesothelioma and occasionally for pancoast tumours, but theoretically may have a place in any unilateral cancer pain below C4. Predicted survival should be less than 2 years, as deafferentation pain and unpleasant and untreatable dysaesthesias may occur after this time period.

10.5.5 Psychological and Physical

Pain is one of the most frequently feared and experienced symptoms for cancer patients and pain that is inadequately managed has a significant negative impact on patients' well-being and overall quality of life. The impact of grief reactions, concurrent treatment, prognosis, and social circumstance all have a significant impact on the individuals' experience of pain and feed into a complex bio-psycho-social model which makes pain problems challenging both to quantify and to treat. A patient's own beliefs, misconceptions, fears, and societal stigma around both pain and its treatments present a significant barrier to patients seeking help to successfully manage their pain. Interventions that are targeted to increase a patient's own knowledge and support them in managing their own condition can go some way towards overcoming these difficulties.

10.5.5.1 Self-Management

Self-management of cancer pain can be defined as "the process in which patients with cancer pain make the decision to manage their pain, enhance their self-efficacy by solving problems caused by the pain and incorporate pain-relieving strategies into daily life" [14]. When successful, this approach empowers the patient in the development of their own strategies that are unique to each individual. The focus of self-management is on improving the level of function and quality of life, alongside attempts to reduce the intensity of pain experienced. Lorig and Holman [15] described three main tasks or pillars of self-management, which are summarised in Fig. 10.12 below.

Patients will require the support of health professionals to achieve these tasks and reach their own goals. Self-management interventions assume the patient is an active part of the process, with an emphasis on the application of knowledge and skills to treat one's own condition, rather than the mere provision of knowledge of skills. In order to empower patients with problem-solving skills, self-management interventions should:

- increase patients' skills and confidence,
- include regular assessments of problems and progress towards solutions,

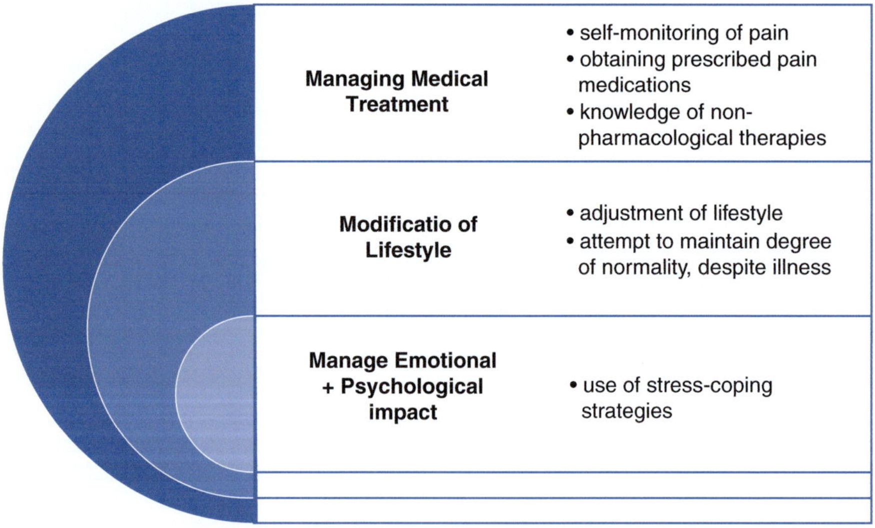

Fig. 10.12 Tasks in the self-management of cancer pain

- utilise goal setting.
- provide problem-solving support.

10.5.5.2 Theoretical Framework

Michie et al. [16] created a framework for characterising and designing behaviour change interventions. Their work suggests that behaviour change interventions work by affecting change in one or more of three key domains to bring about a change in behaviour. Figure 10.13 below describes how an individual's capability "C", opportunities "O" and motivation "M", interact to generate behaviour "B", which is described as the "COM-B" system.

10.5.5.3 Interventions to Support Cancer Pain Self-Management

Self-management interventions should focus on patients' knowledge and skills (enhancing "capability") and attitudes (enhancing "motivation"). Complex interventions that target all three domains (capability, motivation and opportunity) have been shown to be more efficacious reducing pain intensity than those targeting only two areas [17]. Interventions must include the following key components:

1. *Individualised, patient-centred care:* Pain is a complex, individualised experience, so the intervention must be patient centred, focusing on areas that will have a significant impact on that individual's quality of life. Education and training should be individualised to each patient's needs and knowledge gaps.
2. *Address patient's knowledge, skills and attitudes towards their pain:* Aim to improve the patients' and carers' knowledge and skills and encourage a positive attitude towards managing pain. Provide information on the nature of pain, phar-

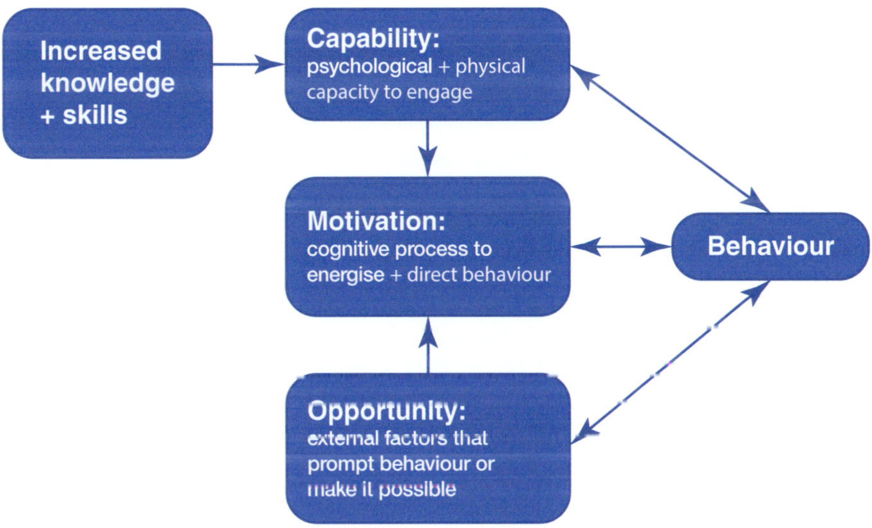

Fig. 10.13 The COM-B system—a framework for understanding behaviour, adapted from *The Behaviour Change Wheel: a new method for characterising and designing behaviour change interventions.* S Michie, M van Stralen & R West. Implementation science (2011): IS. 6.42

macological and non-pharmacological management techniques. Education on optimal timing of medication doses, involving care-givers to increase adherence to analgesic regimes.

3. *Enablement approach:* Increasing means and reducing barriers to optimise the patient's capability to manage their pain. Ensuring active patient engagement through participation in decision making. Improving patient communication by providing patients with prompt lists of questions, provision of a helpline, and improving knowledge of when and how to seek additional medical advice.
4. *Healthcare providers as educators*: Clinicians should receive appropriate training in how to educate patients on self-management. Pain specialists, specialist nurses and palliative care physicians and nurse are often highly skilled in this area.

10.5.5.4 Integrating Self-Management Support into Routine Clinical Practice

Integration of self-management support into existing clinical practice requires clinicians to have the knowledge to design interventions that are compatible within existing clinical frameworks. Pain assessment, re-assessment and identification of any barriers to effective management should be a routine part of each consultation with a cancer patient. Additional support and advice should be provided to patients depending on their varying needs, which requires cooperation,integration and strong communication within the whole multi-disciplinary team; including pre-assessment, pain specialists, oncologists, surgeons, specialist nurses, psychologists and palliative care.

10.5.5.5 Cancer Pain Outcomes

Evidence of efficacy of self-management interventions has been largely evaluated based on a reduction of pain intensity on a numerical rating scale. By this measure, a systematic review of 26 randomised control trials [18] found only one-third of self-management interventions to be efficacious. There was however evidence to suggest improvement in patient knowledge, self-efficacy, and adherence to medications, despite lack of effect of numerical pain rating scales. Future studies should focus potentially on more patient-centred outcomes such as improvements in quality of life or functional status, rather than solely on pain intensity, areas which may be of greater importance to patients in their day-to-day lives.

10.5.6 Complementary Treatments

Complementary therapies are integral to many cancer care treatments. They offer holistic management and boost the overall behaviour and attitude of cancer patients. These have been used along with medical management to boost the overall well-being. The common ones used are massage, aromatherapy, spas and acupuncture.

10.6 Acute Cancer Pain Syndromes and their Management

10.6.1 Tumour-Related Nociceptive Pain Including Bone Pain and Visceral Obstruction

If a tumour invades somatic or visceral structures such as bone, muscle or connective tissue, pain can result [19]. Invasion into bone, or distal bony metastases resulting in bone pain is one of the most common pain syndromes in cancer patients. The bony pain may be due to marrow infiltration, invasion of the periosteum, lytic lesions destroying the structural integrity resulting in pathological fractures, or release of chemical mediators that activate nociceptors. The movement of these bones may further worsen pain. If the vertebra are involved, neurological compromise and even spinal cord compression may occur as the disease progresses. Hypercalcaemia caused by the release of bone calcium stores also results in pain. Targeted treatment with bone modifying agents such as bisphosphonates is the first-line treatment for bone pain. Radiotherapy may also be required to target bony metastases and relieve local bone pain. In some situations surgery such as vertebroplasty is required to provide stabilisation and relief of pain, ideally prior to development of pathological fractures. (See also Sect. 10.5.3 Non-opioids, treatment of bone pain).

Invasion into the visceral organs or surrounding connective tissue may cause compression or obstruction of hollow structures, resulting in visceral pain. Malignant bowel obstruction is a common pain syndrome in patients with abdominal or pelvic cancer. Initial management of these patients should involve imaging and evaluation of the cause of obstruction. Chemotherapy and radiotherapy can both be utilised in this setting to reduce tumour mass and relieve obstruction, though commonly surgery may be required either to excise the tumour mass, bypass or stent the obstruction. In the interim bowel rest, NG drainage, anticholinergics, corticosteroids and octreotide can provide symptomatic relief [10].

10.6.2 Tumour-Related Neuropathic Pain

Neuropathic pain may be related to tumour compression or invasion of neural tissues, including compression of nerve, plexus, roots or spinal cord [19] (from vertebral involvement, see above). Timely management of these acute pain syndromes is essential as acute pain in cancer patients induces neuronal remodelling and sensitisation which may progress to chronic pain. Neuropathic pain is typically less responsive to opioid-based analgesia, adjuvant therapy with antidepressants, anticonvulsants or interventional approaches should be considered early.

10.6.3 Chemotherapy Associated Pain Syndromes

Chemotherapy drugs have associated adverse effects, many of which are dose limiting. Drugs such as vincristine, platinum, taxanes, thalidomide and bortezomib are known to cause painful dysesthesias, which may progress to polyneuropathy. Paclitaxel is a plant alkaloid taxane used for breast, ovarian, lung, and head and neck cancers. Paclitaxel-associated acute pain syndrome occurs within days after each dose and steadily increases in severity with increasing total dose. The pain may be generalised, or localised to the large axial muscles in the shoulders, paraspinal regions, pelvis and thighs. Patients with worse paclitaxel-associated acute pain syndrome may progress to chemotherapy-induced peripheral neuropathy.

Mucositis is a painful side effect which affects around 20–40% of patients undergoing cytotoxic chemotherapy. It can lead to several problems including pain, nutritional deficiencies, and increased risk of infection due to open sores. It is characterised by inflammation or ulceration of the mucous membranes anywhere along the GI tract. Good oral care can help prevent or decrease the severity of mucositis, the mainstay of which is mouth rinses. Topical anaesthetics, in gel or spray form, can be used to numb the mouth and ice chips can be placed in the mouth to help treat stomatitis during administration of chemotherapy. Benzydamine, artificial saliva or corticosteroids may also help with mouth pain.

Other chemo-associated pain syndromes include high-dose steroids leading to osteonecrosis, and intra-peritoneal chemotherapy causing acute abdominal pain.

10.6.4 Radiotherapy Associated Pain Syndromes

Many tumours require radiotherapy either as an adjunct to other treatments, or as a primary treatment modality. The tissue toxicity due to radiation exposure depends on the site and dose of radiation. Radiation can result in osteonecrosis of bone causing bony pain (see previous), oral mucositis (head and neck cancer) or an acute abdomen (radiotherapy to the abdomen).

Radiotherapy may result in neuropathy due to the direct effect of radiation in nervous tissue or by causing fibrosis of the surrounding nervous plexus. Radiotherapy for breast cancer and Hodgkin's lymphoma can cause radiation-induced brachial plexopathy. Neurogenic pain is present almost in all cases which can vary from mild to incapacitating. In severe cases surgical exploration with neurolysis should be considered, and may be effective in over 80% of patients with refractory pain, though at the expense of potentially worsening motor function.

10.6.5 Surgical Associated Pain Syndromes

Acute post-surgical pain commonly exists after major cancer surgery and its severity is based on extent and site of surgical intervention [20]. Tissue damage leads to nociceptive pain and nerve injury leads to neuropathic pain. Post-surgical pain syndromes have been described for various specific interventions [18] including post-mastectomy, post-amputation, post-thoracotomy, and post radical neck surgery (see Fig. 10.14.) These pain syndromes are often preceded by acute pain and poorly controlled post-operative pain. Provision of optimal pain control post-operatively

Pain syndrome	Features
Post thoracotomy pain	Results from intercostal nerve injury from rib traction and resection Immediate post-op pain, aching sensation and sensory loss in distribution of incision
Post mastectomy pain	Results from surgical damage to the intercostal brachial nerve. Presentation may be delayed Presents with tight, contracting burning pain in the posterior arm and axilla, radiating across chest wall. Increases with arm movement
Post amputation pain	Pain in distribution of absent limb extremity, often leads to chronic pain
Post radical neck surgery pain	Usually presents late with burning dysasthesia, shock-like shooting and laminating pain

Fig. 10.14 Post-surgical pain syndromes

with regional anaesthesia may reduce the risk of persistent post-surgical pain (see Sect. 10.7 Perioperative implications of pain control).

10.7 Perioperative Implications of Pain Control

Effective preoperative pain control may have additional benefits in the perioperative period such as improving post-operative pain scores and reducing post-operative opioid requirements, although the evidence is limited. Minimising post-operative opioid requirements is desirable, as excessive opioid intake may adversely impact the immune system and even increase the risk of cancer recurrence.

10.7.1 Preoperative Implications of Pain Control

Optimum pain management should begin before surgery. This is a necessity for all of the reasons already discussed, improving levels of physical activity, mood, sleep, quality of life, and enabling participation in prehabilitation programmes. Preoperative pain which is poorly controlled may predict increased levels of post operative pain and increased opioid consumption in the perioperative period, which may, in turn, confer an increased risk of developing persistent post-surgical pain and potentially increased risk of cancer recurrence. Many of the risk factors for poorly controlled post-operative pain are prevalent in the population undergoing cancer surgery and are listed below.

Preoperative assessment of pain is an essential part of perioperative planning and allows patient education regarding potential strategies employed in the perioperative management of their pain. Patients with complex pain issues, such as cancer patients with mixed pain syndromes, or patients on high doses of preoperative opioids can be identified. Liaising with pain specialists and the inpatient pain team at this stage allows development of a plan for optimal pain management in the preoperative period, with appropriate allocation of resources. For instance a patient with complex cancer pain on high-dose opioids preoperatively may require a bed in a high observation area due to potential for opioid tolerance higher dose requirement, which is linked to a higher risk of adverse events. Depending on the type of surgery performed, these patients may also require an alternative route of administration for their baseline opioid requirement, particularly if they cannot resume eating and drinking post-operatively (Table 10.1).

10.7.2 Post-Operative Pain, Enhanced Recovery and Cancer Recurrence

Post-operative pain has well recognised physiological consequences; it increases the neuroendocrine stress response, baseline oxygen requirements, and places cardio-respiratory stress on the body. Poorly controlled post-operative pain is still very common, as the UK Peri-operative Quality Improvement (PQIP) data has shown; almost one in five patients reported severe pain within the first 24 h following surgery [20]. Poorly controlled pain following surgery causes decreased patient satisfaction, delays in mobilisation, delayed discharge, and increased length of stay. Moreover, the intensity and duration of pain experienced increase the likelihood of patients developing chronic or persistent post-surgical pain, which results in longer-term psychological, social and economic adversity.

Optimising post-operative analgesia is an essential part of enhanced recovery (ERAS) pathways. ERAS pathways aim to minimise the post-operative stress response and minimise the time taken for the patient to return to normal function. The adverse effects of opioids in the immediate post-operative period are documented and dose-dependent. Higher doses of opioids are associated with excessive sedation, respiratory complications, and increased nausea and vomiting. The use of multimodal analgesia including regional anaesthesia as part of opioid minimisation is strongly advocated.

High-dose opioids have been implicated in increased risk of cancer recurrence [21]. It has been shown that many different cancer types inherently express

Table 10.1 Risk factors for development of poorly controlled post-operative pain

Patient demographics	Psychological factors	Pre-op pain- related factors	Surgical factors
Female gender	Pre-existing anxiety	Poorly controlled pre-op pain	Extent of surgery/major surgery
Younger age	Depression	Use of pre-op opioids	Abdominal surgery
	Negative affect		Emergent surgery
	Sleep disorders		Surgical technique, extent of nerve damage

mu-opioid receptors, their activation leads to production of factors such as VEG-F which promotes tumour survival, and deletion of the mu-receptor gene within animal models reduces the chance of metastasis [22]. A small study women with advanced breast cancer patients showed taking the opioid antagonist conferred a small advantage in median length of survival [23]. Women whose breast cancer expressed a mutant variant of the mu-receptor gene had reduced analgesia from opioids but prolonged survival from their cancer [24]. It seems biologically plausible high doses of opioids perioperatively may have negative implications for cancer recurrence and survival.

Different pain management strategies may have implications that reach far beyond the hospital stay. Cancer surgery creates a "perfect storm" in which cancer cells are disseminated through the bloodstream and given the opportunity to survive and metastasise [21]. The stress response to surgery causes immunosuppression and release of pro-inflammatory cytokines which increase the chances of cancer cell survival and hence increase the recurrence of a tumour. Over the past decade, there has been an increased research focus on how different anaesthetic techniques impact this response. Figure 10.15 below summarises the impact of anaesthetic technique on possible cancer recurrence [21].

Opioid reduction strategies within ERAS protocols, such as utilisation of NSAIDs and regional anaesthesia, may additionally lower the risk of cancer

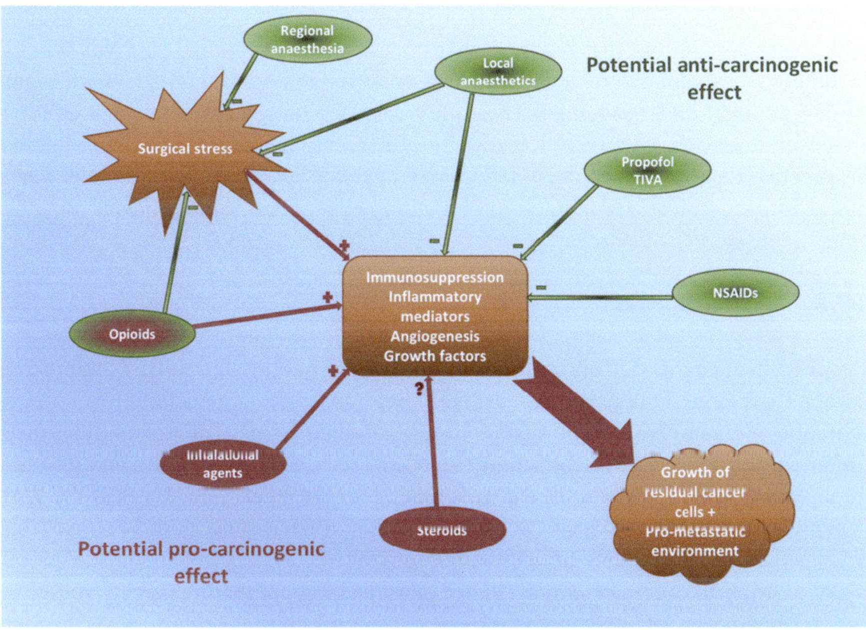

Fig. 10.15 Summary of the potential impact of commonly used anaesthetic agents upon cancer progression, metastasis and recurrence. *The impact of anaesthetic technique upon outcome in oncological surgery.* M.T. Evans,T. Wigmore and L.J.S. Kelliher. BJA Educ. 2019;19(1):14–20

recurrence. As detailed previously, NSAIDs act via their inhibition of the cyclo-oxygenase (COX) enzymes that produce prostaglandins. The net effect of prostaglandins on the immune response is to increase interleukins 4, 6 and 10, reduce TNFa, and inhibit NK cell activity [22]. These actions favour the progression of neoplasia, whilst allowing it to evade the host's innate immune defence. The use of NSAIDS to inhibit COX, reduce the synthesis of prostaglandins, and potentially reduce the risk of cancer recurrence is supported by epidemiological studies, which demonstrate an association between NSAID use with reduced risk of colorectal cancer [22] and breast cancer [25]. Although prospective trial data is lacking, it would seem the administration of NSAIDs perioperatively is a useful adjunct, both in terms of opioid reduction and potentially reducing COX-2 immune-mediated effects on cancer growth.

Regional anaesthesia techniques have become key components of many ERAS pathways. Potential benefits include opioid minimisation, attenuation of the stress response to surgery (and hence reduced immunosuppression) and perhaps direct immunomodulatory effects of the local anaesthetic agents [21] themselves. In vitro studies have shown local anaesthetics have cytotoxic effects on lymphoma cells [22], and inhibit the proliferation of adenocarcinoma cells in a concentration-dependent manner.

Retrospective cohort studies have reported benefits with the use of regional anaesthesia including prolonged overall and disease-free survival for breast, prostate, colorectal, ovarian, and head and neck cancers. Further studies, both prospective and retrospective undertaken in more recent years have yielded mixed results, with many concluding that regional anaesthesia offers no overall survival benefit, including a systematic review and meta-analysis incorporating 28 studies and 67,577 patients undergoing cancer surgery across a range of sub-specialties [26]. However, due to the relatively low quality of existing data and lack of high-quality prospective data it is difficult to definitively evaluate whether regional anaesthesia has an impact on long-term outcomes including cancer recurrence and survival.

10.8 Conclusions

Despite advances in our understanding, cancer pain continues to be a significant burden for a large number of patients, including those who may benefit from prehabilitation preoperatively. Optimising control of pain as part of prehabilitation is important to improve physical activity levels, as well as quality of life and psychological well-being. Patients should be screened for complex pain issues at the time of pre-assessment and referred to a pain specialist if necessary, as early as possible in their preoperative course (as shown in Fig. 10.16).

In addition to opioid- and non-opioid pharmacological therapies, psychological support including self-management of pain has an important role to play through empowering patients to participate in decisions and maximising their quality of life by achieving a better balance between pain and the adverse effects of analgesics. Physical interventions may be of benefit in complex patients with refractory pain.

Liaising with the in-hospital acute pain team perioperatively can be beneficial in complex patients with high opioid requirements. A strategy involving multimodal analgesia, to minimise opioids and aid enhanced recovery is important to attenuate the perioperative stress response and minimise the time taken for the patient to

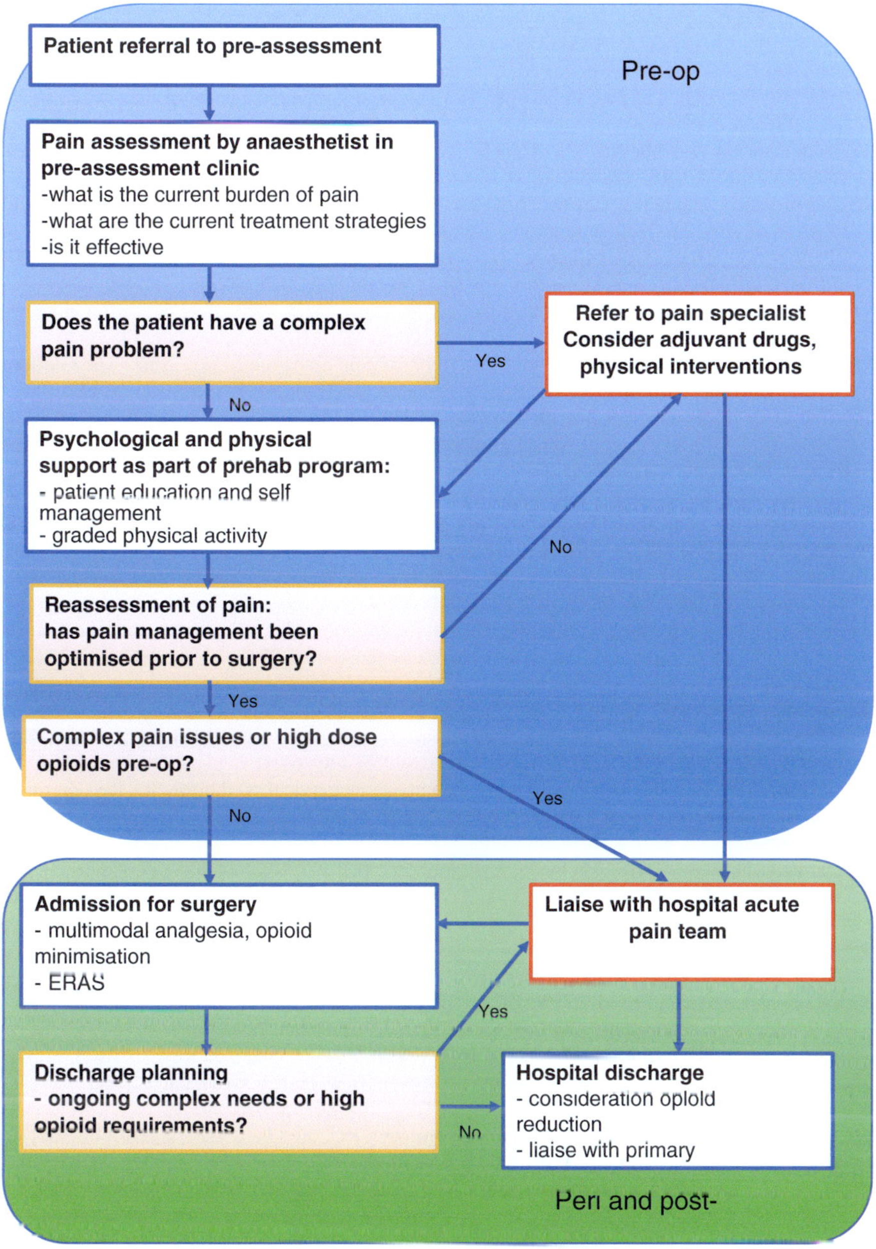

Fig. 10.16 Flowchart of suggested pain management pathway during prehabilitation

return to their baseline function. Perioperative pain management may also have a role to play in the reduction of cancer recurrence risk and improvement of long-term survival, though strong evidence supporting this hypothesis is yet to be elucidated.

References

1. van den Beuken-van Everdingen MH, de Rijke JM, Kessels AG, Schouten HC, van Kleef M, Patijn J. Prevalence of pain in patients with cancer: a systematic review of the past 40 years. Ann Oncol. 2007;18(9):1437–49.
2. Scott-Warren J, Bhaskar A. Cancer pain management—part I: general principles. CEACCP. 2014;14(6):278–84.
3. Nersesyan H, Slavin KV. Current approach to cancer pain management: availability and implications of different treatment options. Ther Clin Risk Manag. 2007;3(3):381–400.
4. Fallon M, Hanks G, Cherny N. Principles of control of cancer pain. BMJ. 2006;332(7548):1022–4. https://doi.org/10.1136/bmj.332.7548.1022.
5. Oxberry SG, Simpson KH. Pharmacotherapy for cancer pain, continuing education in anaesthesia. Crit Care Pain. 2005;5(6):203–6. https://doi.org/10.1093/bjaceaccp/mki053.
6. Cleeland C. The brief pain inventory handbook of pain assessment. New York: The Guilford Press; 1991. pp. 378-382
7. Cancer Pain Management, The British Pain Society, 2010.
8. Ventafridda V, Saita L, et al. WHO guidelines for the use of analgesics in cancer pain. Int J Tissue React. 1985;7(1):93–6.
9. Drewes AM, Jensen RD, Nielsen LM, et al. Differences between opioids: pharmacological, experimental, clinical and economical perspectives. Br J Clin Pharmacol. 2013;75(1):60–78. https://doi.org/10.1111/j.1365-2125.2012.04317.x.
10. Lussier D, Huskey AG, Portenoy RK. Adjuvant analgesics in cancer pain management. Oncologist. 2004;9:571–91. https://doi.org/10.1634/theoncologist.9-5-571.
11. WHO guidelines for the pharmacological and radiotherapeutic management of cancer pain in adults and adolescents. Geneva: World Health Organization; 2018. Licence: CC BY-NC-SA 3.0 IGO.
12. Bell RF, Eccleston C, Kalso EA. Ketamine as an adjuvant to opioids for cancer pain. Cochrane Database of Systematic Reviews 2017, Issue 6. Art. No.: CD003351. DOI: https://doi.org/10.1002/14651858.CD003351.pub3. Accessed 27 July 2021.
13. Jackson MB, Pounder D, Price C, et al. Percutaneous cervical cordotomy for the control of pain in patients with pleural mesothelioma. Thorax. 1999;54:238–41.
14. ElMokhallalati Y, Mulvey MR, Bennett MI. Interventions to support self-management in cancer pain. Pain Rep. 2018;3(6):e690. https://doi.org/10.1097/PR9.0000000000000690.
15. Lorig KR, Holman HR. Self-management education: history, definition, outcomes, and mechanisms. Ann Behav Med. 2003;26(1):1–7.
16. Michie S, van Stralen M, West R. The Behaviour Change Wheel: a new method for characterising and designing behaviour change interventions. Implementation Sci. 2011;6:42.
17. Marie N, Luckett T, Davidson PM, et al. Optimal patient education for cancer pain: a systematic review and theory-based meta-analysis. Support Care Cancer. 2013;21:3529–37.
18. Oldenmenger WH, Geerling JI, Mostovaya I, Vissers KCP, de Graeff A, Reyners AKL, van der Linden YM. A systematic review of the effectiveness of patient-based educational interventions to improve cancer-related pain. Cancer Treat Rev. 2018;63:96–103.
19. Garg R. Acute pain syndromes in cancer. J Anesth Crit Care Open Access. 2016;4(3):00136. https://doi.org/10.15406/jaccoa.2016.04.00136.
20. Small C, Laycock H. Acute postoperative pain management. Br J Surg. 2020;107:e70–80.
21. Evans MT, Wigmore T, Kelliher LJS. The impact of anaesthetic technique upon outcome in oncological surgery. BJA Educ. 2019;19(1):14–20. https://doi.org/10.1016/j.bjae.2018.09.008.

22. Heaney A, Buggy DJ. Can anaesthetic and analgesic techniques affect cancer recurrence or metastasis? Br J Anaesth. 2012;109(Suppl 1):i17–28. https://doi.org/10.1093/bja/aes421.
23. Janku F, Johnson LK, Karp DD, Atkins JT, Singleton PA, Moss J. Treatment with methylnaltrexone is associated with increased survival in patients with advanced cancer [published correction appears in Ann Oncol. 2018 Apr 1;29(4):1076]. Ann Oncol. 2016;27(11):2032–8. https://doi.org/10.1093/annonc/mdw317.
24. Bortsov AV, Millikan RC, Belfer I, Boortz-Marx RL, Arora H, McLean SA. μ-Opioid receptor gene A118G polymorphism predicts survival in patients with breast cancer. Anesthesiology. 2012;116(4):896–902. https://doi.org/10.1097/ALN.0b013e31824b96a1.
25. Harris RE. Cyclooxygenase-2 (cox-2) blockade in the chemoprevention of cancers of the colon, breast, prostate, and lung. Inflammopharmacology. 2009;17(2):55–67. https://doi.org/10.1007/s10787-009-8049-8.
26. Grandhi RK, Lee S, Abd-Elsayed A. The relationship between regional anesthesia and cancer: a meta-analysis. Ochsner J. 2017;17(4):345–61.

Part III

Cancer specific Prehabilitation

Prehabilitation for Hepatobiliary-Pancreatic Cancer Surgery

11

Sim Ming Ann, Glenn Kunnath Bonney, and Ashokka Balakrishnan

11.1 The Hepato-Pancreatico-Biliary Cancer Patient Profile

11.1.1 The Hepatobiliary Cancer Patient Going for Surgery

Hepatobiliary cancers encompass cancers involving the gallbladder, liver, and bile ducts.

Hepatocellular carcinomas are the most common form of primary hepatobiliary cancer, where patients frequently present with anorexia, jaundice, weight loss, and malaise [1]. These patients frequently have risk factors including hepatitis, liver cirrhosis, alcoholism, diabetes, and obesity [2]. A subpopulation of patients may also present with secondary liver metastasis and therefore present for surgical resection or radiofrequency ablation of lesions in early stages of disease [3]. In younger patients, breast and colorectal cancers make up the most common primary sites presenting with synchronous liver metastasis. In contrast, for older patients, a more heterogenous distribution of primaries is noted, including stomach, melanoma, and esophageal cancers [4]. Patients presenting with metastatic liver disease may therefore present with more advanced oncological disease burden and inherently be associated with poorer outcomes and survival rates [4].

Biliary tract cancers consist of carcinomas of the gallbladder, extrahepatic bile duct, and the ampulla of Vater. Based on a recent epidemiological study, they are the sixth most diagnosed cancers in the USA [5]. For gallbladder cancers,

S. M. Ann (✉) · A. Balakrishnan
Department of Anesthesia, National University Hospital, Singapore, Singapore
e-mail: ming_ann_sim@Nuhs.edu.sg

G. K. Bonney
Division of Hepatobiliary & Pancreatic Surgery, Department of Surgery, National University Hospital, Singapore, Singapore
e-mail: glenn_bonney@nuhs.edu.sg

A. Chakraborty, A. Balakrishnan (eds.), *Prehabilitation for Cancer Surgery*,
https://doi.org/10.1007/978-981-16-6494-6_11

adenocarcinomas consist of up to 80% of cases, with female gender, age, and congenital biliary tract anomalies being common risk factors [1, 6]. Due to the rapid nature of gallbladder cancer progression, these are often detected once in their advanced stages, with a mean survival of merely 6 months and dismal 5-year survival rates of 5% [6, 7]. Bile duct cancers (cholangiocarcinomas) are also predominantly adenocarcinomas. Their presentation differs from that of gallbladder cancers as they grow slowly and frequently present with delayed metastasis. Therefore, they are commonly diagnosed often only in advanced stages of disease [8]. Cholangiocarcinomas may be associated with parasitic infections, biliary duct cysts, primary sclerosing cholangitis, and hepatolithiasis [9].

11.1.2 The Pancreatic Cancer Patient Going for Surgery

Pancreatic cancer patients present with a unique pathophysiological profile which differentiates them from majority of patients undergoing intra-abdominal surgery. Pancreatic cancer is associated with mass effect on the gastric outlet, generalized catabolic state, pain, anorexia, and pancreatic insufficiency. Therefore, these patients commonly present with jaundice, malnutrition, infections, diabetes, and exocrine deficits. Up to 60–70% of patients may be cachexic at the time of diagnosis, with significant sarcopenia on presentation [10]. Patients are also likely to be malnourished with new onset diabetes due to the associated endocrine and exocrine deficiencies. Surgical resection for curative disease typically involves a pancreaticoduodenectomy, which is associated with notoriously high morbidity rates of 40–50%, despite ongoing advancements made to perioperative care and surgical technique. [11] This therefore underscores the importance of optimizing these patients who are at inherently high risk for surgical morbidity and mortality.

11.2 Potential Role and Barriers of Prehabilitation

Prehabilitation programs involve a multi-faceted approach to optimize the functional health and physiological reserve of patients before surgery (Fig. 11.1). This multimodal approach involves: (1) optimization of physical fitness through resistance training, aerobic exercise, flexibility exercises, and balance training; (2) dietary interventions aimed at improving the catabolic state and supporting anabolism; (3) psychological interventions to reduce stress, improve resilience, and improve self-efficacy; and (4) correction of modifiable risk factors such as optimization of comorbids and smoking and alcohol cessation [12].

Current literature demonstrates that prehabilitation enhances functional capacity, does not worsen outcomes, and is applicable to multiple types of major abdominal cancer surgery even in elderly frail patients [12–15]. Prehabilitation is also associated with improved postoperative clinical outcomes such as length of stay, readmissions, and postoperative complications [15–18]. Improvements in aerobic fitness and anaerobic fitness have also been reported, which is associated with a lower

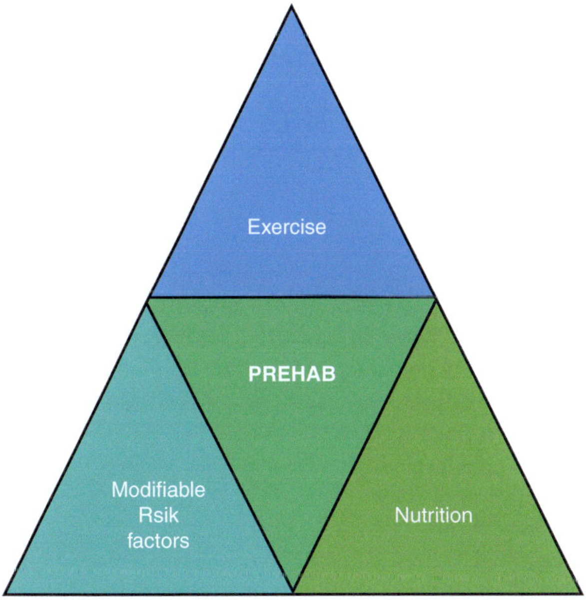

Fig. 11.1 Components of prehabilitation

severity of complications, shorter length of stay, and lower morbidity [19, 20]. Potential healthcare cost savings have also been achieved with the implementation of successful prehabilitation programs. [16]

However, cautious interpretation of these results should be advised in view of the heterogeneity of methods, small sample sizes, and variability in outcome measures. Furthermore, it is also unclear with regard to the applicability of these findings to the patient undergoing HPB cancer surgery in view of its unique patient profile as described above. The results from currently ongoing large prospective randomized controlled prehabilitation trials will shed greater insight into these areas in the future [21].

Barriers to the implementation of prehabilitation regimes most notably include poor compliance to therapy, especially in the setting of an unsupervised home-based program. This could be due to multiple factors, including the physical difficulties of these patients in undertaking prehabilitation regimes at home, variances in home-based setups, and poor patient understanding of physician instructions and rationale for prehabilitation programs. This may be especially relevant to patients undergoing HPB cancer surgery, as these patients are frequently elderly, frail, malnourished, and cachectic with multiple medical co-morbidities both related and unrelated to the disease. A heavily supervised prehabilitation regime may aid to mitigate these although this must be balanced against the resource burden required to enact such a program and its application in a clinically timely manner. However, a recent study involving 20 patients with pancreatic cancer showed promising rates of up to 80% compliance with a home-based exercise regime, leading to a significant improvement in baseline physical activity [22].

11.3 Specific Aspects of Prehabilitation for the Hepato-Pancreatico-Biliary Patient

A suggested perioperative framework for prehabilitation for the HPB patient is presented in Fig. 11.2.

11.3.1 Exercise

Patients with hepatobiliary and pancreatic cancers are frequently malnourished, cachectic, and sarcopenic. Sarcopenia is also a known risk factor for postoperative short-term outcomes following pancreatic surgery. In the longer term, sarcopenia is also an adverse indicator of poor prognosis and overall survival rates in both surgical and non-surgical candidates [23, 24]. In addition, the perioperative fluid shifts, surgical blood loss, anesthesiologic stressors (i.e. respiratory depression, ciliary dysfunction with general anesthesia), and use of sedative agents may predispose these patients to be at further risk of decreased aerobic physical fitness postoperatively [25]. Patients with decreased preoperative aerobic fitness may thus be at risk of tissue hypoxia and its complications, due to an expected decline in aerobic fitness postoperatively. Therefore, patients with HPB cancers are ideally suited to prehabilitation regimes to optimize these areas.

Evidence from multiple studies supports the emerging role for exercise prehabilitation in this population [13, 26–30]. Previously reported prehabilitation exercise regimes for HPB surgical cancer range from 2 to 4 weeks in length for patients presurgical resection and 2 to 6 months for those planned for neoadjuvant therapy. These involved 2–5 sessions per week of exercise programs involving aerobic, strengthening, and resistance components. The individual duration of the aerobic, resistance, and strengthening components ranged from 20 minutes per session to one hour [31]. Adherence to exercise regimens was higher for fully supervised exercise programs as compared to unsupervised or partially supervised regimes. These exercise interventions were associated with improvements in lean muscle mass, Cardiopulmonary Exercise Testing (CPET) scores, walking speed, and inflammatory markers (ie. C-reactive protein, serum albumin). At the systems-based level, this translated to shorter length of stay, improved preoperative quality of life, and decreased rates of delayed gastric emptying. However, these gains did not translate to an improvement in other major complication rates or mortality, which could also have been contributed by insufficient study power to detect a significant difference in these areas [32].

11.3.2 Nutrition

Patients with HPB cancer frequently present with obstructive symptoms including jaundice and weight loss and, less commonly, gastric outlet obstruction. The metabolic effects frequently result in weight loss, sarcopenia, and diabetes [33]. Exocrine

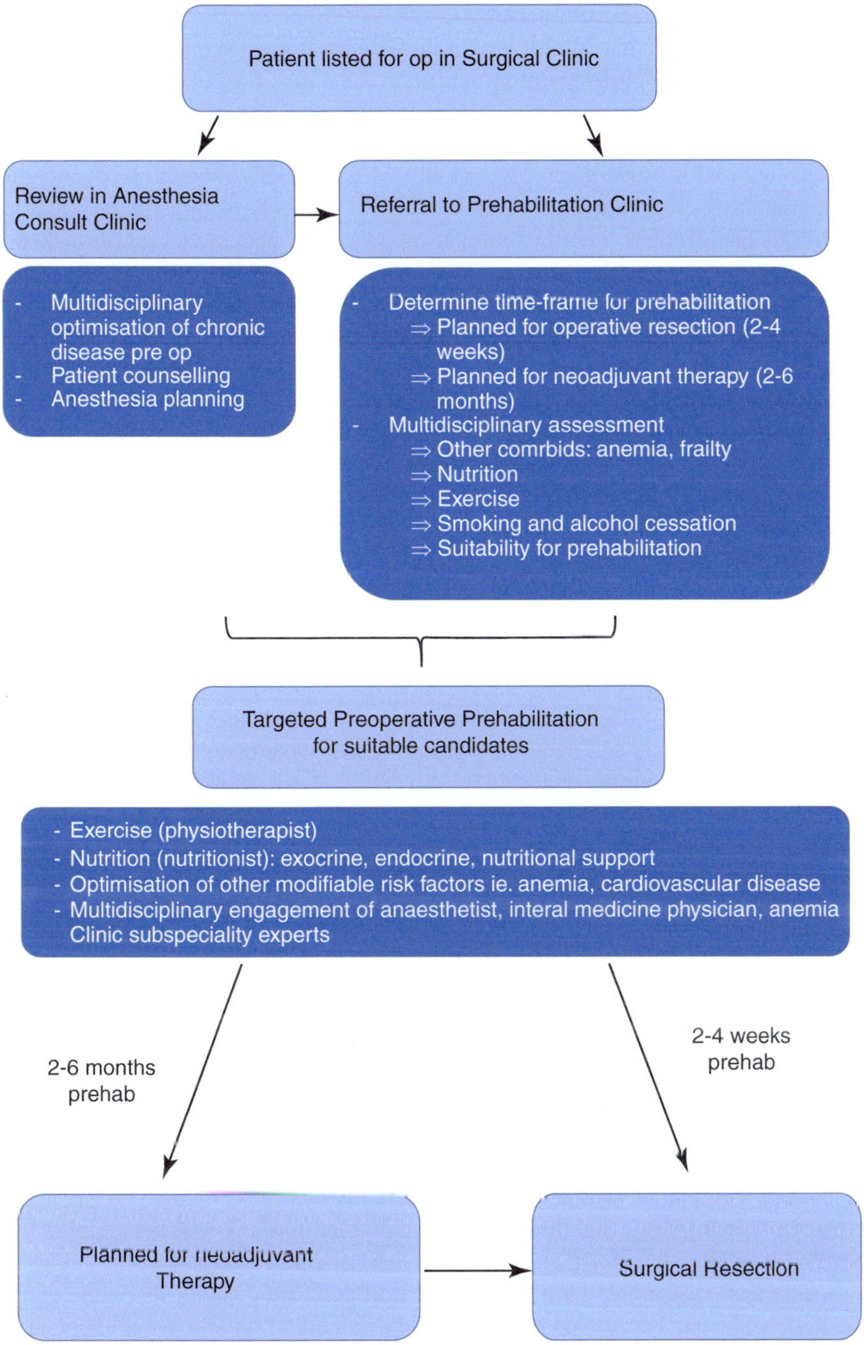

Fig. 11.2 Suggested perioperative framework for prehabilitation in HPB surgical patients

enzymatic deficiencies from pancreatic cancer further increase the risk of nutritional malabsorption. In addition, recent studies involving pancreatic cancer patients have demonstrated improvement in long-term outcomes with the use of pancreatic enzyme supplementation; such as survival, nutritional status, quality of life, and reduction in malabsorption symptoms such as pain and diarrhea. [34–36] Moreover, patients with HPB cancers may also present with obstructive symptoms due to gastric outlet obstruction and may require nutritional supplementation via parenteral or enteral means. Current literature comparing parenteral and enteral nutritional supplementation for patients with gastric outlet obstruction has demonstrated more favorable outcomes with enteral nutritional supplementation [37]. Between the two, up to two weeks of preoperative enteral nutrition have been reported to be associated with greater improvements in nutrition status, gastrointestinal function, immune function, and hospital cost savings when compared to parenteral nutrition [38]. Malnutrition is also an established risk factor for poor wound healing [39]. Therefore, when taken in combination, these factors if not optimized would further increase the risk of preoperative malnutrition and hence worsen perioperative morbidity [40]. Prehabilitation may therefore confer benefit in optimizing the nutritional status of these patients preoperatively, reversing sarcopenia, therefore potentially improving postoperative morbidity and long-term patient outcomes.

However, this must be balanced against the time frame required to yield meaningful improvements in nutritional status, as compared to the risk of disease progression without timely surgical intervention. Two studies to date have studied the role of nutritional prehabilitation interventions in HPB patients, with Ausania's providing both endocrine and exocrine support, while Nakajima et al. prescribed leucine rich essential amino acids [13, 30]. These have shown improvements in outcomes including shorter length of stay and delayed gastric emptying rates. They have also demonstrated an improvement in lean muscle mass and reduction in systemic inflammatory markers.

11.3.3 Anemia, Smoking, and Alcohol Cessation

Anemia is a common modifiable risk factor for major morbidity and death for HPB surgery [41]. This therefore underscores the need and potential benefit of correcting these risk factors prior to elective surgical resection [42]. The potential causes of anemia in patients include nutritional deficiencies (iron, B12, folate), marrow suppression due to chemotherapy, anemia of chronic disease, and occult tumor bleeding.

Prehabilitation interventions to correct preoperative anemia should be targeted at the underlying etiology and time frame available for correction of hemoglobin levels. For example, nutritional deficiencies such as B12 and folate should be replaced. The treatment of patients with established iron deficiency should be with supplementation of iron. The choice between oral or parenteral options would depend on the time required for correction, with oral replacements achieving a response in 4–6 weeks, while parenteral formulations are able to achieve results in days [43]. Erythropoiesis stimulating agents may also aid to improve red cell mass and hemoglobin levels, although this should be weighed against the risk of venous thromboembolism and disease progression; a particular concern in pancreatic cancer [44]. Blood transfusions should be considered only in the event of severe anemia with risk of organ ischemia.

Preoperative smoking and alcohol cessation may also yield potential benefits to the prehabilitation of these patients. The provision of a comprehensive smoking cessation regimen involving behavioral support and nicotine replacement therapy may reduce postoperative complications and is also currently recommended by anesthesia best practice guidelines [45]. Being a well-established risk factor for liver cancers, it is unsurprising that alcoholism is commonly encountered among the HPB surgical patient population [46]. Hence, preoperative alcohol cessation interventions such as psychological support, relapse prophylaxis, and pharmacological support strategies may aid in the reduction of postoperative complications [47]. Therefore, cessation of smoking and alcohol may also potentially benefit these patients who are at inherently high operative risk.

11.3.4 Timing: Prehabilitation and Neoadjuvant Chemotherapy

Patients planned for hepato-pancreatico-biliary surgery differ from the major abdominal surgical cohort as they generally fall into 2 groups: with some requiring neoadjuvant chemotherapy, while others will be planned for direct surgery. This bears implications in terms of the time frame and regimen of prehabilitation applicable to these two groups of patients. Patients who are planned for direct surgical resection would typically undergo surgery within 4 weeks, while those planned for neoadjuvant chemotherapy would be planned for 2–6 months duration of chemotherapy prior to surgical resection [31].

Preoperative chemotherapy is a recognized treatment strategy for localized pancreatic cancer patients and involves neoadjuvant regimes of approximately 2–6 months duration [31, 48]. This is noteworthy because this predictable time frame offers a unique opportunity to implement prehabilitation regimes. There is therefore an emerging role for prehabilitation in patients undergoing neoadjuvant therapy with recent studies reporting that aerobic exercise prehabilitation combined with neoadjuvant therapy may confer benefits in terms of tumor regression and modulation [27, 49]. However, the effects of prehabilitation during neoadjuvant therapy on postoperative outcomes following surgical resection remains unknown. Furthermore, neoadjuvant treatments are frequently associated with fatigue, decline in physical fitness, and depletion of muscle tissue which may impair patients' incentive to participate in prehabilitation regimes [50, 51]. However, small studies have shown promising results, with good adherence rates to home-based preoperative exercise regimes for pancreatic cancer patients despite undergoing neoadjuvant chemotherapy [22]. Further study is warranted, with regard to the optimal prehabilitation regime in this population with inherently decreased physiological reserve, who may still benefit from prehabilitation, despite concerns for limited participation.

11.3.5 Other HPB Surgical Specific Challenges

Pancreatic cancer presents with a host of preoperative challenges as described above. Specifically, patients with biliary obstruction may firstly present for biliary stenting prior to elective surgical resection via a Whipple's Surgery (Pancreaticoduodenectomy) [52, 53]. While there may be limited time to prehabilitate patients presenting for emergent biliary stenting, preoperative chemotherapy frequently prescribed for such locally advanced lesions provides a unique window of opportunity for prehabilitation measures. A pancreaticoduodenectomy involves extensive resection of the proximal pancreas, distal stomach, bile duct, gallbladder, and duodenum, with intestinal continuity then re-established via a pancreaticojejunostomy, hepaticojejunostomy, and gastrojejunostomy [52, 53]. Therefore, the importance of optimizing nutrition preoperatively in these patients cannot be further emphasized due to the expected challenges with postoperative nutrition in these patients with extensive gastrointestinal resection.

For hepatectomies of metastatic liver disease, several unique considerations for prehabilitation should be highlighted. Firstly, a multidisciplinary discussion between medical oncologists and surgeons is required to determine the need for neoadjuvant or adjuvant chemotherapy and the urgency of surgery, which would influence the time window available for perioperative prehabilitation. Secondly, the systemic effects of common neoadjuvant chemotherapy for colorectal metastasis to the liver are to be considered. Common agents used include oxaliplatin, irinotecan, and F-fluorouracil derivatives, which are known to result in hepatotoxicity, steatosis, and sinusoidal obstruction syndrome in its end stages of progression [54]. This should be evaluated for preoperatively in suitable patients. Sinusoidal obstruction syndrome is associated with venous congestion, potentially increases the risk and detrimental effects of perioperative transfusions and should be considered during formulation of prehabilitation programs. [55]

Lastly, the potential for intraoperative blood loss in major HPB surgeries remains a persistent challenge despite advances in surgical technique over the years. Perioperative transfusions may be associated with generalized immune dysregulation predisposing to adverse cancer outcomes, reduced surgical and poor surgical outcomes [56–58]. Patients presenting for such surgeries are frequently cachexic and malnourished as detailed above and hence are at increased risk of perioperative anemia. Hence, the importance of multidisciplinary preoperative optimization of anemia as part of the prehabilitation strategy needs to be underscored, which may aid to avoid the need for perioperative blood transfusions and its associated complications. Continual improvements to surgical technique such as intraoperative hepatic segmental or inflow vascular occlusion are also vital to further mitigate these risks, the specific details of which lie beyond the scope of this publication [59].

11.4 Conclusions

Prehabilitation programs developed for hepato-pancreatico-biliary surgery specifically addressing the pathophysiological issues associated with HPB surgery and cancer are urgently needed. Current prehabilitation programs for major abdominal surgery are heterogenous, and caution is advised in the translation of these results to the unique challenges faced by the HPB cancer surgical population. Emerging evidence has demonstrated possible benefit of multimodal prehabilitation for HPB cancer surgery patients. However, further study is warranted with regard to the optimal regime, time frame, and duration of prehabilitation for these patients.

References

1. Benson AB, Abrams TA, Ben-Josef, et al. Hepatobiliary cancers - clinical practice guidelines in oncology. J Natl Compr Cancer Netw. 2009;7(4):350–91.
2. Janevska D, Chaloska-Ivanova V, Janevski V. Hepatocellular carcinoma: risk factors, diagnosis and treatment. Open Access Macedonian J Med Sci. 2015;3(4):732–6. https://doi.org/10.3889/oamjms.2015.111.
3. Evrard S, Rivoire M, Arnaud J. 6011 ORAL Unresectable colorectal liver metastases treated by intraoperative radiofrequency ablation with or without resection: the ARF2003 study. Eur J Cancer. 2011;47:S394–5.
4. Horn S, Stoltzfus K, Lehrer E, et al. Epidemiology of liver metastases. Cancer Epidemiol. 2020;67:101760.
5. Castro F, Koshiol J, Hsing A, et al. Biliary tract cancer incidence in the United States-demographic and temporal variations by anatomic site. Int J Cancer. 2013;133(7):1664–71.
6. Hundal R, et al. Gallbladder cancer: epidemiology and outcome. Clin Epidemiol. 2014;
7. Bartoli E, Capron JP. Epidemiology and natural history of cholelithiasis. Rev Prat. 2000;50(19):2112–6.
8. Fernández-Ruiz M, Guerra-Vales J, Colina-Ruizdelgado F. Comorbidity negatively influences prognosis in patients with extrahepatic cholangiocarcinoma. World J Gastroenterol. 2009;15(42):5279–86.
9. Gia L. Tyson, et al. Risk factors of cholangiocarcinoma. Hepatology; 2011.
10. Rollins K, Tewari N, Ackner A, et al. The impact of sarcopenia and myosteatosis on outcomes of unresectable pancreatic cancer or distal cholangiocarcinoma. Clin Nutr. 2016;35(5):1103–9.
11. Søreide K, Stättner S. Textbook of pancreatic cancer. Springer Nature Switzerland, pp. 2021:567–92.
12. Carli F. Prehabilitation for the anesthesiologist. Anesthesiology. 2020;133(3):645–52.
13. Nakajima H, Yokoyama Y, Inoue T, Nagaya M, Mizuno Y, Kadono I, Nishiwaki K, Nishida Y, Nagino M. Clinical benefit of preoperative exercise and nutritional therapy for patients undergoing hepato-pancreato- biliary surgeries for malignancy. Ann Surg Oncol. 2019;26:264–72.
14. Santa Mina D, Hilton WJ, Matthew AG, Awasthi R, Bousquet-Dion G, Alibhai SMH, Au D, Fleshner NE, Finelli A, Clarke H, Aprikian A, Tanguay S, Carli F. Prehabilitation for radical prostatectomy: a multicentre randomized controlled trial. Surg Oncol. 2018;27:289–98.
15. Minnella EM, Awasthi R, Loiselle SE, Agnihotram RV, Ferri LE, Carli F. Effect of exercise and nutrition prehabilitation on functional capacity in esophagogastric cancer surgery: a randomized clinical trial. JAMA Surg. 2018;153:1081–9.
16. Barberan-Garcia A, Ubré M, Roca J, et al. Personalised prehabilitation in high-risk patients undergoing elective major abdominal surgery: a randomized blinded controlled trial. Ann Surg. 2018;267:50–6.
17. Hughes MJ, Hackney RJ, Lamb PJ, et al. Prehabilitation before major abdominal surgery: a systematic review and meta-analysis. World J Surg. 2019;43:1661–8.
18. Howard R, Yin YS, McCandless L, et al. Taking control of your surgery: impact of a prehabilitation program on major abdominal surgery. J Am Coll Surg. 2019;228:72–80.
19. Lai CW, et al. Patients' inability to perform a preoperative cardiopulmonary exercise test or demonstrate an anaerobic threshold is associated with inferior outcomes after major colorectal surgery. Br J Anaesth. 2013;111(4):607–11.

20. West MA, et al. Cardiopulmonary exercise variables are associated with postoperative morbidity after major colonic surgery: a prospective blinded observational study. Br J Anaesth. 2014;112(4):665–71.
21. van Rooijen S, Carli F, Dalton S, et al. Multimodal prehabilitation in colorectal cancer patients to improve functional capacity and reduce postoperative complications: The first international randomized controlled trial for multimodal prehabilitation. BMC Cancer. 2019;19:98.
22. Ngo-Huang A, Parker N, Wang X, et al. Home-based exercise during preoperative therapy for pancreatic cancer. Langenbeck's Arch Surg. 2017;402(8):1175–85.
23. Mintziras I, et al. Sarcopenia and sarcopenic obesity are significantly associated with poorer overall survival in patients with pancreatic cancer: systematic review and meta-analysis. Int J Surg. 2018;59:19–26.
24. Tan BH, et al. Sarcopenia in an overweight or obese patient is an adverse prognostic factor in pancreatic cancer. Clin Cancer Res. 2009;15(22):6973 9.
25. Bongers B, Dejong C, den Dulk M, et al. Enhanced recovery after surgery programmes in older patients undergoing hepatopancreatobiliary surgery: what benefits might prehabilitation have? Eur J Surg Oncol. 2021;47(3):551–9.
26. Dunne D, Jack S, Jones R, et al. Randomized clinical trial of prehabilitation before planned liver resection. Br J Surg. 2016;103(5):504–12.
27. Ngo-Huang A, Parker NH, Bruera E, et al. Home-based exercise prehabilitation during preoperative treatment for pancreatic cancer is associated with improvement in physical function and quality of life. Integr Canc Ther. 2019;18
28. Parker NH, Ngo-Huang A, Lee RE, et al. Physical activity and exercise during preoperative pancreatic cancer treatment. Support Care Canc. 2019;27(6):2275e84.
29. Marker RJ, Peters JC, Purcell WT, Jankowski CA. Effects of preoperative exercise on physical fitness and body composition in pancreatic cancer survivors receiving neoadjuvant therapy: a case series. Rehabilitation Oncology. 2018;36(4):9.
30. Ausania F, Senra P, Melendez R, Caballeiro R, Ouvina R, Casal-Nunez E. Prehabilitation in patients undergoing pancreaticoduodenectomy: a randomized controlled trial. Rev Esp Enferm Dig. 2019;111(8):603e8.
31. Bundred J, Kamarajah S, Hammond J, et al. Prehabilitation prior to surgery for pancreatic cancer: a systematic review. Pancreatology. 2020;20(6):1243–50.
32. Lambert J, Hayes L, Keegan T, et al. The impact of Prehabilitation on patient outcomes in hepatobiliary, colorectal, and upper gastrointestinal cancer surgery. Ann Surg. 2020;
33. Ozola Zalite I, et al. Influence of cachexia and sarcopenia on survival in pancreatic ductal adenocarcinoma: a systematic review. Pancreatology. 2015;15(1):19–24.
34. Bruno MJ, Haverkort EB, Tijssen GP, Tytgat GNJ, van Leeuwen DJ. Placebo controlled trial of enteric coated pancreatin microsphere treatment in patients with unresectable cancer of the pancreatic head region. Gut. 1998;42:92–6.
35. Landers A, Brown H, Strother M. The effectiveness of pancreatic enzyme replacement therapy for malabsorption in advanced pancreatic cancer, a pilot study. Palliat Care. 2019;12
36. Domínguez-Muñoz JE, Nieto-Garcia L, López-Díaz J, Lariño-Noia J, Abdulkader I, Iglesias-Garcia J. Impact of the treatment of pancreatic exocrine insufficiency on survival of patients with unresectable pancreatic cancer: a retrospective analysis. BMC Cancer. 2018;18:534.
37. Xin F, Mzee S, Botwe G., et al. Short-term evaluation of immune levels and nutritional values of EN versus PN in gastric cancer: a systematic review and a meta-analysis. World J Surg Oncol. 2019;17(1).
38. Chen Z, Lin S, Dai Q, et al. The effects of pre-operative enteral nutrition from nasal feeding tubes on gastric outlet obstruction. Nutrients. 2017;9(4):373.
39. Molnar J, Underdown M, Clark W. Nutrition and chronic wounds. Adv Wound Care. 2014;3(11):663–81.
40. Tzeng CW, et al. Morbidity and mortality after pancreaticoduodenectomy in patients with borderline resectable type C clinical classification. J Gastrointest Surg. 2014;18(1):146–55. discussion 155–6

41. Tohme S, Varley P, Landsittel D. Preoperative anemia and postoperative outcomes after hepatectomy. HPB. 2016;18(3):255–61.
42. Muñoz M, Acheson AG, Auerbach M, Besser M, Habler O, Kehlet H, et al. International consensus statement on the peri-operative management of anaemia and iron deficiency. Anaesthesia. 2017;72(2):233–47.
43. Bohlius J, Schmidlin K, Brillant C, Schwarzer G, Trelle S, Seidenfeld J, et al. Recombinant human erythropoiesis-stimulating agents and mortality in patients with cancer: a meta-analysis of randomised trials. Lancet. 2009;373(9674):1532–42.
44. Bartoszko J, Thorpe KE, Laupacis A, Wijeysundera DN. METS study investigators; international and national coordinators; central project office operations committee; CPET methods committee; outcome adjudication committee; international steering committee. Association of preoperative anaemia with cardiopulmonary exercise capacity and postoperative outcomes in noncardiac surgery: a substudy of the measurement of exercise tolerance before surgery (METS) study. Br J Anaesth 2019;123(2):161e9.
45. Testino G, Leone S, Borro P. Alcohol and hepatocellular carcinoma: a review and a point of view. World J Gastroenterol. 2014;20(43):15943.
46. Oppedal K, Møller AM, Pedersen B, Tønnesen H. Preoperative alcohol cessation prior to elective surgery. Cochrane Database Syst Rev. 2012;7:CD008343.
47. Khorana AA, Mangu PB, Berlin J, et al. Potentially curable pancreatic cancer: American Society of Clinical Oncology clinical practice guideline. J Clin Oncol. 2016;34(21):2541–56.
48. Florez Bedoya CA, Cardoso ACF, Parker N, et al. Exercise during preoperative therapy increases tumor vascularity in pancreatic tumor patients. Sci Rep. 2019;9(1):13966.
49. McLachlan SA, Fisher RJ, Zalcberg J, et al. The impact on health-related quality of life in the first 12 months: a randomised comparison of preoperative short-course radiation versus long-course chemoradiation for T3 rectal cancer (trans-Tasman radiation oncology group trial 01.04). Eur J Cancer. 2016;55:15–26.
50. West MA, Loughney L, Barben CP, et al. The effects of neoadjuvant chemoradiotherapy on physical fitness and morbidity in rectal cancer surgery patients. Eur J Surg Oncol. 2014;40(11):1421–8.
51. Awad S, Tan BH, Cui H, et al. Marked changes in body composition following neoadjuvant chemotherapy for oesophagogastric cancer. Clin Nutr. 2012;31(1):74–7.
52. Bond-Smith G, Banga N, Hammond TM, Imber CJ. Pancreatic adenocarcinoma. BMJ. 2012;344:e2476.
53. Kosuri K, Muscarella P, Bekaii-Saab TS. Updates and controversies in the treatment of pancreatic cancer. Clin Adv Hematol Oncol. 2006;4:47–54.
54. Page AJ, Kooby DA. Perioperative Management of Hepatic Resection. J Gastrointest Oncol. Mar. 2012;3(1):19–27.
55. Nakano H, Oussoultzoglou E, Rosso E, Casnedi S, Chenard-Neu MP, Dufour P, Bachellier P, Jaeck D. Sinusoidal injury increases morbidity after major hepatectomy in patients with colorectal liver metastases receiving preoperative chemotherapy. Ann Surg. Jan. 2008;247(1):118–24.
56. Kooby DA, Stockman J, Ben-Porat L, et al. Influence of transfusions on perioperative and long-term outcome in patients following hepatic resection for colorectal metastases. Ann Surg. 2003;237:860–70.
57. Schriemer PA, Longnecker DE, Mintz PD. The possible immunosuppressive effects of perioperative blood transfusion in cancer patients. Anesthesiology. 1988;68:422–8.
58. Yeh JJ, Gonen M, Tomlinson JS, Idrees K, Brennan MF, Fong Y. Effect of blood transfusion on outcome after pancreaticoduodenectomy for exocrine tumour of the pancreas. Br J Surg. 2007;94:466–72.
59. Smyrniotis V, Farantos C, Kostopanagiotou G, Arkadopoulos N. Vascular control during hepatectomy: review of methods and results. World J Surg Nov. 2005;29(11):1384–96.

Prehabilitation for Colorectal Cancer Surgery

12

Henry Stuart Watson, Dibyendu Bandyopadhyay, and Saikat Sengupta

12.1 Background

Colorectal cancer (CRC) is the commonest gastrointestinal malignancy worldwide and the second most common cause of cancer deaths in the United Kingdom [1]. There are an estimated 41,000 new cases diagnosed each year, resulting in approximately 16,000 cancer deaths across the United Kingdom (UK) [2]. Epidemiological data suggests that across western society the incidence of CRC diagnoses is steadily increasing [3]. Interestingly, this increase has also been mirrored in the developing world where the adoption of a western style diet has been implicated [3]. From 2004 to 2014, CRC incidence rates in India increased by 20%. During 2004–2005, the incidence rate of CRC was 5.8 per 100,000 persons. It increased to 6.9 during 2012–2014 [4]. In the UK, CRC incidence started to fall in the 1990s but has again increased since the advent of CRC screening where there is detection of earlier asymptomatic cancers [5, 6]. Across both genders CRC is predominantly a disease of the over 50s with incidence rates rising steeply between the ages of 50 and 54 years and peak incidence between the ages of 80 and 84 years [2]. Therefore, with an ever-increasing elderly population it is predicted that incidence rates will continue to rise, which in turn is likely to lead to increased numbers of patients undergoing major colorectal resectional surgery. Despite significant improvements there is still a drive to improve colorectal surgical outcomes. Major abdominal

H. S. Watson
General Surgery, Yorkshire Deanery, London, UK
e-mail: henrywatson@doctors.org.uk

D. Bandyopadhyay
York & Scarborough Teaching Hospitals, York, UK

S. Sengupta (✉)
Department of Anaesthesiology, Apollo Multispecialty Hospitals (formerly Apollo Gleneagles Hospitals), Kolkata, India

A. Chakraborty, A. Balakrishnan (eds.), *Prehabilitation for Cancer Surgery*,
https://doi.org/10.1007/978-981-16-6494-6_12

surgery is associated with post-operative complications in approximately 30% of cases and even in the absence of complications is associated with a significant reduction in both functional and physiological capacity post-operatively [7, 8]. In respect of both patient outcomes and health economics there is renewed interest in optimising colorectal peri-operative care.

The benefits of post-operative interventions on improving patient outcomes are well documented. There is a multitude of evidence highlighting the significant benefits of colorectal enhanced recovery programmes (ERAS) on a range of outcome measures including mortality, morbidity, post-operative complications, and length of hospital stay [9, 10]. There is also emerging evidence that ERAS may even be associated with improved overall and disease-free survival in colorectal cancer surgery [11]. ERAS programmes include a variety of preoperative and post-operative interventions and are most successfully utilised in institutions with a dedicated enhanced recovery nurse specialist. ERAS protocols often run counter to "traditional/historic" surgical thinking and include preoperative carbohydrate loading, specific anaesthetics and regional analgesics, minimally invasive surgery, the introduction of diet early in the immediate post-operative period, and early mobilisation. Other preoperative interventions include smoking cessation and optimisation of haemoglobin levels prior to surgery.

12.2 Prehabilitation for Colorectal Surgery

The success of ERAS programmes in enhancing post-operative recovery has garnered further interest in the preoperative optimisation of patients undergoing colorectal surgery. Poor preoperative physical fitness is detrimental to post-operative outcomes and has been shown to increase mortality, post-operative complications, and to also delay post-operative recovery [12–14].

12.2.1 Definition

Prehabilitation is defined as the preoperative optimisation of patients in order to enhance overall post-operative recovery. Prehabilitation employs a variety of exercise and nutritional programs to improve functional capacity and recovery following colorectal surgery. This may also impact on a patient's ability to receive either neoadjuvant or adjuvant treatment as an adjunct to surgery in appropriate clinical situations which is not uncommon in colorectal cancer.

12.2.2 Prehabilitation Plan: Trimodal Approach

There is significant variation as to the components of a successful prehabilitation programme. Although early prehabilitation programmes focused on the physiological aspects of optimising functional capacity, there is now recognition of a multimodal approach. A trimodal model of prehabilitation encompasses physical exercise, nutritional/dietary, and psychosocial domains. Needless to say some of the aspects and domains of prehabilitation and ERAS come under a common umbrella.

Physical exercise programmes are designed to improve preoperative physiological capacity in order to both preserve and improve post-operative functional capacity. Functional capacity is a key concept in the utilisation of prehabilitation. With respect to cardiovascular physiology, it reflects an individual's ability to undertake normal daily activities that require sustained aerobic metabolism [15]. Major abdominal surgery is associated with a significant post-operative reduction in physiological functional capacity (20–40%), even in the absence of complications [7].

Nutritional optimisation through dietary interventions is of paramount importance in reducing post-operative complications and improving long-term outcomes. Cachexia, sarcopenia, and myopenia are all associated with impairment of long-term outcomes in colorectal cancer patients [16]. Conservative measures estimate that between 20 and 50% of patients undergoing major abdominal surgery are undernourished [17, 18]. The body enters a catabolic state post-operatively and therefore undernourished patients are more prone to impaired recovery and post-operative complications.

Many of the early prehabilitation programmes were uni- or bi-modal, concentrating primarily on exercise and dietary interventions. However, it was noted that even in patients undergoing exercise and dietary prehabilitation programmes, the desired outcomes were not achieved or there was poor compliance with prehabilitation regimens [19]. High anxiety and psychological stress were among the factors identified that appeared to impede successful implementation of prehabilitation programmes. Therefore, inclusion of psychological support is a recommended component of any successful prehabilitation model.

12.2.3 Baseline Measurements

To achieve optimal outcomes from the implementation of prehabilitation programmes baseline measures of functional capacity, nutrition and psychological evaluation are required.

Subjective measures of functional capacity are commonplace but lack both validity and standardisation. They include enquiries regarding an individual's ability to undertake simple tasks such as climbing the stairs or distances walked without impairment.

More formalised measures of functional capacity include cardiopulmonary exercise testing (CPET) which is an objective measure of cardiac pulmonary and circulatory function. A key parameter of CPET is the anaerobic threshold (AT), which marks the switch from aerobic to anaerobic metabolism, when there is insufficient oxygenation delivery to tissues. It is therefore an individualised risk assessment of an individual's ability to respond to the physiological stresses of major surgical procedures and is a predictor of morbidity and mortality. The AT guides operative risk stratification of patients and aids in the identification of patients that require higher level post-operative care [20]. Other physiological measures of functional capacity include the maximum rate of oxygen consumption measured during incremental exercise (VO2 peak). Less invasive tests like the 6 min walk test (6MWT) which quantifies the distance walked over a 6 min period, incremental shuttle walk test (ISWT), or the stair-climbing test are an assessment of aerobic capacity. An ISWT distance greater than 400 m (40 × 10 m shuttles) has correlated with a maximum oxygen uptake (VO2max) ≥15 mL/kg/min. Patients with such capability have been shown to undergo major thoracic surgery and do not need a CPET [21]. Similarly, patients who have an exercise ability equal to or above 22 m on the stair-climbing test are considered low risk. However, patients who cannot reach the designated cut-off of 22 m should undergo CPET. They are at increased risk for peri-operative death and cardiopulmonary complications. Performance at symptom-limited stair-climbing test is associated with increased cardiopulmonary complications, mortality, and costs after major lung resection [22]. The aforementioned measures are predictive of post-operative mortality and morbidity [23, 24].

There are a variety of nutritional measures that may be undertaken at baseline including anthropometric measurements of body fat composition, hand grip strength, and body mass index. There are also a number of validated food diaries that assess dietary intake including quantification of calories and protein.

Validated assessment of a patient's psychological state includes the hospital anxiety and depressions score (HADS), GAD-7 score, and PHQ-9 score. Psychosocial parameters may also be assessed with health-related quality of life (QOL) assessments such as the 36-item short-list questionnaire (SL-36).

12.3 Evaluation, Planning, and Consideration

The optimal duration of the prehabilitation program should be determined by the best compromise between compliance and effectiveness. A prehabilitation program between 2 and 4 weeks seems to be ineffective [25] whereas to exceed 3-month duration is associated with a very poor compliance [26]. If allowed by the underlying disease, duration ranging from 6 to 8 weeks seems to be a good compromise between feasibility and effectiveness [27]. There is robust evidence to show that measured and calculated delays to surgery do not affect long-term cancer outcomes and therefore there should be sufficient scope for the delivery of prehabilitation programmes [28].

12.3.1 Dietary Interventions

Given the heterogeneous nature of prehabilitation programmes across colorectal surgery there is no single recommended regime. Provision of a specialist dietician to assess nutritional requirements is desirable. Key to optimisation is identification of cachectic and sarcopenic patients, in order to provide protein supplementation, thereby switching the body to an anabolic state to increase lean muscle mass. This in part helps counter the catabolic state that follows major abdominal surgery. Provision of vitamin D and other micronutrients may also be appropriate in order to increase muscle mass. There is also a synergistic effect of providing both carbohydrate and protein supplementation immediately prior to or following the prehabilitation exercise routines, where there may be up to a 25% increase in dynamic muscle strength [29–31].

12.3.2 Exercise Regimes

Again, there is widespread variation across the delivery of exercise regimes in prehabilitation programmes, partly due to the inherent variation across patient's baseline fitness. There is a balance to be struck between achieving optimal improvements in cardiorespiratory physiology and ensuring compliance in a population of patients that will exhibit varying motivation. Broadly speaking exercise regimes should be complementary, focussing on a combination of endurance exercises to optimise cardiorespiratory functional capacity and strength and conditioning exercises, to improve muscle strength. Engaging patients in exercise regimes may be more successful in a supervised hospital environment with a suitably qualified health professional. However economic considerations may preclude this. Provision of exercise equipment at home may improve compliance, but again in the absence of supervision this cannot be ensured.

Exercise regimes tailored to individual patients can be developed using the VO2 and AT measurements taken from CPET testing. Hereby interval training can be designed to achieve 85% of the VO2 peak [32]. More basic exercise regimes to improve cardiovascular fitness include set walking and cycling exercises where aerobic exercise targets are based on reaching a set percentage of maximal heart rate. The 6 min walk test can also be done at intervals to ascertain meaningful increase in exercise capacity. Studies suggest that an improvement of about 30 m in distance walked from the previous test denotes the minimally important difference (MID) [33].

12.3.3 Improving Psychological Outcomes

The primary goal of psychological interventions is to achieve compliance with prehabilitation programmes. Again, there is an array of interventions available, with a combination of counselling with a trained psychologist, relaxation exercises, and provision of audio-visual material. It is also appropriate to manage individual expectations in what can be realistically achieved when undergoing prehabilitation.

12.4 Effects

The outcomes following implementation of prehabilitation regimes in colorectal surgery vary significantly, in part due to the heterogeneous nature of study design. Overall, there appears to be an improvement in physiological functional capacity, but this does not always translate to reduction in the occurrence of post-operative complications. A single study focussed on patients over the age of 65, classified as frail, found no improvement on surgical outcomes, specifically complications, re-admissions, and length of stay [34]. There was also no marked improvement in either preoperative physiological capacity or return to functional capacity post-operatively after following a prehabilitation programme. This may be partly explained by the need for a longer duration of prehabilitation to take effect, particularly dietary interventions to increase lean muscle mass. Although prehabilitation programmes may not improve surgical outcomes there is some evidence that individuals who exhibit an improvement in physiological functional capacity preoperatively were more likely to recover to baseline levels of functional capacity post-operatively, which in the context of patients requiring adjuvant chemotherapy may be of benefit [35].

There is limited data exploring long-term outcomes following implementation of prehabilitation regimes in colorectal cancer surgery. A pooled study of two separate randomised controlled trials and a cohort study determined that patients that underwent prehabilitation exhibited improved disease-free survival; this was mostly relevant in patients with stage III disease, where there was lymph node spread. There was no effect on overall survival [36].

There is no evidence that prehabilitation influences an individual's ability to undergo chemotherapy following colorectal cancer surgery. However, one might infer that if prehabilitation reduces the risk of post-operative complications and also helps to maintain physical fitness, then in a subset of patients prehabilitation may increase the likelihood that eligible individuals may receive adjuvant chemotherapy.

Across most studies there is no evidence to indicate a reduction in complications following implementation of a prehabilitation regime. Interestingly, in one study, patients whose functional capacity deteriorated during the prehabilitation intervention were at higher risk of complications (Grade IIIb Clavien-Dindo or higher) [37]. In turn this may facilitate the development of a risk scoring system and help to take measures proactively in the peri-operative period to obtain an optimal outcome. In reality it may translate into pre-emptive avoidance of high-risk bowel anastomosis and adoption of high dependency or equivalent level care. Further studies are required to explore whether a patient's ability to make a full and rapid recovery following a complication is facilitated by undergoing prehabilitation.

There is significant heterogeneity across studies assessing whether prehabilitation improves quality of life following colorectal cancer surgery. Many studies have not explored impacts on quality of life. Two studies suggest an improvement post-operatively as measured by the SF-36 questionnaire [38, 39].

Looking at the desired time scale of prehabilitation for 6–8 weeks, it makes every sense to offer this to the colorectal cancer patients undergoing neoadjuvant radiotherapy, chemotherapy, or a combination. This group of patients are oncologically at higher risk and the period between their neoadjuvant treatment and major surgery is the appropriate period for a multimodal prehabilitation to make these patients better prepared for surgery resulting in improved outcomes [40].

In cases of rectal cancer two opposite spectra of patients with early and advanced rectal cancer would benefit from prehabilitation. In early rectal cancer there is increasing interest in organ preservation and this encompasses treatment with either short course radiotherapy and delay or long course chemo radiotherapy. Various trials (e.g., STAR-TREC) [41] are looking into the feasibilities and possibilities.

Following assessment at an interval after non-surgical treatment, some of these patients will require local excision or even major surgery if they remain poor responders to radiotherapy. Preparing these patients with prehabilitation from the outset would be beneficial. Conversely, results of the RAPIDO trial [42] showed benefit of neoadjuvant chemotherapy following radiotherapy in locally advanced rectal cancer in reducing disease related treatment failure. Hence, these patients can maximise the beneficial effects of prehabilitation prior to their major resection.

12.5 Prehabilitation Multidisciplinary Team/Facility

At present there is no recommendation as to the constituent members of a prehabilitation team. It should be a multidisciplinary approach. In a trimodal model the presence of a dietitian and psychologist is necessary. A dietitian can identify the nutritional requirements to optimise the patient to an anabolic state. A psychologist enables the setting of realistic goals and identifies areas of concerns and anxiety, which once addressed may improve compliance with prehabilitation regimes. Anaesthetic input is of significant importance especially when trying to ascertain the baseline physiological parameters such as aerobic threshold and functional capacity and also its subsequent assessment. Considering the prevalent age group of colorectal cancer, involvement of the care of the elderly medicine physician would be of significant value in optimisation of these patients. In hospital based supervised exercise regimes the presence of a sports scientist is appropriate. The input from the surgeon and the colorectal nurse specialist are important in forming management plans and continuity of care and support. The provision of team members for a prehabilitation programme will be dictated by the economic conditions within the setting of individual institutions.

12.6 Delivery of Prehabilitation

The mode of delivery of a prehabilitation programme is very much dependent on the local resources available. A supervised trimodal programme is likely to improve patient compliance. A programme of approximately 6–8 weeks duration is sufficient and should consist of:

- Dietary/nutritional intervention.
  - Assessment of baseline dietary requirements/nutritional status (sarcopenia/cachexia/muscle mass)
  - Provision of protein supplementation and carbohydrates in conjunction with exercise to increase lean muscle mass
  - Supplementation of trace elements where appropriate need identified
  - Optimisation of haemoglobin
- Psychological intervention
  - Baseline assessment of mood/anxiety/quality of life

  - Provision of audio-visual/reading material to explain concept of prehabilitation in order to alleviate anxiety and improve compliance
  - Relaxation techniques
- Exercise regimes
  - Baseline assessment of functional capacity using either CPEX or 6-min walking test
  - Cessation of smoking
  - Strengthening exercises to increase muscle mass
  - Daily walking or cycling regimes (stationary if preferred)
  - Exercise regimes may increase in intensity and be developed to target a particular physiological parameter such as increasing heart rate

12.7 Current Barriers to Prehabilitation and Future Work

Perhaps the most significant barrier to delivering prehabilitation in colorectal surgery is the lack of level I evidence of the exact modes of its implementation. Most studies exhibit significant heterogeneity, particularly with respect to the design of prehabilitation programmes. There is also no agreement in assessing the baseline capacity and other parameters.

There are also economic considerations when trying to set up a prehabilitation programme. There is significant investment required in both staffing and equipment. Furthermore, there is a lack of staff trained in the field of prehabilitation. Health economic study is essential to look at the benefit and cost analysis to ascertain any economic benefit. If so, this may drive the move towards investment in prehabilitation services. The present insurance premium in the private sectors does not cover the cost of prehabilitation. However, in the setting of private insurance-based systems, prehabilitation may be seen as an accepted tool to reduce surgical risks, its complications, and the associated costs.

In summary a trimodal model of prehabilitation would appear to confer most benefit with regard to maintaining functional capacity. There is however a lack of evidence pointing to uniform clinical benefits. At present the foremost benefit is likely in patients who undergo neoadjuvant treatment. It seems that customised or individualised prehabilitation programmes are the way forward.

There is a need for more robust evidence and a multicentre randomised controlled trial with standardised prehabilitation protocol will hopefully provide more answers [32].

References

1. Bray F, Ferlay J, Soerjomataram I, Siegel RL, Torre LA, Jemal A. Global cancer statistics 2018: GLOBOCAN estimates of incidence and mortality worldwide for 36 cancers in 185 countries. CA Cancer J Clin. 2018;68(6):394–424.

2. Cancer Research UK. https://www.cancerresearchuk.org/health-professional/cancer-statistics/statistics-by-cancer-type/bowel-cancer. Accessed February 2019.
3. Center MM, Jemal A, Ward E. International trends in colorectal cancer incidence rates. *Cancer Epidemiol.* Biomarkers Prev. 2009;18(6):1688–94.
4. Thomas VM, Baby B, Wang K, Lei F, Chen Q, Huang B, Mathew A. Trends in colorectal cancer incidence in India. J Clin Oncol. 2020;38(15_suppl):e16084.
5. Jones AM, Morris E, Thomas J, Forman D, Melia J, Moss SM. Evaluation of bowel cancer registration data in England, 1996-2004. Br J Cancer. 2009;101(8):1269–73.
6. Logan RFA, Patnick J, Nickerson C, Coleman L, Rutter MD, von Wagner C. On behalf of the English bowel cancer screening evaluation committee. Outcomes of the bowel cancer screening Programme (BCSP) in England after the first 1 million tests. Gut. 2012;61(10):1439–4.
7. Christensen T, Kehlet H. Postoperative fatigue. World J Surg1993;17(2):220—5.: Lawrence VA, Hazuda HP, Cornell JE, Pederson T, Bradshaw PT, Mulrow CD,et al. Functional independence after major abdominal surgery in the elderly. J Am Coll Surg. 2004;199:762–72.
8. Schilling PL, Dimick JB, Birkmeyer JD. Prioritizing quality improvement in general surgery. J Am Coll Surg. 2008;207(5):698–704.
9. Greco M, Capretti G, Beretta L, Gemma M, Pecorelli N, Braga M. Enhanced recovery program in colorectal surgery: a meta-analysis of randomized controlled trials. World J Surg. 2014;38(06):1531–41.
10. Varadhan KK, Neal KR, Dejong CH, Fearon KC, Ljungqvist O, Lobo DN. The enhanced recovery after surgery (ERAS) pathway for patients undergoing major elective open colorectal surgery: a meta-analysis of randomized controlled trials. Clin Nutr. 2010;29(04):434–40.
11. Gustafsson UO, Oppelstrup H, Thorell A, et al. Adherence to the eras protocol is associated with 5-year survival after colorectal cancer surgery: a retrospective cohort study. World J Surg. 2016;40:1741–7. https://doi.org/10.1007/s00268-016-3460-ypmid:http://www.ncbi.nlm.nih.gov/pubmed/26913728.
12. Lawrence VA, Hazuda HP, Cornell JE, Pederson T, Bradshaw PT, Mulrow CD, et al. Functional independence after major abdominal surgery in the elderly. J Am Coll Surg. 2004;199(5):762–72.
13. Robinson TN, Wu DS, Pointer L, Dunn CL, Cleveland JC. MossM. Simple frailty score predicts postoperative complications across surgical specialties. Am J Surg. 2013;206(4):544–50.
14. Wilson RJT, Davies S, Yates D, Redman J, Stone M. Impaired functional capacity is associated with all-cause mortality after major elective intra-abdominal surgery. Br J Anaesth. 2010;105(3):297–303.
15. Arena R, Myers J, Williams MA, Gulati M, Kligfield P, Balady GJ, Collins E, Fletcher G, American Heart Association Committee on Exercise, Rehabilitation, and Prevention of the Council on Clinical Cardiology; American Heart Association Council on Cardiovascular Nursing. Assessment of functional capacity in clinical and research settings: a scientific statement from the American Heart Association Committee on Exercise. Rehabilitation, and Prevention of the Council on Clinical Cardiology and the Council on Cardiovascular Nursing. Circulation. 2007 Jul 17;116(3):329–43.
16. Schwegler I, von Holzen A, Gutzwiller J-P, Schlumpf R, Müh-lebach S, Stanga Z. Nutritional risk is a clinical predictor of postoperative mortality and morbidity in surgery for colorectal cancer. Br J Surg. 2010;97(1):92–7.
17. Correia MITD, Waitzberg DL. The impact of malnutrition on morbidity, mortality, length of hospital stay and costs evaluated through a multivariate model analysis. Clin Nutr. 2003;22(3):235–9.
18. Corish CA, Kennedy NP. Protein-energy undernutrition in hospital in-patients. Br J Nutr. 2000;83(6):575 91.
19. Gillis C, Li C, Lee L, Awasthi R, Augustin B, Gamsa A, Liberman AS, Stein B, Charlebois P, Feldman LS, Carli F. Prehabilitation versus rehabilitation: a randomized control trial in patients undergoing colorectal resection for cancer. Anesthesiology. 2014 Nov;121(5):937–47. https://doi.org/10.1097/ALN.0000000000000393.

20. Agnew N, MBBS FRCA. Preoperative cardiopulmonary exercise testing. Contin Educ Anaesth Crit Care Pain. April 2010;10(2):33–7. https://doi.org/10.1093/bjaceaccp/mkq001.
21. Brunelli A, Kim AW, Berger KI, Addrizzo-Harris DJ. Physiologic evaluation of the patient with lung cancer being considered for resectional surgery: diagnosis and management of lung cancer, 3rd ed: American College of Chest Physicians evidence-based clinical practice guidelines. Chest. 2013;143(5 Suppl):e166S–90S.
22. Brunelli A, Refai M, Xiumé F, Salati M, Sciarra V, Socci L, Sabbatini A. Performance at symptom-limited stair-climbing test is associated with increased cardiopulmonary complications, mortality, and costs after major lung resection. Ann Thorac Surg. 2008;86(1):240.
23. Carlisle J, Swart M. Mid-term survival after abdominal aor-tic aneurysm surgery predicted by cardiopulmonary exercise testing. Br J Surg. 2007;94(8):966–9.
24. Hennis PJ, Meale PM, Grocott MPW. Cardiopulmonary exercise testing for the evaluation of perioperative risk in non-cardiopulmonary surgery. Postgrad Med J. 2011;87(1030):550–7.
25. Dronkers JJ, Lamberts H, Reutelingsperger IMMD, Naber RH, Dronkers-Landman CM, Veldman A, et al. Preoperative therapeutic programme for elderly patients scheduled for elective abdominal oncological surgery: a randomized controlled pilot study. Clin Rehabil. 2010;24(7):614–22.
26. Carli F, Zavorsky GS. Optimizing functional exercise capacity in the elderly surgical population. Curr Opin Clin Nutr Metab Care. 2005;8(1):23–32.
27. Le Roy B, Selvy M, Slim K. The concept of prehabilitation: what the surgeon needs to know? J Visc Surg. 2016 Apr;153(2):109–12. https://doi.org/10.1016/j.jviscsurg.2016.01.001.
28. Curtis NJ, West MA, Salib E, Ockrim J, Allison AS, Dalton R, Francis NK. Time from colorectal cancer diagnosis to laparoscopic curative surgery-is there a safe window for prehabilitation? Int J Color Dis. 2018 Jul;33(7):979–83. https://doi.org/10.1007/s00384-018-3016-8.
29. Burke LM, Hawley JA, Ross ML, Moore DR, Phillips SM, Slater GR, et al. Preexercise aminoacidemia and muscle protein synthesis after resistance exercise. Med Sci Sports Exerc. 2012;44(10):1968–77.
30. Esmarck B, Andersen JL, Olsen S, Richter EA, Mizuno M, Kjaer M. Timing of postexercise protein intake is important for muscle hypertrophy with resistance training in elderly humans. J Physiol. 2001;535(1):301–11.
31. Hargreaves M. Pre-exercise nutritional strategies: effects on metabolism and performance. Can J Appl Physiol. 2001;26:S64–70.
32. van Rooijen S, Carli F, Dalton S, et al. Multimodal prehabilitation in colorectal cancer patients to improve functional capacity and reduce postoperative complications: the first international randomized controlled trial for multimodal prehabilitation. BMC Cancer. 2019;19:98. https://doi.org/10.1186/s12885-018-5232-6.
33. Du Bois RM, Weycker D, Albera C, Bradford WZ, Costabel U, Kartashov A, Lancaster L, Noble PW, Sahn SA, Szwarcberg J, Thomeer M, Valeyre D, King TE Jr. Six-minute-walk test in idiopathic pulmonary fibrosis: test validation and minimal clinically important difference. Am J Respir Crit Care Med. 2011;183(9):1231.
34. Carli F, Bousquet-Dion G, Awasthi R, et al. Effect of multimodal Prehabilitation vs postoperative rehabilitation on 30-day postoperative complications for frail patients undergoing resection of colorectal cancer: a randomized clinical trial. JAMA Surg. 2020;155(3):233–42. https://doi.org/10.1001/jamasurg.2019.5474.
35. Mayo NE, Feldman L, Scott S, Zavorsky G, Kim DJ. CharleboisP, et al. impact of preoperative change in physical function on postoperative recovery: argument supporting prehabilitation for colorectal surgery. Surgery. 2011;150(3):505–14.
36. Trépanier M, Minnella EM, Paradis T, Awasthi R, Kaneva P, Schwartzman K, Carli F, Fried GM, Feldman LS, Lee L. Improved disease-free survival after Prehabilitation for colorectal cancer surgery. Ann Surg. 2019 Sep;270(3):493–501. https://doi.org/10.1097/SLA.0000000000003465.
37. Carli P, Charlebois B, Stein L, Feldman G, Zavorsky D, Kim, et al. Randomized clinical trial of prehabilitation in colorectal surgery. Br J Surg. 2010;97(8):1187–97.

38. Dunne R, Jones D, Lythgoe H, Malik G, Poston S. Jack, et al., 111. Prehabilitation before liver surgery. Eur J Surg Oncol. 2014;40(11):S52.
39. Li F, Carli L, Lee P, Charlebois B, Stein AS, Liberman, et al. Impact of a trimodal prehabilitation program on functional recovery after colorectal cancer surgery: a pilot study. Surg Endosc. 2013;27(4):1072–82.
40. West MA, Loughney L, Lythgoe D, Barben CP, Sripadam R, Kemp GJ, Grocott MP, Jack S. Effect of prehabilitation on objectively measured physical fitness after neoadjuvant treatment in preoperative rectal cancer patients: a blinded interventional pilot study. Br J Anaesth. 2015 Feb;114(2):244–51. https://doi.org/10.1093/bja/aeu318.
41. Rombouts AJM, Al-Najami I. Abbott NL for STAR-TREC collaborative group, et al can we save the rectum by watchful waiting or TransAnal microsurgery following (chemo) radiotherapy versus Total mesorectal excision for early REctal cancer (STAR-TREC study)?: protocol for a multicentre, randomised feasibility study. BMJ Open. 2017;7:e019474. https://doi.org/10.1136/bmjopen-2017-019474.
42. Bahadoer RR, Dijkstra EA, van Etten B, Marijnen CAM, Putter H, et al. Short-course radiotherapy followed by chemotherapy before total mesorectal excision (TME) versus preoperative chemoradiotherapy, TME, and optional adjuvant chemotherapy in locally advanced rectal cancer (RAPIDO): a randomised, open-label, phase 3 trial. Lancet Oncol. 2021;22(1):29–42.

Prehabilitation for Thoracic and Oesophageal Resection Surgery

13

Chao Tong Teo and Theng Wai Foong

13.1 Introduction

Lung cancer is one of the most common cancers, especially in the developing countries [1]. It is also the leading cause of cancer mortality worldwide [1, 2]. Surgical resection and radical lymph node dissection remain an important curative option for lung cancer. Oesophageal cancer is another relatively deadly cancer, being one of the top ten causes of mortality [1]. However, thoracic and oesophageal resection surgery is a high-risk surgery, and careful assessment of the patient's health condition is important for safe delivery of treatment.

Surgical and anaesthetic risk is influenced significantly by cardiorespiratory comorbidities and cardiopulmonary function. About 40–70% of lung cancer patients suffer from chronic obstructive pulmonary disease (COPD) [3], 26% with coronary artery disease, and diabetes in 13% [4]. A patient stratified as high risk has 2.6 times more postoperative complications and 7.7 times more likely to die compared to another considered as low risk [5]. Oesophageal cancer is also frequently associated with smoking and COPD, leading to greater risk of malnutrition and hypoxaemia [6]. After risk–benefit profiling and stratification, some patients are deemed inoperable due to their excessively high risk.

Prehabilitation has been shown to improve physiological reserves prior to the surgery [7, 8]. It plays an important role particularly in high-risk patients who may otherwise be deemed inoperable, improving their preoperative function, risk–benefit profile, and chance of survival with surgery. Prehabilitation has also

C. T. Teo · T. W. Foong (✉)
Department of Anaesthesia and Surgical Intensive Care Unit, National University Health System Singapore, Singapore, Singapore
e-mail: theng_wai_foong@nuhs.edu.sg

A. Chakraborty, A. Balakrishnan (eds.), *Prehabilitation for Cancer Surgery*,
https://doi.org/10.1007/978-981-16-6494-6_13

been shown to decrease postoperative morbidity and mortality [9], improve postoperative quality of life, and shorten duration of hospital stay [10].

13.2 Preoperative Assessment and Risk Stratification for Thoracic Surgery

Preoperative assessment and risk stratification for patients undergoing lung resection surgery have been well described [11, 12]. These risk stratification tools allow us to identify moderate to high-risk patients who may greatly benefit from prehabilitation. Cardiopulmonary tests such as pulmonary function tests (PFT), shuttle walk test (SWT), and cardiopulmonary exercise testing (CPET) are commonly used. These are important to ascertain the cardiac and pulmonary reserves of the patient prior to surgery.

13.2.1 Cardiopulmonary Function Tests

The PFT is a simple but valuable tool that provides information of the airways and pulmonary parenchyma via spirometry and the diffusing capacity of the lung for carbon monoxide (DLCO), respectively [13].

Various lung volumes and capacities can be obtained from spirometry testing. The forced expiratory volume in 1 s (FEV1) and forced vital capacity (FVC) are the results of more value. The spirometry curve and the FEV1/FVC ratio can help determine obstructive and/or restrictive disease and its severity.

The DLCO measures the uptake of carbon monoxide (CO) after a single 10 s vital capacity breath hold with 10% helium and 0.3% CO. It helps elucidate the integrity and function of the alveoli and parenchyma and therefore estimates the percentage of alveoli and lung parenchyma with effective diffusion function.

The shuttle walk test (SWT) is a low technology, easily performed exercise tolerance test that involves the patient walking a 10 m circuit, in time to beeps of increasing pace. The patient is tasked to walk for as long as they can, until they are too breathless to continue, reaches 85% of the predicted maximal heart rate (maximum HR = 220-age) or cannot keep up with the pace of the beeps. The heart rate and pulse oximetry (SpO_2) are recorded during the test. This is a reliable and valid test to assess exercise capacity of individuals, with correlation of results to peak oxygen consumption being 0.67–0.95 [14].

Lastly, the CPET is an objective clinical assessment of a patient's exercise, musculoskeletal and cardiopulmonary capacity. Various parameters such as the ECG, SpO_2, spirometry, end tidal oxygen (ETO_2) and carbon dioxide ($ETCO_2$), blood pressure, and arterial blood gases are obtained during a standardised exercise cycle ergometer regime with increasing resistance. O_2 consumption and CO_2 production during various exercise intensities are recorded, and peak O_2 consumption (VO_2max) and anaerobic threshold are then calculated. This is one of the most objective measures to predict cardiopulmonary reserves in patients [15].

13.2.2 Preoperative Risk Assessment

Figure 13.1 shows the American College of Chest Physicians (ACCP) clinical practice guideline recommendations on preoperative risk stratification algorithm for lung resection [11]. Patients who are considered for lobectomies or pneumonectomies should have their predicted postoperative (PPO) FEV1 and ppoDLCO calculated.

$$\text{PPO values} = \text{preoperative values} \times \left(1 - \text{fraction of total perfusion for the resected lung}\right)$$

Predicted postoperative values of >60% in both FEV1 and DLCO indicate low risk of perioperative death and cardiopulmonary complications, and no further investigation is required. Patients with ppoFEV1 or ppoDLCO between 30 and 60% should undergo a stair-climbing test or shuttle walk test (SWT) to ascertain their cardiopulmonary function. Patients who failed the shuttle walk test (<400 m) or stair-climbing test (<22 m) or have either ppo values <30% should have a formal cardiopulmonary exercise testing (CPET) to determine the maximum oxygen consumption (VO_2max) value. Patients with VO_2max <10 ml/kg/min are deemed as high-risk and are advised not to proceed with surgery as risk of complications and

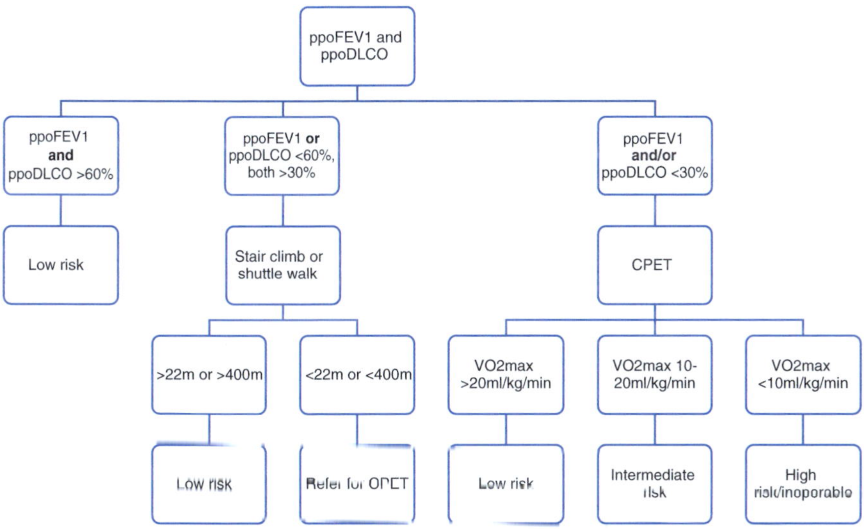

Fig. 13.1 Preoperative risk stratification algorithm for lung resection. *Ppo* Predicted postoperative value (PPO values = preoperative values x (1 – fraction of total perfusion for the resected lung)), *FEV1* Forced expiratory volume in 1 s, *DLCO* Diffusing capacity of lung for carbon monoxide, *CPET* Cardiopulmonary exercise testing, *SCT* Stair climb test, SWT Shuttle walk test, *VO_2max* Maximum oxygen consumption. Adapted from the ACCP guidelines [10]. For patients in consideration for lobectomies or pneumonectomies, ppoFEV1 and ppoDLCO should be calculated. Either segmental counting or perfusion scans can be used for calculation

mortality may outweigh the benefits. The European Respiratory Society (ERS)/ European Society of Thoracic Surgeons (ESTS) recommends a similar risk stratification algorithm [12]. In these high-risk patients, considerable risk of severe cardiopulmonary morbidity and residual functional loss is expected. Patients should then be counselled on alternative surgical, i.e. minor resections or minimally invasive surgery, or nonsurgical options.

These risk stratification guidelines all fall on three main parameters, namely respiratory mechanics (FEV1), lung parenchymal function (DLCO), and cardiopulmonary reserve (VO_2max). These make up the colloquial three-legged stool of thoracic risk profiling, where a deficit in one will portend poorer outcomes [16].

Nevertheless, these high-risk patients can potentially improve their VO_2max[17] or FEV1 values through prehabilitation [18–20]. Prehabilitation plays a vital role in this group of patients by improving physiological reserves and risk profile from high-risk to moderate-risk, thus enabling surgery with a more acceptable risk. This is demonstrated in a few prospective studies [21, 22] and randomised controlled trials [19, 23, 24], where prehabilitation programmes improved their physiologic parameters.

This is especially crucial in thoracic surgery, as there will be a definite reduction in lung volumes and function postoperatively, and patients are at higher risk of postoperative pulmonary complications because of this unique consideration. By targeting and improving one or more of these physiologic parameters through prehabilitation, the perioperative morbidity and mortality risk will then be reduced.

13.3 Prehabilitation in Thoracic Surgery

Prehabilitation is a multidisciplinary programme involving multiple stakeholders including the anaesthetist, surgeon, nursing staff, physiotherapist, dietician, and psychologist. The implementation of prehabilitation into thoracic enhanced recovery after surgery (ERAS) has been recommended by the ERAS® Society and the European Society of Thoracic Surgeons (ESTS) [25]. It reduces risk for the patient by targeting modifiable risk factors via exercise, nutritional support, and smoking cessation programme.

Thoracic surgery is a high-risk operation which entails one-lung ventilation (OLV), and all patients will have significant reduction in functional status postoperatively [26]. This is evident even in segmentectomies [27]. The risk of greater fall in functional status to below the dependent threshold is also higher in patients with low cardiopulmonary reserves, poor effort tolerance [5, 28], malnutrition [29] and who are currently smoking [28]. This can be circumvented with a comprehensive prehabilitation programme.

Figure 13.2 demonstrates the effect of prehabilitation on the functional status and recovery. Patients with prehabilitation have improved preoperative functional status and remain above the functional dependent threshold even with the reduction

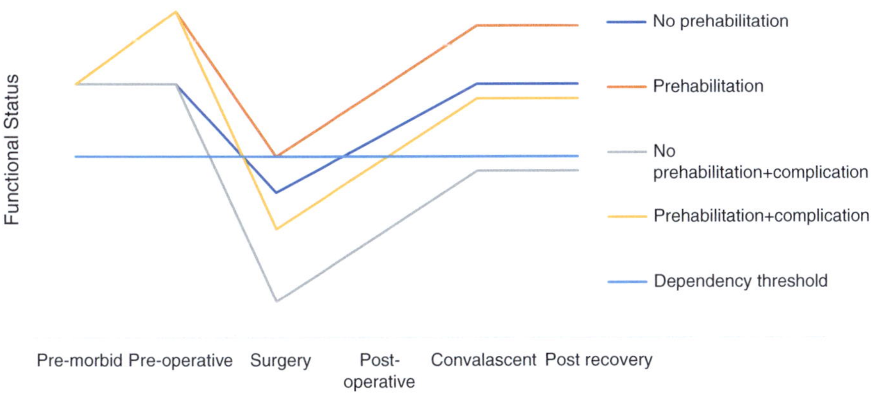

Fig. 13.2 Effects of prehabilitation on functional status and recovery. Thoracic surgery is a high-risk operation, and all patients will have significant reduction in functional status postoperatively *(blue line)*. Patients with prehabilitation have improved preoperative functional status and remain above the functional dependent threshold even with the reduction in postoperative functional status *(orange line)*. Patients who suffer complications perioperatively may have further reductions in their functional status. Prehabilitation is crucial in such patients by shortening the duration of time spent below the dependent threshold and enabling rehabilitation and recovery *(yellow line)*. Those who have poor physiologic reserves and do not undergo prehabilitation may be at a higher risk of being dependent for long term, even after recovery *(grey line)*

in postoperative functional status. Patients who suffer complications perioperatively may have further reductions in their functional status. Prehabilitation is crucial in such patients by shortening the duration of time spent below the dependent threshold and enabling rehabilitation and recovery. Those who have poor physiologic reserves and do not undergo prehabilitation may be at a higher risk of being dependent for long term, even after recovery. Better postoperative physiologic function can also enable rehabilitation, resulting in enhanced recovery. Thus, prehabilitation has been shown to improve quality of life postoperatively [9, 10].

However, the adoption of an ERAS protocol for thoracic surgery is less widespread, much less prehabilitation. This may be due to limitations in the centres or preconceived ideas of potential delay in lung cancer surgery. Nevertheless, studies and centres that implemented prehabilitation programmes for thoracic lung resection have shown reductions in postoperative complications [18, 30]. Varying programmes have been implemented in these centres, common components include preoperative high intensity exercise regimens, smoking cessation, nutrition optimisation, and correction of premorbid statuses. Table 13.1 summarises the various components of prehabilitation that have been implemented for patients undergoing thoracic lung resection surgery. Benefits include decreased incidence of postoperative lung infection, atelectasis, lowered mortality in high-risk patients [9], and increased patient satisfaction and quality of life [10]. As such, it is postulated that prehabilitation programmes can potentially decrease healthcare cost, conserve intensive care resources, and improve patient outcomes.

Table 13.1 Types of prehabilitation programmes

Prehabilitation programmes	
Exercise	Endurance type exercises • Treadmill running • Resistance ergocycle • Walking exercises
	Resistance type exercises • Resistance band training • Free weight training • Upper limb: Bicep curls, wall push-ups, etc • Lower limb: Wall squats, hips raised • Abdominal wall: Sit-ups
	High intensity interval training
	Respiratory muscle training • Inspiratory muscle training • Expiratory muscle training
Smoking cessation programmes	Addiction programmes
	Psychological support
	Nicotine replacement therapy
Nutritional support	Dietician review
	Caloric supplementation
	Immunomodulating diet therapy
Optimisation of comorbidities	COPD control
	Anaemia correction
	Cardiac optimisation

There are many prehabilitation programmes that can be instituted for thoracic surgical patients. Within these programmes, there is a myriad of therapies, each with specific goals and benefits for the patient. These programmes are synergistic and complement each other and may be of increased advantage to the patient if combined together

13.3.1 Preoperative Exercise

A common form of prehabilitation is physiotherapy and preoperative exercise. There have been reports of numerous benefits that can be obtained from preoperative exercise regimens. The benefits of preoperative exercise are summarised in Table 13.2.

Two randomised control trials (RCTs) that implemented short term intense physical exercise for patients planning for lung cancer surgery have shown that those who underwent intensive preoperative exercise regimes have improvements in various parameters important for preoperative risk stratification [18–20].

Licker et al. [18] reported an RCT involving 151 non-small cell lung cancer patients showed that preoperative exercise improves cardiopulmonary function with:

- 15% median increase in their 6MWT distance
- 8% increase in their anaerobic threshold
- 15% increase in their VO_2max.

Table 13.2 Benefits of preoperative exercise

Preoperative	Intraoperative	Postoperative
Improved respiratory mechanics: FEV1	Better tolerance of one-lung ventilation	Reduced risk of postoperative pulmonary complications: Lung infection, atelectasis
Improved lung parenchyma function: DLCO		Potentially reduce admission to high-dependency/ICU
Improved cardiorespiratory reserve: 6MWT, walking speed, walking distance, VO_2max		Potentially reduce healthcare cost

Esra et al. [19] also showed similar results in the cardiopulmonary function and also in their lung mechanics and parenchymal functions such as:

- increase in walking distance of 60%,
- increase in walking speed of 23%,
- 5% improvement of their DLCO
- increase of 7.6% of their FEV1.

A cohort study by Boujibar et al. which included 38 patients with VO_2max <20 ml/min/kg on CPET undergo a programme consisting of exercise retraining, muscle strengthening, and smoking cessation also improved their cardiopulmonary function:

- All participants increased their VO_2max post prehabilitation
- One particular patient from VO_2max 9.2 ml/min/kg to 12.8 ml/min/kg, thus upgraded from excessively high risk to operable status [17].

As these parameters are used for preoperative risk profiling, these improvements should then potentially decrease the patient's perioperative risk and also increase fitness to operation. Studies also showed that exercise confers improved post-surgical outcomes, which likely mirrors the lowered perioperative risk from improved preoperative parameters.

The above cardiopulmonary improvements could be attributed to increased muscle strength and possible bronchodilation and shunting of blood to the non-diseased lung from exercise. This potentially is helpful during the one-lung ventilation intraoperatively during thoracic surgery. Furthermore, improved muscle strength and VO_2max can also help in preparing for postoperative chest physiotherapy that is important in the recovery of thoracic surgery. Gao et al. showed via a 342 patient prospective study that entails prehabilitation with breathing exercises and power bicycle exercise training. Postoperative complication rate is significantly reduced post-prehabilitation (16.9% vs 83.3%), and lung infection rates were also decreased (2.81% vs 17.9%) [30]. Total cost and hospital stay were not increased despite the implementation of prehabilitation. This is also reproduced in the study by Licker et al. involving HIIT regimes; incidence of pulmonary complications was lower in patients who underwent prehabilitation compared to those who did not (23% versus 44%), owing to a significant reduction in atelectasis (12.2% versus 36.4%) [18]. By preventing respiratory complications, patients will then have lower likelihood of requiring prolonged ICU stays or ventilatory support.

However, most studies only focused on pulmonary complications. Other important factors such as cardiovascular complications and postoperative physical function are not well studied and warrant future investigation. Nonetheless, prehabilitation can lead to reduced morbidity in patients, therefore could potentially save cost for individual patients and for the healthcare system and should be encouraged.

Many different exercise regimes have been described, but most studies showed that a combination of endurance exercises and resistance training to be the most sensible approach and showed more significant results. HIIT regimes are also growing in popularity, owing to their perceived efficiency. Duration of prehabilitation is another important factor; time is required for building up physiologic reserves. A duration of 2–6 weeks of exercise is most commonly used, due to the urgency of curative lung resection surgery. The type and duration of exercise are detailed as below:

13.3.1.1 Type of Exercise

There exist several types of exercise regimes, such as endurance or aerobic exercise, resistance or weight exercises, and high intensity interval training (HIIT), summarised in Table 13.3. Endurance training was viewed as a preferred method to increase muscle endurance and aerobic threshold from higher cardiac outputs and enhanced oxygen extraction efficiency. These exercises include running, resistance cycling, or swimming. Conversely, resistance exercises are thought to be more effective in increasing muscle strength and mass. Free weight training, resistance bands, weight lifting machines are examples of resistance training.

Table 13.3 Types of exercise regimes and effects

Type of exercise	Examples	Theorised effects
Endurance training	Treadmill running Resistance ergocycle Walking exercises	Increase muscle endurance Increase aerobic threshold Enhanced oxygen extraction efficiency
Resistance exercises	Resistance band training Free weight training Upper limb: Bicep curls, wall push-ups, etc. Lower limb: Wall squats, hips raised Abdominal wall: Sit-ups	Increase muscle strength Increase muscle mass
High intensity interval training	Repeated sessions of brief intermittent exercises	Increase VO_2max Increase inspiratory and general muscle strength

Various exercise regimes have been designed for thoracic patients to build their physiologic reserves, and these all can target various parts of the "three-legged stool" of thoracic risk profiling. Increased muscle strength and endurance are likely a manifestation of improvement of all "3-legged stool" parameters

More recent studies in healthy individuals have shown that HIIT is also effective in increasing VO_2max and inspiratory muscle strength [31, 32]. Such exercises refer to repeated sessions of brief intermittent high intensity exercise close to VO_2max, with pauses in between for rest and a cool down period for recovery. HIIT appears to be comparable to endurance training in improving physiologic parameters, but possibly using a shorter period (2 weeks vs 7–8 weeks) [33, 34].

The improved muscle strength, improved anaerobic threshold, and VO_2max derived from the various exercise types are also reproduced in patients with COPD and with lung cancer for thoracic surgery [9]. Thus, thoracic patients can participate in any of the above-mentioned exercise regimens, and centres can tailor their prehabilitation programme according to their physiotherapy expertise and equipment available.

If there is urgency to perform the surgery, HIIT can be considered, as it seems to improve muscular fitness and VO_2max more efficiently than the other programmes, albeit at the expense of patient's comfort levels; most HIIT participants will experience a sense of immense fatigue lasting at least 10–20 min following each bout of high-level exercise. This would require great motivation on the patient's part.

However, a retrospective observational study showed a possible increase in injury incidence with HIIT. A report of 125–127% increase in lower extremity strains and sprains and 124% increase in upper extremity strains corresponded to a period where HIIT participation increased 274%. However, this study only showed a possible correlation and may not be generalisable to HIIT in supervised settings [35]. Nonetheless, this might still be of concern for the more frail patients in consideration for thoracic surgery, who might be predisposed to injury. Close supervision and correct techniques can prevent such injuries.

There have been no studies that show superiority of one exercise type over another. Until further studies are done to compare efficacy, one can only surmise that HIIT appears to be the most time effective. However, as all types can increase the cardiopulmonary function to the benefit of the patient, the exercise form chosen should be tailored to the patient's abilities, local culture and resources available to the individual healthcare system.

13.3.1.2 Duration of Exercise

To build up muscular strength and endurance, time and effort need to be invested, and patients need to be motivated and participate in the exercise regimes and interventions prescribed. There is no fixed recommended duration for prehabilitation, but most centres implemented 2–6 weeks of prehabilitation to meet predetermined timeframes from diagnosis of cancer to surgery.

Many centres bemoan the length of time required for exercise prehabilitation, potentially delaying a semi-urgent cancer surgery, thereby risking progression of the malignancy. Indeed, exercise prehabilitation requires time to complete; however, a randomised control trial involving 60 lung cancer patients have shown that even a short 1-week course of high intensity exercise regimen can improve cardiopulmonary function and reduce postoperative complications [19]. After a week of physical therapy, it was found that non-diseased lung's V/Q distribution was improved, and FVC, FEV1, and DLCO also improved. PaO_2 was increased, and $PaCO_2$ was decreased. Total walking distance and maximum speed were also increased. All these might have contributed to a significant decrease in postoperative morbidity (16.7% vs 3.3%) and decrease in hospital stay (9.66 days vs 5.4 days). As such HIIT can be a good consideration for centres who prefer to have a limited time to surgery from diagnosis.

Furthermore, a cohort study involving 38 patients also illustrates that the time taken for prehabilitation did not increase the time taken to surgery as compared to their controls [17]. They noted that preoperative assessment before lobectomy took a similar amount of time as prehabilitation. Consequently, proper planning and early institution of prehabilitation can thus circumvent the issue of urgency of surgery. Concurrent investigations and surgical planning will save time and limit the number of visits that the patient will need to take to the hospital, thus further increasing patient satisfaction and reducing cost.

Home-based exercise programmes were also investigated by Coats et al. [36] A 4-week self-monitored and supervised home exercise programme comprising aerobic (resistance ergocycle) and resistance training with free weights was imposed to 20 participants. Supervision included individual coaching by a physiotherapist and weekly telephone follow-up. It showed relatively high adherence rates and also eventual improvements in the 6-min walk test distance (improved by 28 m compared to before intervention) and greater strength of the upper and lower limb muscles (increase in strength by 14–27% compared to baseline). The participants also reported improvements in dyspnoea, and to be having more energy post-intervention, thus also having a reduction in the mean depression scores. Time and cost savings are additional benefits scored by the home-based technique. However, of the 40 eligible participants, only 20 patients agreed to participate. The rest cited a lack of interest or time or felt too anxious about their diagnosis. Thus, the high adherence rates could be a selection bias to motivated individuals.

In order to have an effective home-based programme, motivational supervision may be important to avoid dropouts and non-adherence to the prescribed exercises, which will diminish the benefits that the programme accords. Nonetheless, home exercise techniques, if implemented well, are helpful to increase the volume and duration of exercise that a thoracic patient can undergo prior to their time-sensitive surgery.

Therefore, the above studies have shown that a well thought out and administered prehabilitation programme does not lengthen the time from diagnosis to surgery, and urgency to excision is not a strong reason to omit prehabilitation. Even a 1-week course can provide benefits as well. Individualised prehabilitation exercise and motivational programmes may need to be concurrently prescribed to improve compliance and safety.

13.3.2 Smoking Cessation

Smoking is the most important risk factor for lung cancer and predisposes to other cardiorespiratory comorbidities. Perioperative complications are increased by six-fold in those who smoke [24]. Smoking cessation reduces postoperative complications and mortality. A retrospective study involving 7990 patients who underwent lung cancer resection showed that smoking cessation for more than a year prior to surgery lowers the odd of dying postoperatively by 28.5% compared to current smokers and 4% compared to those who stopped less than a year [37].

The risk of respiratory complications steadily declined as the interval between smoking cessation and the operation increased, 20% in those who stopped within a month, and 55% in those who ceased smoking for more than a year [37]. Another retrospective study involving 271 pneumonectomy patients showed that after smoking cessation for more than a month, the odds of developing pneumonia or ARDS postoperatively decreased by 2.7 times [38].

This decrease in complication and mortality rate is likely from the improvements in ciliary clearance and pulmonary function. These lead to improved ventilation during OLV in thoracic surgery and prevent barotrauma and volutrauma in patients with poorer lung mechanics.

Smoking cessation also appears to have the potential to improve quality of life postoperatively. A prospective cohort study of 70 patients for lung cancer resection showed former smokers (those who stopped prior to diagnosis) had shorter periods of physical function impairments than recent quitters (those who stopped after diagnosis prior to surgery).

Compared to recent quitters, former smokers reported less dyspnoea 1- and 3-months post-surgery, less incidence of chronic pain up to a year post-operation, shorter duration of persistent decrease in physical and social function (1–3 months vs 12 months) [10]. This shows that a smoking cessation programme can aid in increasing patients' postoperative recovery and quicker return to baseline function.

The optimal timing of smoking cessation was never well defined by various studies, but Nakagawa et al. showed that at least 4 weeks of cessation of smoking was required for any meaningful decrease in respiratory complications [39]. However, as lung cancer surgery is recommended by some centres to be done within 4 weeks of diagnosis, smoking cessation programmes might not have sufficient time to create any meaningful impact. Nonetheless, it is still beneficial to advise patients to join a smoking cessation programme as soon as possible to help reduce complications and mortality. Information about the advantages of stopping smoking should be shared with the patients during early clinic consults to reap more benefits.

13.3.3 Nutrition Support

Malnutrition is commonly observed in cancer patients and can contribute to poorer wound healing, muscle wasting, and increased pulmonary complications postoperatively. The European Society for Clinical Nutrition and Metabolism (ESPEN) guidelines recommend that all patients to be screened preoperatively for their nutritional status, and those at high risk of malnutrition to be given caloric support 1–2 weeks prior to surgery [40].

A retrospective observational study by Thomas et al. of 19,625 patients undergoing lobectomies for primary lung cancer reported a significantly higher mortality rate in patients whose BMI is <18.5 (odds ratio 1.89) and also an increased incidence of pulmonary, surgical, and infectious complications, 21.1%, 23.2%, 5.1%, respectively [29]. This highlights the importance of identifying at risk population groups to institute nutritional interventions in order to prevent postoperative issues. A dietician review and caloric supplementation for weight gain can potentially reduce mortality and morbidity in lung cancer patients. They can also enhance effort tolerance preoperatively.

Nutritional support and caloric supplementation usually entail a high protein supplement to prevent sarcopenia and enhance protein stores within the body. This prevents protein catabolism arising from surgical stress and inflammation. Muscle strength can then be preserved, and thus allowing better postoperative rehabilitation, mobilisation, and incentive spirometry.

Studies evaluating the effect of nutrition on thoracic cancer surgery are currently lacking. However, one can extrapolate results from those involving gastrointestinal surgery. A randomised control trial involving 48 colorectal cancer patients receiving whey protein supplementation showed a mean improvement in functional walking capacity before surgery of +20.8 m vs 1.2 m in the control group [41]. This pilot trial shows promise in protein supplementation in increasing muscle strength and effort tolerance in preoperative patients. This may mean improved pulmonary mechanics and cardiopulmonary function, therefore improving perioperative risk in thoracic surgery. Further investigation may be warranted to observe if similar outcomes can be obtained for lung resection surgery.

Nutritional support with protein can be in the form of immunomodulating therapy as well. A prospective study by Kaya et al. involving 58 lung cancer patients had 31 of them undergo a 10-day nutritional intervention with an immune modulating diet enriched with arginine, omega-3 fatty acids, and nucleotides [42]. There was a significant decrease in complication rates in the intervention group (16.6% vs 44.4%). The group with diet intervention also had a lower mean chest tube drainage time (4 days vs 6 days).

Overall, nutritional support is shown to be an important pillar of prehabilitation to reduce postoperative morbidity and should not be neglected. It can be potentially synergistic with exercise to help replenish and build muscle mass and optimise recovery postoperative as well [43]. Nonetheless, more targeted studies to investigate the effect of both exercise and nutrition are required.

13.3.4 Anaemia Optimisation

Preoperative anaemia is a common finding in patients with lung cancer, similar to many other oncologic patients. It is defined as a haemoglobin level of less than 13 g/dL for males and less than 12 g/dL for females. Presence of anaemia portends poorer outcomes in patients, regardless of severity.

A retrospective cohort study investigating data from 227,435 patients undergoing major non-cardiac surgery in 2008 from the American College of Surgeons' National Surgical Quality Improvement Program database, of which 69,299 patients were found to have anaemia, showed that 30-day postoperative mortality was 1.42 times higher in patients with anaemia (odds ratio [OR] 1.42, 95% CI 1.31–1.54). This was seen in the patients with mild anaemia as well (OR 1.41, CI 1.3–1.54) [44]. The 30-day morbidity also mirrored mortality outcomes; patients with anaemia were 1.35 times more likely to have any type of postoperative complication than those without anaemia. Similarly, even those with mild anaemia had raised morbidity (OR 1.31, CI 1.26–1.36) [44]. Although these data are from all non-cardiac surgery, it is likely to be reproduced in the thoracic surgery subgroup as well.

As such, it may be prudent to investigate for and correct any degree of anaemia in patients undergoing thoracic surgery, in order to avoid the increased mortality and morbidity associated with anaemia. For mild to moderate anaemia, with haemoglobin levels of more than 8 g/dL, main strategies include haematinics such as iron supplementation, replacement of vitamin B12 or folate, and erythropoietin. These therapies are not associated with the immunologic or infective transfusion reactions that may accompany packed cell transfusions. Furthermore, most thoracic patients do not tolerate large fluid loads due to the deleterious effect on pulmonary mechanics and ventilation. With the reduction in lung volume and lymphatic drainage following more extensive thoracic surgery, the concomitant increase in pulmonary pressures and increased permeability of capillary membranes can predispose to pulmonary oedema and thus poorer respiratory outcomes [45].

In longer term views, perioperative blood transfusions appear to reduce overall survival and increase recurrence of tumours. A meta-analysis of 18 studies involving 5915 thoracic patients showed a higher risk of death (RR: 1.25, 95% CI: 1.13–1.38) and cancer recurrence (RR: 1.42, 95% CI: 1.20–1.67), for patients who underwent transfusion [46].

As such, preoperative anaemia screening and optimisation have been implemented as part of Patient Blood Management which is endorsed by World Health Organization [47].

13.4 Prehabilitation in Oesophageal Resection Surgery

Oesophageal carcinoma remains a relatively common cancer in Asia, with an incidence of 5.2 and 0.7 per 100,000 for oesophageal squamous cell carcinoma (SCC) and adenocarcinoma (AC), respectively [48]. SCC is more common in central and southeast Asia, while AC burden is higher in Europe and North America. Males are of higher risk. Both variants of oesophageal carcinoma are associated with the highest amount of weight loss among all cancers, stemming from dysphagia and odynophagia from the disease. This is further worsened by neoadjuvant chemoradiotherapy that is a mainstay in oesophageal carcinoma treatment.

Malnutrition and cachexia can affect up to 80% of these patients, leading to greater morbidity [49]. The profound muscle and fat loss, with systemic inflammation from the cancer, is a major determinant of post-treatment morbidity and mortality.

On top of the exercise therapies, smoking cessation, and anaemia optimisation mentioned above, there are some considerations specific to oesophagectomy that warrant further discussion.

13.4.1 Nutrition Support

Nutritional intervention has been shown to improve outcomes in oesophageal surgery. A case control study of 65 patients by Ligthart-Melis showed that patients with intensive nutritional support gained an average of 4.8% more weight than controls, and they are at lower odds of 0.23 (95% confidence interval: 0.053–0.97; $P = 0.045$) of developing complications postoperatively with intensive nutritional support [50]. This is postulated to be due to increased muscle mass, glycogen, and fat stores to withstand the stress of surgery and treatment. This mirrors the effect of nutritional supplementation mentioned in the section above.

Immunomodulating nutrition therapy using arginine and omega-3 fatty acid enriched diets preoperatively is also shown to be beneficial to a myriad of cancer surgery, oesophageal carcinoma included. A randomised control trial of 123 patients for oesophagectomy showed that those with immune enhancing nutrition had lower rates of infectious complications as compared to those with normal nutrition therapy (18% vs 38%) [51]. This result is reproduced in a later randomised control trial involving 40 patients by Kanekiyo et al. that showed reduced postoperative infections and shorter antibiotic duration [52]. All these are supported in meta-analyses of gastrointestinal surgeries of 2730 patients [53] and general major elective surgery involving 1918 patients [54], where both showed decreased postoperative infections, wound complications, and possibly mortality.

13.4.2 Route of Enteral Nutrition

A major consideration for preoperative feeding is its route. Various enteral feeding routes have been used, including nasogastric tubes (NGT), percutaneous gastrostomy, and oesophageal stenting. Logic might suggest that stenting is most ideal as it provides dysphagia relief and allows oral feeding; however, evidence showed otherwise.

A prospective study by Yu et al. of 81 patients showed that NGT and gastrostomy were comparatively more effective than oesophageal stenting [55], with less pain, higher serum albumin levels (as a marker of nutrition), and better quality of life. European Society of Gastrointestinal Endoscopy guidelines [56], endorsed by

ESPEN, also reviewed oesophageal stent use versus NGT/gastrostomy and have noted that stenting confers a much higher complication rate and morbidity such as stent migration and pain. Another review article by de la Mora Levy et al [57] also supports this finding. Thus, stenting is not recommended as the first line for oesophageal cancer patients to alleviate dysphagia, and the more traditional routes of NGT and gastrostomy insertions are preferred.

13.4.3 Analgesia for Oral Mucositis

Oral mucositis is a common side effect from the neoadjuvant chemoradiotherapy that oesophageal cancer patients have to undergo prior to their surgery. Quality of life is much affected from the pain that accompanies it. This can contribute to the poorer oral intake and systemic inflammation.

As such, various therapies have been used to alleviate pain from mucositis. However, no widespread studies have investigated or compared efficacy of such treatment. This may be a potential area of future study.

Opioids are commonly utilised and are effective in reducing pain. Fentanyl is commonly used and may be administered transdermal and via a patient controlled analgesia (PCA) device. An investigation involving 46 patients showed that transdermal fentanyl is effective in lowering pain scores significantly [58] and eliminated the pain in 67.4% of patients by day 6 of treatment. Quality of life is thus greatly improved, with manageable side effects.

Various studies also showed that topical morphine mouthwash can be helpful to reduce mucositis pain. A systematic review of RCT on topical morphine for patients undergoing chemoradiotherapy for various cancers by Saunders et al [59] showed a consistent analgesic effect of topical morphine, thus recommends the usage of morphine mouthwash as a therapeutic agent for mucositis.

Topical local anaesthetics (LA) are another commonly utilised group of drugs. However, only a few studies have investigated them in isolation. Nonetheless, systemic review by Saunders et al. [59] showed clinical benefit in reducing pain. Therefore, topical LA can be considered to mitigate the pain from mucositis to allow temporary relief for eating or oral hygiene.

There are other agents such as sucralfate, which is postulated to act as a mucosal coating to protect against mucositis. However, an RCT involving 30 patients who developed mucositis showed no significant benefit over a soda mouthwash. This is supported by a Multinational Association of Supportive Care in Cancer and International Society of Oral Oncology (MASCC/ISOO) clinical practice guideline [60]. They also do not support the use of antimicrobial lozenges to prevent or treat mucositis, as they do not show any clinical benefit [60].

Therefore, the mainstay of mucositis treatment still lies upon topical and systemic opioids and topical LA solutions. These should be readily available to alleviate the mucositis pain in oesophageal cancer patients.

13.5 Conclusion

Prehabilitation for thoracic and oesophageal surgery includes preoperative exercise, smoking cessation, nutrition support, and anaemia optimisation. In addition, oesophageal carcinoma carries unique challenges, and nutritional supplementation is highly important to counter its associated malnutrition and cachexia. NGT and gastrostomy feeding appears to be preferred routes for enteral feeding if possible, and the pain from mucositis arising from neoadjuvant chemoradiotherapy should be aggressively treated to improve quality of life of these patients.

Patients who undergo well organised prehabilitation programmes can benefit greatly, with significant decrease in postoperative mortality and morbidity, better quality of life, and potentially lower health care cost. Targeted regimens based on individual patient profile and health care resources available may be required to make full use of the limited time available between diagnosis of cancer and surgery. Also, the frailest may benefit the most from such programmes, as they may experience greater decrease in risk or improve their risk profile from inoperable status to operable. Psychological profiling and motivational supervision can help increase adherence to the various prehabilitation programmes. Nonetheless, great coordination between the various healthcare stakeholders (physiotherapists, dieticians, medical, surgical, anaesthetic teams, etc.) and the patients is required to execute a successful programme.

References

1. Ferlay J, et al. Estimating the global cancer incidence and mortality in 2018: GLOBOCAN sources and methods. Int J Cancer. 2019;144:1941–53.
2. Torre LA, Siegel RL, Jemal A. Lung cancer statistics. Adv Exp Med Biol. 2016;893:1–19.
3. Young RP, et al. COPD prevalence is increased in lung cancer, independent of age, sex and smoking history. Eur Respir J. 2008;34:380–6.
4. Boffa DJ, et al. Data from the Society of Thoracic Surgeons general thoracic surgery database: the surgical management of primary lung tumors. J Thorac Cardiovasc Surg. 2008;135:247–54.
5. Stanzani F, et al. Mortalidade, morbidade e categorização de risco para complicações perioperatórias em pacientes com câncer de pulmão. J Bras Pneumol. 2014;40:21–9.
6. Krzystek-Korpacka M, et al. Respiratory insufficiency related to copd accelerates systemic inflammation, under-nutrition, and angiogenesis in esophageal malignancies. Exp Oncol. 2008;30(1):75–80. http://dspace.nbuv.gov.ua/xmlui/handle/123456789/139020
7. Li T-C, Yang M-C, Tseng AH, Lee HH-C. Prehabilitation and rehabilitation for surgically treated lung cancer patients. J Cancer Res Pract. 2017;4:89–94.
8. Sebio Garcia R, Yáñez Brage MI, Giménez Moolhuyzen E, Granger CL, Denehy L. Functional and postoperative outcomes after preoperative exercise training in patients with lung cancer: a systematic review and meta-analysis. Interact Cardiovasc Thorac Surg. 2016;23:486–97.
9. Sanchez-Lorente D, et al. Prehabilitation in thoracic surgery. J Thorac Dis. 2018;10:S2593–600.
10. Balduyck B, et al. The effect of smoking cessation on quality of life after lung cancer surgery. Eur J Cardio-Thoracic Surg. 2011;40:1432–8.
11. Brunelli A, Kim AW, Berger KI, Addrizzo-Harris DJ. Physiologic evaluation of the patient with lung cancer being considered for resectional surgery: diagnosis and management of lung cancer, 3rd ed: American college of chest physicians evidence-based clinical practice guidelines. Chest. 2013;143:e166S–90S.

12. Brunelli A, et al. ERS/ESTS clinical guidelines on fitness for radical therapy in lung cancer patients (surgery and chemo-radiotherapy). Eur Respir J. 2009;34:17–41.
13. Hirai T. Pulmonary function tests. In: Medical radiology. Berlin: Springer Science and Business Media Deutschland GmbH; 2021. p. 11–20. https://doi.org/10.1007/978-3-030-43539-4_2.
14. Parreira VF, et al. Measurement properties of the incremental shuttle walk test: a systematic review. Chest. 2014;145:1357–69.
15. Levett DZH, et al. Perioperative cardiopulmonary exercise testing (CPET): consensus clinical guidelines on indications, organization, conduct, and physiological interpretation. Br J Anaesth. 2018;120:484–500.
16. Slinger P, Darling G. Preanesthetic assessment for thoracic surgery. In: *Principles and practice of anesthesia for thoracic surgery*. Cham: Springer International Publishing; 2019. p. 13–41. https://doi.org/10.1007/978-3-030-00859-8_2.
17. Boujibar F, et al. Impact of prehabilitation on morbidity and mortality after pulmonary lobectomy by minimally invasive surgery: a cohort study. J Thorac Dis. 2018;10:2240–8.
18. Licker M, et al. Short-term preoperative high-intensity interval training in patients awaiting lung cancer surgery: a randomized controlled trial. J Thorac Oncol. 2017;12:323–33.
19. Pehlivan E, Turna A, Gurses A, Gurses HN. The effects of preoperative short-term intense physical therapy in lung cancer patients: a randomized controlled trial. Ann Thorac Cardiovasc Surg. 2011;17:461–8.
20. Vagvolgyi A, Rozgonyi Z, Kerti M, Vadasz P, Varga J. Effectiveness of perioperative pulmonary rehabilitation in thoracic surgery. J Thorac Dis. 2017;9:1584–91.
21. Bobbio A, et al. Preoperative pulmonary rehabilitation in patients undergoing lung resection for non-small cell lung cancer. Eur J Cardio-Thoracic Surg. 2008;33:95–8.
22. Cesario A, et al. Pre-operative pulmonary rehabilitation and surgery for lung cancer. Lung Cancer. 2007;57:118–9.
23. Morano MT, et al. Preoperative pulmonary rehabilitation versus chest physical therapy in patients undergoing lung cancer resection: a pilot randomized controlled trial. Arch Phys Med Rehabil. 2013;94:53–8.
24. Stefanelli F, et al. High-intensity training and cardiopulmonary exercise testing in patients with chronic obstructive pulmonary disease and non-small-cell lung cancer undergoing lobectomy. Eur. J. Cardio-Thoracic Surg. 2013;44:e260–5.
25. Batchelor TJP, et al. Guidelines for enhanced recovery after lung surgery: recommendations of the enhanced recovery after surgery (ERAS®) society and the European Society of Thoracic Surgeons (ESTS). Eur J Cardio-thoracic Surg. 2019;55:91–115.
26. Weissman C. Pulmonary function after cardiac and thoracic surgery. Anesth Analg. 1999;88:1272–9.
27. Gu Z, et al. Pulmonary function changes after different extent of pulmonary resection under video-assisted thoracic surgery. J Thorac Dis. 2018;10:2331–7.
28. Smetana GW, Lawrence VA, Cornell JE. Preoperative pulmonary risk stratification for noncardiothoracic surgery: systematic review for the American College of Physicians. Ann Intern Med. 2006;144:581–95.
29. Thomas PA, et al. National perioperative outcomes of pulmonary lobectomy for cancer: the influence of nutritional status†. Eur. J. Cardio-thoracic Surg. 2014;45:652–9.
30. Gao K, et al. Cardiopulmonary exercise testing screening and pre-operative pulmonary rehabilitation reduce postoperative complications and improve fast-track recovery after lung cancer surgery: a study for 342 cases. Thorac Cancer. 2015;6:443–9.
31. Menz V, et al. Functional vs. Running low-volume high-intensity interval training: Effects on vo2max and muscular endurance. J Sport Sci Med. 2019;18:497–504.
32. Astorino TA, Allen RP, Roberson DW, Jurancich M. Effect of high-intensity interval training on cardiovascular function, &OV0312;o2max, and muscular force. J Strength Cond Res. 2012;26:138–45.
33. Burgomaster KA, Hughes SC, Heigenhauser GJF, Bradwell SN, Gibala MJ. Six sessions of sprint interval training increases muscle oxidative potential and cycle endurance capacity in humans. J Appl Physiol. 2005;98:1985–90.

34. Coyle EF. Very intense exercise-training is extremely potent and time efficient: a reminder. J Appl Physiol. 2005;98:1983–4.
35. Rynecki ND, Siracuse BL, Ippolito JA, Beebe KS. Injuries sustained during high intensity interval training: are modern fitness trends contributing to increased injury rates? J Sports Med Phys Fitness. 2019;59:1206–12.
36. Coats V, et al. Feasibility and effectiveness of a home-based exercise training program before lung resection surgery. Can Respir J. 2013;20:10–6.
37. Mason DP, et al. Impact of smoking cessation before resection of lung cancer: a Society of Thoracic Surgeons general thoracic surgery database study. Ann Thorac Surg. 2009;88:362–71.
38. Vaporciyan AA, et al. Incidence of major pulmonary morbidity after pneumonectomy: association with timing of smoking cessation. Ann Thorac Surg. 2002;73:420–6.
39. Nakagawa M, Tanaka H, Tsukuma H, Kishi Y. Relationship between the duration of the preoperative smoke-free period and the incidence of postoperative pulmonary complications after pulmonary surgery. Chest. 2001;120:705–10.
40. Weimann A, et al. ESPEN guidelines on enteral nutrition: surgery including organ transplantation $. Artic Press Clin Nutr. 2006;25:224–44.
41. Gillis C, et al. Prehabilitation with whey protein supplementation on perioperative functional exercise capacity in patients undergoing colorectal resection for cancer: a pilot double-blinded randomized placebo-controlled trial. J Acad Nutr Diet. 2016;116:802–12.
42. Kaya SO, et al. Is preoperative protein-rich nutrition effective on postoperative outcome in non-small cell lung cancer surgery? A prospective randomized study. J Cardiothorac Surg. 2016;11:14.
43. Payne C, Larkin PJ, McIlfatrick S, Dunwoody L, Gracey JH. Exercise and nutrition interventions in advanced lung cancer: a systematic review. Curr Oncol. 2013;20:e321.
44. Kosmidis P, Krzakowski M. Anemia profiles in patients with lung cancer: what have we learned from the European cancer Anaemia survey (ECAS)? Lung Cancer. 2005;50:401–12.
45. Sengupta S. Post-operative pulmonary complications after thoracotomy. Indian J Anaesth. 2015;59:618–26.
46. Luan H, Ye F, Wu L, Zhou Y, Jiang J. Perioperative blood transfusion adversely affects prognosis after resection of lung cancer: a systematic review and a meta-analysis. BMC Surg. 2014;14:1–8.
47. Goodnough LT, Shander A, Riou B. Patient Blood Manag Anesthesiol. 2012;116:1367–76.
48. Arnold M, Soerjomataram I, Ferlay J, Forman D. Global incidence of oesophageal cancer by histological subtype in 2012. Gut. 2015;64:381–7.
49. Bower MR, Martin RCG. Nutritional management during neoadjuvant therapy for esophageal cancer. J Surg Oncol. 2009;100:82–7.
50. Ligthart-Melis GC, et al. Dietician-delivered intensive nutritional support is associated with a decrease in severe postoperative complications after surgery in patients with esophageal cancer. Dis Esophagus. 2013;26:587–93.
51. Fukuda T, et al. Can immune-enhancing nutrients reduce postoperative complications in patients undergoing esophageal surgery? Dis Esophagus. 2008;21:708–11.
52. Kanekiyo S, et al. Efficacy of perioperative immunonutrition in esophageal cancer patients undergoing esophagectomy. Nutrition. 2019;59:96–102.
53. Cerantola Y, Hübner M, Grass F, Demartines N, Schäfer M. Immunonutrition in gastrointestinal surgery. Br J Surg. 2011;98:37–48.
54. Marik PE, Zaloga GP. Immunonutrition in high-risk surgical patients. J Parenter Enter Nutr. 2010;34:378–86.
55. Yu FJ, et al. Enteral nutrition and quality of life in patients undergoing chemoradiotherapy for esophageal carcinoma: a comparison of nasogastric tube, esophageal stent, and ostomy tube feeding. Gastrointest Endosc. 2018;88:21–31.e4.
56. Spaander MCW, et al. Esophageal stenting for benign and malignant disease: European Society of Gastrointestinal Endoscopy (ESGE) clinical guideline. Endoscopy. 2016;48:939–48.

57. de la Mora Levy J. G. & Manzano-Robleda, M. del C. nutrition before chemoradiotherapy or surgery: temporary esophageal stents or tube feeding? Is the evidence hard to swallow? Gastrointest Endosc. 2018;88:32–4.
58. Xing SZ, Zhang Y. Efficacy and safety of transdermal fentanyl for the treatment of oral mucositis pain caused by chemoradiotherapy in patients with esophageal squamous cell carcinoma. Support Care Cancer. 2015;23:753–9.
59. Saunders DP, et al. Systematic review of antimicrobials, mucosal coating agents, anesthetics, and analgesics for the management of oral mucositis in cancer patients and clinical practice guidelines. Support Care Cancer. 28(5):2473–84. https://doi.org/10.1007/s00520-019-05181-6.
60. Lalla RV, et al. MASCC/ISOO clinical practice guidelines for the management of mucositis secondary to cancer therapy. Cancer. 2014;120:1453–61.

Prehabilitation for Surgery in Urology, Urogynaecology, and Gynaecological Oncology

14

Pradeep Durai, Harvard Z. J. Lin, Jaydip Bhaumik, and Pearl S. Y. Tong

Abbreviations

6MWT	6-minute walk test
BMI	Body mass index
EFD	Erectile function domain
EPR-GO	Enhancing patients' resilience in gynaecological oncology
ERAS	Enhanced recovery after surgery
FACT-B	Functional assessment of cancer therapy-bladder
IIEF	International Index of Erectile Function
NCEPOD	National Confidential Enquiry into Patient Outcome and Death
PFE	Pelvic floor exercises
RC	Radical cystectomy
RP	Radical prostatectomy
SF-12	12 Item short from survey
SHIM	Sexual Health Inventory for Men
VRCD	Very low-calorie diet

P. Durai (✉)
Division of Urology, Ng Teng Fong General Hospital, National University Health System, Singapore, Singapore
e-mail: pradeep_durai@nuhs.edu.sg

H. Z. J. Lin · P. S. Y. Tong
Department of Obstetrics and Gynaecology, National University Hospital, National University Health System, Singapore, Singapore

J. Bhaumik
Department of Gynaecological Oncology, Tata Medical Center, Kolkata, India

A. Chakraborty, A. Balakrishnan (eds.), *Prehabilitation for Cancer Surgery*,
https://doi.org/10.1007/978-981-16-6494-6_14

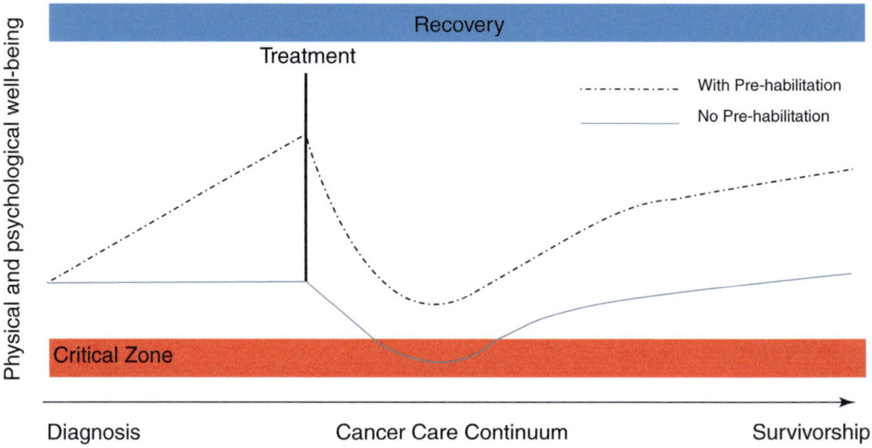

Fig. 14.1 Hypothesized mechanisms of prehabilitation supportive care interventions on patient outcomes

14.1 Introduction

An ageing population with higher life expectancy puts us in some sort of a silver Tsunami wherein we will be dealing with more elderly and frail patients with associated multiple comorbidities who will need major urological surgery [1]. National Confidential Enquiry into Patient Outcome and Death (NCEPOD) report showed that preoperative optimization is important in preventing morbidity and mortality after surgery [2].

Cancer prehabilitation is a process on the continuum of care that occurs between the time of a cancer diagnosis and the beginning of acute treatment [3]. Prehabilitation is a multi-professional concept which has garnered more attention in the recent past. Undergoing a major surgery puts enormous metabolic stress on the body and tilts it towards a catabolic phase. If not managed properly, functional capacity of an individual can decline. There needs to be a process to enhance the ability to withstand the stress, especially a cancer surgery puts on human body [4]. Paterson et al. graphically represented the role of prehabilitation in patient undergoing cancer treatment (Fig. 14.1) [5].

There are studies which have shown that poor preoperative performance status increases morbidity and mortality [6]. Optimizing preoperative functional capacity can improve outcomes. There is paucity of literature in urological oncology on prehabilitation. In this chapter, we will focus on prehabilitation for major uro-oncology surgery, radical cystectomy (RC) with urinary diversion.

14.2 Multi-Professional Care Model

The concept of prehabilitation involves identifying impairments in physical and psychological health and intervening with the aim of reducing peri-operative morbidity and mortality [7]. Prehabilitation in cancer surgery is expanding from the single physical interventions to multi-professional complex programs [4]. Professionals including but not limited to physicians, uro-oncology surgeon, uro-oncology specialist nurse, physiotherapist, psychologist, dietician, medical-social worker will encompass a strong team to assist with prehabilitation.

In a complex urological procedure like radical cystectomy, fitness for surgery is paramount. Bringing all the field experts together with a common goal of prehabilitation helps to improve surgical outcomes.

14.3 Prehabilitation in Urologic Oncology

14.3.1 Role of Prehabilitation in Radical Cystectomy (RC)

14.3.1.1 Physical Strength Optimization

Preoperative exercise program to improve patient fitness has potential to reduce postoperative complications. In a systematic review on the effect of preoperative exercise on patients undergoing lung cancer surgery showed that the postoperative complications rates were halved, and length of stay is also reduced [8].

Functional performance predicts survival in patients undergoing radical cystectomy [9]. Studies have shown preoperative exercise prior to radical cystectomy is beneficial and increases muscle strength and physical performance [4, 10]. Compliance to the exercise program is crucial in achieving the desired outcome in prehabilitation. Simple yet robust program is key as showed in the randomized controlled trial RCT by Jensen, where 66% of study group patients followed more than 75% of the exercise regimen and they showed better muscle strength when compared to controls [10].

Better functional capacity improves postoperative morbidity and improves cystectomy outcomes [11]. CanMore trial used a CanMore exercise program prior to robotic-assisted radical cystectomy. Program involved 12-week (1 h twice a week) standardized and individually adapted exercise intervention and behavioural support [12].

Despite the benefits of an exercise program, there are many challenges in implementing it. Availability of a physiotherapist, time, and travel for each exercise session will pose great challenge, given the limited resources available in many countries.

Interventions:

- Preoperative physiotherapist review at least 4 weeks before surgery to initiate the exercise program.
- Assessment using a 6-min walk test (6MWT) to assess aerobic capacity and endurance.

14.3.1.2 Psychological Health Optimization

Psychological health is often overlooked, and mental distress can lead to poor surgical outcomes. Diagnosing cancer has big toll on patient's mental health and it often goes unidentified. Optimizing psychological health requires identifying patients at risk of depression.

Validated questionnaire like 12-item short from survey (SF-12) is useful to measure patient reported physical and mental health. Lower SF-12 score was independently associated with more significant complications in patients with bladder cancer undergoing radical cystectomy [13].

Anxiety, depression, and mood disorders affect postoperative hospital readmission rates and mortality. Studies have shown poor mental health and increased stress impairs immune system which leads to significant postoperative complications like poor wound healing, anastomotic breakdown, and severe postoperative infections [13]. Preoperative psychological counselling and relaxation exercises have improved surgical outcomes.

Interventions:

- Use SF-12 questionnaire to evaluate patient's physical and mental health.
- If SF-12 is low, psychological evaluation should be obtained before surgery to optimize mental health.

14.3.1.3 Nutrition Optimization

14.3.1.3.1 Immunonutrition

Malnutrition is underreported and underrecognized. Immunonutrition, which aims to improve immune system has been evaluated in several studies on nutrition prior to radical cystectomy [14].

Arginine supplementation prior to major surgery has been shown to improve surgical outcomes in general surgery patients [15]. During major surgery, cell-mediated immunity is impaired as there is imbalance between Th1 and Th2 cells. Also, interleukin-6 (IL-6) was noted to be higher in patients undergoing major surgery [16]. Patients receiving Immunonutrition prior to radical cystectomy have been shown to maintain Th1, Th2 balance and low IL-6 levels. This in turn translates to lesser postoperative infections [16].

Interventions:

Arginine containing supplements is to be given 5–7 days prior to radical cystectomy.

14.3.1.3.2 Enhanced Recovery After Surgery (ERAS)

Studies reporting and evaluating ERAS in major surgery are aplenty. ERAS after RC has been reported in few studies [17, 18]. ERAS was based on the principle that prolonged preoperative fasting can increase insulin resistance and push body into a catabolic phase even before the major surgery has started. This can be mitigated by carbohydrate loading up to 2 h prior to major surgery and resuming enteral feeding as soon as possible after surgery. Carbohydrate loading is not fraught without risks. In patients with poor gastric emptying, carbohydrate loading increases aspiration risk on anaesthetic induction.

Interventions:

- To institute ERAS protocol whenever feasible for patients undergoing RC.
- Use of a nasogastric tube during anaesthesia will reduce the risk of aspiration in patients who have received carbohydrate load prior to surgery.

14.3.1.4 Sexual Health Optimization

14.3.1.4.1 Sexual Dysfunction

Sexual dysfunction after extirpative pelvic surgery is common. Apart from surgical/anatomical reasons, various other psychological and body image related factors play a role in sexual dysfunction after RC. There is paucity of literature on sexual functional outcomes after RC when compared to radical prostatectomy which received much more attention [19].

In one of the studies, cystectomy was shown to negatively impact erectile function compared to other non-cystectomy intervention for bladder cancer and prevalence of erectile dysfunction after RC was 89% [20]. Orthotopic urinary diversion after RC has improved recovery of sexual function but it is confounded by the fact, orthotopic diversion is usually offered to younger and fit patients instead of older patients who have competing risks for organic erectile dysfunction [21].

Various questionnaires were used to assess sexual dysfunction. These include International Index of Erectile Function (IIEF), Erectile Function Domain (EFD or an abbreviated version of this questionnaire known as the Sexual Health Inventory for Men (SHIM). Functional Assessment of Cancer Therapy-Bladder (FACT-B) and EORTC-QOL-B20 are bladder cancer specific questionnaires that include sexual function and dysfunction items [19].

14.3.1.4.2 Prehabilitation

Preoperative erectile dysfunction can be evaluated with questionnaires mentioned above. The most used one is IIEF-5. Studies have shown that penile rehabilitation may be more beneficial in older patients and patients with a diminished preoperative erectile function. Younger patients (<55 yrs) with good preoperative function do not benefit from preoperative counselling or interventions. Identifying at-risk patients is important to tailor the sexual health optimization preoperatively.

Phosphodiesterase type 5 (PDE5) inhibitors are traditionally the first choice of treatment. Daily dose of Tadalafil 5 mg has been used before radical prostatectomy which showed significant improvement in recovery of erectile function after surgery. There are no available studies on preoperative Tadalafil in patients undergoing RC. However, it is reasonable to extrapolate the observations made in radical prostatectomy studies to radical cystectomy too.

Interventions:

- Preoperative evaluation of erectile function using validated questionnaire (IIEF).

- Preoperative tadalafil 5 mg once daily, starting 1 month prior to radical cystectomy, in at-risk patients.
- Preoperative counselling about erectile dysfunction available rehabilitation intervention for erectile dysfunction including pharmacological intervention, vacuum erection devices, etc.

14.3.2 Role of Prehabilitation in Prostate Cancer

Prostate cancer is the second most commonly diagnosed cancer globally. Localized prostate cancer treatment includes surgery and radiotherapy, which affects patients' quality of life. Similar to radical cystectomy, patient undergoing curative treatment for prostate cancer suffers reduced physical function, fatigue, urinary incontinence, erectile dysfunction. Cancer prehabilitation is a process on the continuum of care that occurs between the time of a cancer diagnosis and the beginning of acute treatment.

14.3.2.1 Physical Health Optimization

Urinary incontinence is a common consequence of radical prostatectomy (RP), which can cause a profound negative impact on quality of life. American Urology Association recommends that all men who opt for RP should have a proper assessment prior to pelvic floor muscle training interventions.

Exercise has been shown to improve function, fitness, strength, cognition, and quality of life in cancer patients [22]. For men diagnosed with prostate cancer, a referral to an experienced exercise professional at diagnosis would ensure best health-related outcomes from treatment. There is currently no set prescription of exercise that would be considered evidence-based for all men with prostate cancer. Moderate to high intensity aerobic and resistance-based exercise would be appropriate for most prostate cancer patients [5].

Interventions:

- Pelvic floor exercises (PFE) 4 weeks before RP will improve pelvic floor muscle tone and also improves patient compliance in adopting PFE post-op.
- Early referral and introduction of an exercise program prior to treatment is recommended

14.3.2.2 Psychological Health Optimization

Diagnosis and treatment of prostate cancer often have a lasting impact on a man's quality of life and overall psychosocial well-being. Traditionally, men have the tendency to remain stoic in the face of adversity. This in turn can lead to reduced illness adjustment. They experience a noticeably higher incidence of anxiety and depression. With reported rates of 27% and 17%, respectively [23].

During the prehabilitation period men may be more motivated to address determinants of distress and implementing psychosocial interventions at this point can lead to an overall improvement in mood, well-being, and immune function [24].

Interventions:

- Psychologist opinion can be sought for at-risk patients as mentioned in radical cystectomy segment.

14.3.2.3 Sexual Health Optimization

Sexual counselling helps address patient and partner's anxiety and stress related to sexual well-being and support. Sexual counselling has been associated with lower treatment discontinuation rates compared with those who did not receive sexual counselling [5]. PDE-5 inhibitors can be used as a part of penile rehabilitation. Studies have shown the use of PDE-5 inhibitors along with vacuum erection devices that are considered an effective form of therapy for erectile dysfunction in men with prostate cancer [5].

Interventions:

- PDE-5 inhibitors: low dose tadalafil 5 mg daily to start 4 weeks before RP.
- Education about the use of vacuum erection devices and sexual counselling.

14.3.2.3.1 Prostate Cancer Care Model

Paterson et al. described a care model of consultation in prostate cancer patients where multi-professional care model is conceptualized nicely (Fig. 14.2). Each member of the multidisciplinary team has defined roles in providing optimal care and treatment, but as a collective team their contributions fit together and complement care delivery [5].

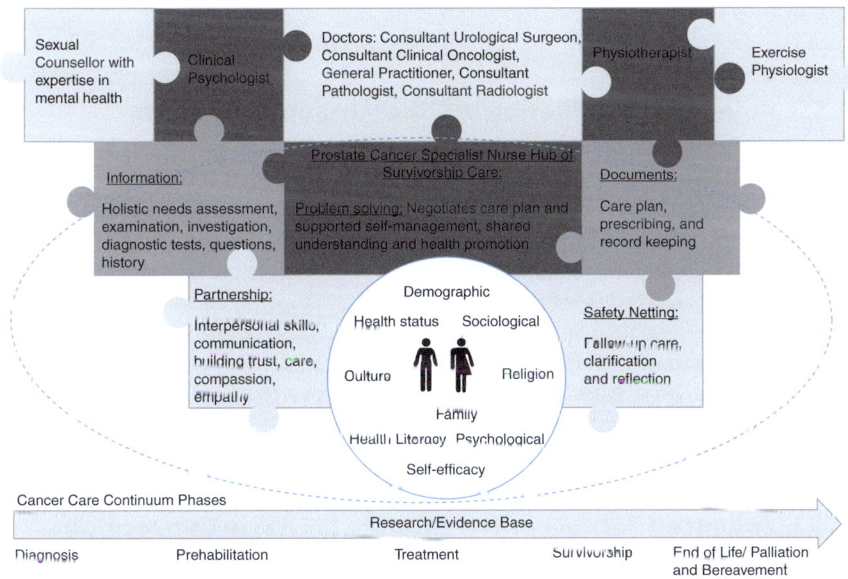

Fig. 14.2 Prostate cancer care model [5]

Table 14.1 Prehabilitation in renal, testicular, and penile cancer

Cancer	Problem	Prehabilitation method	Interventions
Renal cell carcinoma with IVC thrombus	Major surgery requiring hepato-biliary, vascular, and cardio-thoracic surgeon Long postoperative recovery in IVC thrombus extending to atrium Psychological distress	Multi-professional care model Physical therapy optimization Psychological optimization	Multidisciplinary meeting to discuss prehabilitation Physiotherapist referral Psychologist/psychiatrist referral (for at-risk patients)
Advanced testicular cancer with retroperitoneal metastasis	Major surgery with retroperitoneal lymph node dissection (RPLND) which can lead to significant morbidity Younger patients with emotional distress in losing testis Sexual side effects (erectile dysfunction/ejaculatory disorders)	Multi-professional care model Nutritional optimization Sexual health optimization	Multidisciplinary meeting to discuss prehabilitation Dietician referral Psychologist/psychiatrist referral (for at-risk patients)
Penile cancer with lymph node metastasis	Major surgery with radical inguinal node dissection +/− pelvic node dissection which can lead to significant morbidity Psychological side effects Malnutrition due to lymphorrhoea, lymphedema, and infection	Multi-professional care model Psychological optimization Nutritional optimization	Multidisciplinary meeting to discuss prehabilitation Psychologist/psychiatrist referral Dietician referral

14.3.3 Role of Prehabilitation in Other Urological Cancers

The approach to prehabilitation in urological cancers other than the urinary bladder and prostate, depending on the type and grade of the cancer is summarized in Table 14.1.

The overall process of prehabilitation in urological cancer surgery can be summarized in the following flowchart (Fig. 14.3).

14.4 Concept of Enhanced Recovery After Surgery (ERAS) and Prehabilitation in Urogynaecology and Gynaecological Oncology

14.4.1 Enhanced Recovery After Surgery (ERAS) in Gynaecology

The strategies in ERAS in obstetrics and gynaecology have been largely limited to gynaecologic oncology patients, especially for ovarian cancer surgeries due to the extensive nature of surgery. These operations are usually conducted via a generous

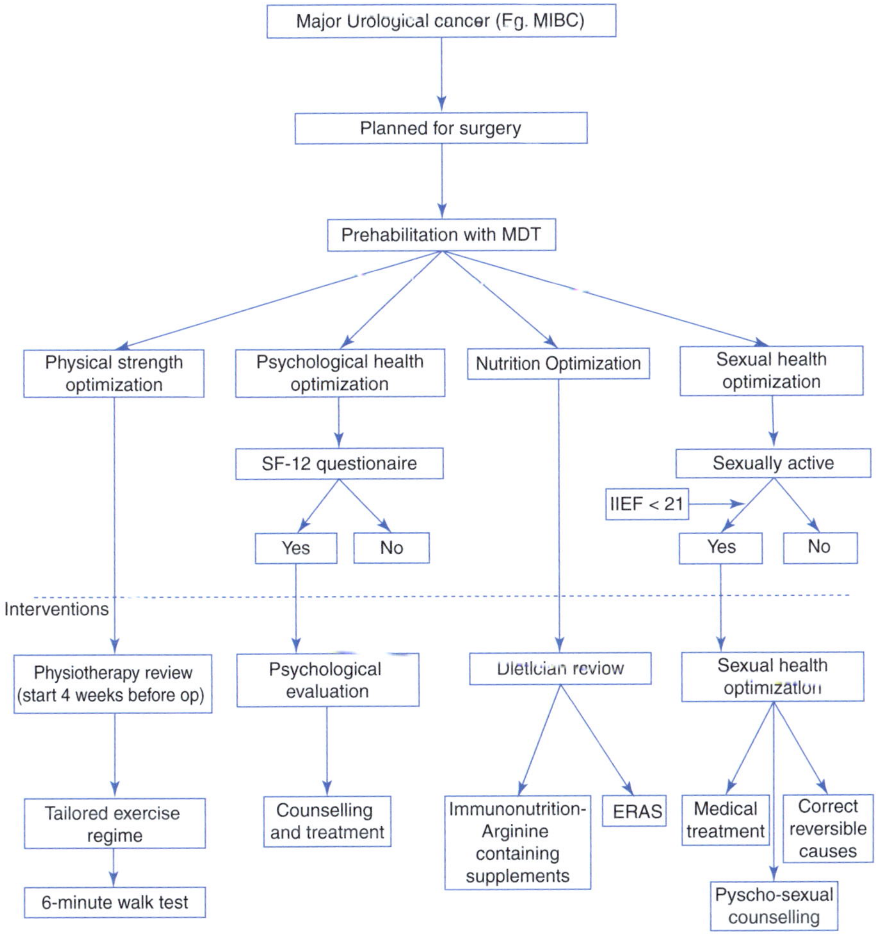

Fig. 14.3 Flowchart showing prehabilitation algorithm in Urologic oncology. Legends: MIBC, Muscle Invasive Bladder Cancer; SF-12, 12-Item Short Form Survey, IIEF, International Index of Erectile Function, ERAS, Enhanced Recovery After Surgery

sized midline laparotomy wound and often include apart from the traditional hysterectomy bilateral salpingo-oophorectomy and omentectomy, appendectomy, retroperitoneal lymphadenectomy, peritonectomy and stripping of the diaphragm, bowel resection, and solid organ resections such as splenectomy and partial hepatectomy. Ovarian cancer patients also tend to present in advanced stages. The diagnosis is delayed due to the nonspecific nature of the clinical presentations, leading to patients being compromised physically, metabolically, psychologically, and nutritionally. These women will not only have extensive peritoneal deposits and involvement of visceral organs, but they will also commonly suffer from large ascites leading to hypo-proteinemia and pleural effusion and associated lung collapse, leading them to a chronic hypoxic state. Prehabilitation in these patients is challenging and needs a multidisciplinary team approach to implement.

Though there are not many studies on this topic, benefits of ERAS for this population have been demonstrated in terms of decrease in length of hospitalization as well as decrease in complication rates. This is well summarized in a comprehensive review by Armbrust et al., of 12 observational studies on PREHAB and ERAS in gynaecological oncology consisting of five studies on prehabilitation [25]. Despite the study protocols being heterogenous and that no study evaluated a pathway for patients with extensive ovarian or cervical cancer, most studies showed fewer complication rates and shorter length of hospital stay. Another observational study from Kochi, India compared the role of implementation of ERAS protocol in a prospectively observed cohort of patients undergoing surgery for ovarian cancer with retrospective data on similar patients operated prior to the implementation of ERAS protocol [26]. This protocol included prehabilitation in terms of patient counselling and education and a loading carbohydrate drink 2 h prior to the surgery. Compliance with the protocol was 90.6%, the length of hospital stay was shorter and complication rates significantly less. The 30-day readmission rates were similar.

The latest guidelines in ERAS for gynaecological oncologic surgery were published in 2019 and cover well established components of pre-admission information, education, counselling, perioperative optimization including bowel preparation, venous thromboembolism prophylaxis, infection prevention, and recommended anaesthetic protocols. Of note, prehabilitation is a new component of these guidelines, which state that "there are no high-quality studies for prehabilitation in gynaecologic oncology patients. Extrapolated work in colorectal surgery shows certain patients benefit clinically from prehabilitation but further work in gynaecologic oncology is needed". The level of evidence available is low and hence corresponding recommendation grade is weak [27].

The concept of ERAS has otherwise not taken off in other aspects of gynaecological surgery largely due to the nature of such surgeries and the relatively younger and generally healthier patient groups, minimizing the mileage to be gained from adopting ERAS strategies.

14.4.2 Prehabilitation in Gynaecology

Prehabilitation (covering the three major components of nutrition, physical, and psychological well-being) in the field of gynaecology and gynaecological oncology is currently a novel concept. There is a paucity of data regarding prehabilitation and cervical/endometrial/vulvar malignancies, gynaecological surgeries as well as obstetrics.

One very important aspect of prehabilitation in gynaecological cancer surgery is the optimization of pulmonary function. Patients with large ascites and pleural effusion who have been otherwise deemed fit for surgery and are likely to undergo diaphragmatic stripping and pleural resection are at a very high risk of difficulty in extubating after surgery and subsequent lung complications. Similarly, morbidly obese patients undergoing minimal access surgery, either laparoscopic or robotic, are also at risk of pulmonary complications when kept in head down position for a prolonged period. Preoperative incentive spirometry and breathing exercises under supervision of a respiratory physiotherapist should improve the postoperative outcome in these patients.

The unique nature of gynaecological cancers must be appreciated to discuss or recommend prehabilitation or ERAS for such patients. Aside from ovarian cancer described above, the typical patient profile for the other common gynaecological cancers such as endometrial and cervical malignancies must be understood. Endometrial cancer is typically known to be common in the affluent populations, majority of whom are obese or morbidly obese and have associated co-morbidities like diabetes and hypertension. While most of the patients will need pelvic surgery only in the form of hysterectomy and pelvic nodal assessment and removal where necessary, there are a significant minority of patients who will also need upper abdominal surgery that includes para-aortic lymph node dissection and omentectomy. Cervical cancer, however, is most common in the underprivileged nations secondary to poor access to cervical cancer screening. Early stages of cervical cancer are amenable to surgery, whereas for tumours larger than 4 cm and cancer in the later stages are typically treated with concurrent chemoradiation. On rare occasions anterior, posterior, or total pelvic exenteration is reserved for patients of cervical cancer who have a central pelvic recurrence or when there is a residual disease after completion of chemoradiation. These surgeries are limited to areas where appropriate surgical resources are available as they require very specific surgical expertise and tertiary perioperative care. Vulvar cancer in early stages does not usually compromise the physical or nutritional function of the patient. However, majority of the patients in the developing countries present late in the disease progression and need quite extensive surgery involving a very wide area of excision at the perineum and plastic reconstruction.

There is some interest in the field of ovarian cancer, for reasons like its progress in the ERAS front as outlined above. It must be appreciated that there is usually a time pressure between presentation of the patient to the gynaecological oncologist with a suspicious and often "finally" symptomatic pelvic mass, to the time of surgery, limiting the time available for prehabilitation. Nevertheless, the "time pressure" is a theoretical perception rather than a real threat that surgery will have to be done within the next few days. Allowing time for prehabilitation even for a week or two is unlikely to cause progression of disease to the extent that will make the outcome different. Conversely, this may assist in better recovery of the patients undergoing extensive surgery for ovarian cancer. There is a subgroup of ovarian cancer patients, who would not be suitable for primary surgery, either due to ill health or extensive disease precluding full oncological clearance. These patients would typically undergo three cycles of neoadjuvant chemotherapy over a period of 9 weeks. In this cohort, prehabilitation is potentially feasible.

Extrapolating the potential advantages of prehabilitation on patient recovery in surgical patients, there are two ongoing studies involving ovarian cancer patients. Miralpeix et al. have proposed a multimodal prehabilitation program for patients undergoing elective gynaecological oncology surgery. It includes medical optimization, physical intervention, nutritional counselling, and psychological support on top of the ERAS protocol. The baseline assessment is performed approximately 2–4 weeks before the scheduled surgery date, while patients are undergoing preoperative investigations. In the baseline assessment, preoperative assessment of nutritional, physical, and psychological status is performed with a prescription home-based program or a supervised program, depending on the results of the screening tests. During the week before surgery (preoperative) and 8 weeks after surgery (postoperative), the patients' compliance is tracked via their daily diaries, and the three aspects of physical, nutritional, and emotional well-being are evaluated. During the perioperative time all patients are enrolled in an ERAS program. Patients restart their multimodal prehabilitation immediately after surgery (during their hospital stay) and continue it following discharge for up to 8 weeks. The outcome of this program is evaluated using the Short Form 12-item Survey (SF-12) questionnaire to evaluate their general health status at baseline, before surgery, and 8 weeks after surgery. The schema of their prehabilitation program is outlined in Fig. 14.4 [28].

Armbrust and his group proposed a bicentric study including patients with ovarian cancer and planned surgical intervention (primary diagnosis and first platinum-sensitive relapse) [25]. Patients classified ASA > 3 or with severe complications during the prehabilitation phase are excluded. The EPR-GO (enhancing patients' resilience in gynaecological oncology) algorithm has the main goal to enhance patients' resilience and improve patients care in gynaecological oncology. The pathway is presented in Fig. 14.5 [25]. It mainly consists of three different parts: Prehabilitation Phase I, Phase II (hospital stay with planned surgery and postoperative care), and Phase III (second PREHAB program prior chemotherapy). After each phase, a standardized evaluation will be performed. Within the hospital stay for surgery, ERAS elements will be implemented with high attention to protocol

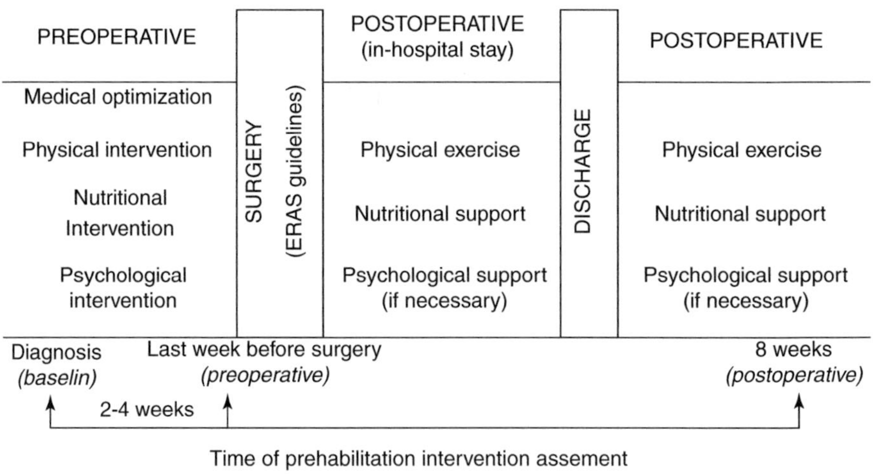

Fig. 14.4 Prehabilitation program combined with an ERAS approach. [*Miralpeix, E.*, et al., *Role and impact of multimodal prehabilitation for gynecologic oncology patients in an Enhanced Recovery After Surgery (ERAS) program. Int J Gynecol Cancer, 2019.* ***29****(8): p. 1235–1243*]

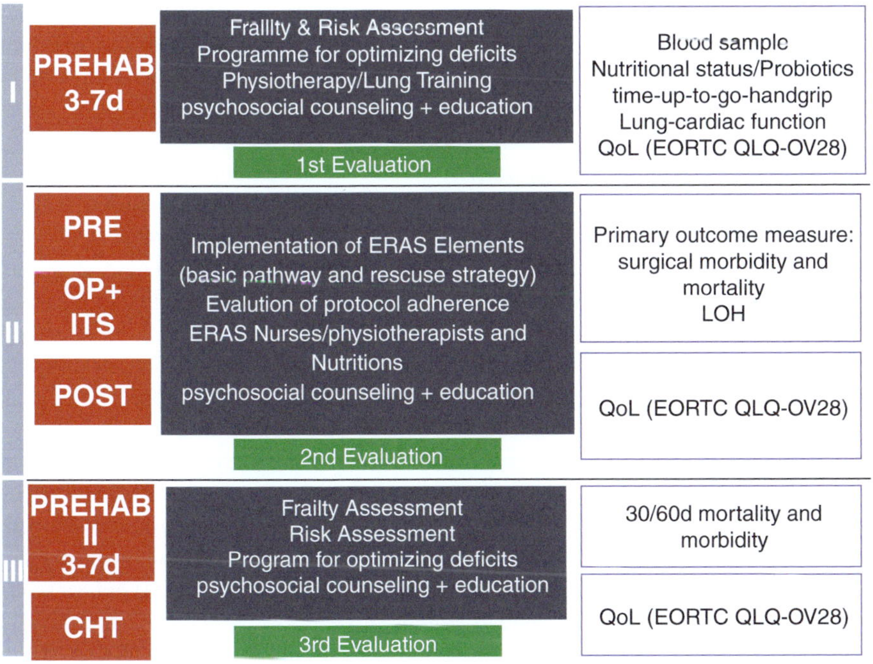

Fig. 14.5 The enhancing patient's resilience in gynaecological oncology (EPR-GO) Algorithm. [*Armbrust, R.*, et al., *Prehabilitation programs and ERAS protocols in gynecological oncology: a comprehensive review. Archives of Gynecology and Obstetrics, 2020. **301**.*]. Weight optimization as part of prehabilitation for endometrial cancer patients

adherence. If adjuvant treatment (chemotherapy) is necessary, patients will enter Phase III. Patients will be assessed regarding physical and psychological status again and will be trained again [25].

Interestingly, one aspect of gynaecological cancers, early-stage type 1 endometrial cancer, may be amenable to a special aspect that could fall under the category of prehabilitation. It is known that the gold standard treatment for endometrial cancer is surgery (hysterectomy +/− salpingo oophorectomy and nodal assessment), via a minimally invasive route if possible. This cancer typically affects women with raised body mass indices with cardiovascular risk factors, due to the excessive endogenous oestrogen from adipose tissues stimulating the endometrial lining. With the current epidemic of obesity, the number of younger women being afflicted with this condition is on the rise, leading to a recognition of alternative interventions such as progestogen therapy (oral Megestrol acetate or medroxyprogesterone acetate, or levonorgestrel intrauterine system, and/or metformin) for fertility sparing cases [29]. These strategies are understandably limited to those with apparent early stage and low-grade endometrial malignancies and the success rates for regression of malignancy exceeds 50%, although the durability of such responses is uncertain.

This leads to extrapolation of using these strategies for obese, especially the morbidly obese, or patients unfit or at high risk of surgery, to "buy time" and optimize them for surgery. This possibly gives patients time for referral to weight management services, where multimodal weight loss strategies could be employed. These weight loss strategies have been adopted in bariatrics surgery and can possibly be applied to gynaecological surgery without compromising its oncological outcome. These include nutritional intervention such as very low-calorie diet (VLCD), physiotherapy interventions to increase physical activity, psychological assessments to explore and address barriers to weight loss, screening for associated medical conditions such as hypertension, diabetes mellitus, hyperlipidaemia, obstructive sleep apnoea and treatment by dedicated specialist doctors, as well as bariatrics surgery. These strategies aim to achieve a reasonable degree of weight loss to allow them to have a successful outcome at surgery, especially minimally invasive surgery, where a Trendelenburg position is necessary, without affecting respiratory function in a manner prohibiting surgery of such nature. This weight reduction may also help improve oncological outcomes for these patients. Moreover, it is well known that the prognosis for this group of patients following definitive treatment is generally good, and the long-term survival is unrelated to malignancy. There are currently no known studies in this area.

The recently concluded feMME trial is a multicentre, three-armed, randomized, Phase II trial for obese patients with early stage of endometrial cancer to investigate the effectiveness of conservative treatment options focused on the weight loss intervention along with anti-hormonal treatment (levonorgestrel intra-uterine device) with or without metformin. The authors suggest that the results of this trial could benefit patients and reduce health costs through a reduction in hospitalizations and a lower incidence of adverse events currently observed with standard treatment. However, the final paper did not address this issue, but focused on the oncological outcomes of the three arms, which demonstrated complete response rates at 6 months were encouraging for patients with endometrial cancer across the three groups [30].

14.4.3 Prehabilitation for Pelvic Floor Prolapse Surgery

Female pelvic reconstruction surgery can be divided into incontinence and prolapse surgery. Pelvic floor failure is contributed mainly from pelvic trauma including pregnancy, obstetric trauma, prolonged increases in intra-abdominal pressure such as coughing and constipation. Pelvic tissue also starts to undergo degeneration after menopause. Prehabilitation aims to correct the possible contributory factors prior to surgery.

For incontinent surgery, pelvic floor exercise should be offered as first line treatment for at least 3 months before surgery is offered [30]. A pelvic floor training program comprises at least eight contractions performed three times a day. In women who cannot activate their pelvic floor muscles adequately, electrical stimulation or biofeedback should be added to aid motivation and adherence to therapy [30]. In patients with a concurrent element of urgency symptoms, bladder training should be offered for a minimum of 6 weeks and overactive bladder medication be added should training be inadequate to control symptoms. Consider lifestyle changes that reduce intra-abdominal pressure such as losing weight to a target BMI of 30 kg/m^2. Minimizing weightlifting and treating constipation will also help to reduce contributory factors towards weakening the pelvic floor support. In patients with uterovaginal prolapse, consider vaginal oestrogen especially in patients with signs of vaginal atrophy.

The need for prehabilitation for benign gynaecological conditions such as uterine fibroids, ovarian cysts, and endometriosis, as well as obstetrics cases is limited due to the relatively younger and healthier population. The nature of such surgical procedures is also usually less complex and may even be deferred for months due to its non-urgent nature as well as alternative effective medical therapies available. Also, an increasing number of such cases are performed in a minimally invasive manner, or via limited abdominal incisions, with a corresponding decrease in surgical stress to the patient. Any concurrent medical conditions should still be optimized accordingly without any specific need for application of "prehabilitation". Keeping in mind the definition of prehabilitation, which is to establish baseline components such as nutrition, physical, psychological functions, identify deficits and working towards optimizing these aspects prior to an anticipated surgical stressor to reduce its potential repercussions, it is not surprising that this concept has not attracted much interest in obstetrics and gynaecology except for ovarian malignancies.

14.5 Conclusion

Prehabilitation is yet to be embedded as a standard of care in most urological and gynaecological procedures. However, emerging evidence conducted in prehabilitation interventions appears to have merit. An evidence-based and logical approach to prehabilitation can lead to improved, clinically significant surgical outcomes.

References

1. Hamel MB, et al. Surgical outcomes for patients aged 80 and older: morbidity and mortality from major noncardiac surgery. J Am Geriatr Soc. 2005;53(3):424–9.
2. Cui HW, Turney BW, Griffiths J. The preoperative assessment and optimization of patients undergoing major urological surgery. Curr Urol Rep. 2017;18(7):54.
3. Molenaar CJL, et al. Prehabilitation, making patients fit for surgery - a new frontier in perioperative care. Innov Surg Sci. 2019;4(4):132–8.
4. Jensen BT, Lauridsen SV, Jensen JB. Prehabilitation for major abdominal urologic oncology surgery. Curr Opin Urol. 2018;28(3):243–50.
5. Paterson C, et al. Prostate cancer Prehabilitation and the importance of multimodal interventions for person centred care and recovery. Semin Oncol Nurs. 2020;36(4):151048.
6. Wilson RJ, et al. Impaired functional capacity is associated with all-cause mortality after major elective intra-abdominal surgery. Br J Anaesth. 2010;105(3):297–303.
7. Silver JK. Integrating rehabilitation into the cancer care continuum. PM R. 2017;9(9 Suppl 2):S291–s296.
8. Steffens D, et al. Preoperative exercise halves the postoperative complication rate in patients with lung cancer: a systematic review of the effect of exercise on complications, length of stay and quality of life in patients with cancer. Br J Sports Med. 2018;52(5):344.

9. Bolenz C, et al. Management of elderly patients with urothelial carcinoma of the bladder: guideline concordance and predictors of overall survival. BJU Int. 2010;106(9):1324–9.
10. Jensen BT, et al. Exercise-based pre-habilitation is feasible and effective in radical cystectomy pathways-secondary results from a randomized controlled trial. Support Care Cancer. 2016;24(8):3325–31.
11. Kaye DR, et al. The feasibility and impact of a Presurgical exercise intervention program (Prehabilitation) for patients undergoing cystectomy for bladder cancer. Urology. 2020;145:106–12.
12. Porserud A, et al. The CanMoRe trial - evaluating the effects of an exercise intervention after robotic-assisted radical cystectomy for urinary bladder cancer: the study protocol of a randomised controlled trial. BMC Cancer. 2020;20(1):805.
13. Sharma P, et al. Preoperative patient reported mental health is associated with high grade complications after radical cystectomy. J Urol. 2016;195(1):47–52.
14. Oberle AD, et al. Optimizing nutrition prior to radical cystectomy. Curr Urol Rep. 2018;19(12):99.
15. Drover JW, et al. Perioperative use of arginine-supplemented diets: a systematic review of the evidence. J Am Coll Surg. 2011;212(3):385–99.
16. Hamilton-Reeves JM, et al. Perioperative Immunonutrition modulates inflammatory response after radical cystectomy: results of a pilot randomized controlled clinical trial. J Urol. 2018;200(2):292–301.
17. Deibert CM, et al. A prospective randomized trial of the effects of early enteral feeding after radical cystectomy. Urology. 2016;96:69–73.
18. Daneshmand S, et al. Enhanced recovery protocol after radical cystectomy for bladder cancer. J Urol. 2014;192(1):50–5.
19. Modh RA, Mulhall JP, Gilbert SM. Sexual dysfunction after cystectomy and urinary diversion. Nat Rev Urol. 2014;11(8):445–53.
20. Allareddy V, et al. Quality of life in long-term survivors of bladder cancer. Cancer. 2006;106(11):2355–62.
21. Hedgepeth RC, et al. Body image and bladder cancer specific quality of life in patients with ileal conduit and neobladder urinary diversions. Urology. 2010;76(3):671–5.
22. Papadopoulos E, et al. Effects of six months of aerobic and resistance training on metabolic markers and bone mineral density in older men on androgen deprivation therapy for prostate cancer. J Geriatr Oncol. 2020;11(7):1074–7.
23. Vartolomei L, Shariat SF, Vartolomei MD. Psychotherapeutic interventions targeting prostate cancer patients: a systematic review of the literature. Eur Urol Oncol. 2018;1(4):283–91.
24. Orom H, et al. Factors associated with emotional distress in newly diagnosed prostate cancer patients. Psychooncology. 2015;24(11):1416–22.
25. Armbrust R, et al. Prehabilitation programs and ERAS protocols in gynecological oncology: a comprehensive review. Arch Gynecol Obstet. 2020;301
26. Agarwal R, et al. A prospective study evaluating the impact of implementing the ERAS protocol on patients undergoing surgery for advanced ovarian cancer. Int J Gynecol Cancer. 2019;29(3):605–12.
27. Nelson G, et al. Guidelines for perioperative care in gynecologic/oncology: enhanced recovery after surgery (ERAS) society recommendations-2019 update. Int J Gynecol Cancer. 2019;29(4):651–68.
28. Miralpeix E, et al. Role and impact of multimodal prehabilitation for gynecologic oncology patients in an enhanced recovery after surgery (ERAS) program. Int J Gynecol Cancer. 2019;29(8):1235–43.
29. Janda M, et al. Complete pathological response following levonorgestrel intrauterine device in clinically stage 1 endometrial adenocarcinoma: results of a randomized clinical trial. Gynecol Oncol. 2021;161(1):143–51.
30. *Urinary incontinence and pelvic organ prolapse in women: management*. NICE guideline 2019 [cited 2021 30 May]; Available from: https://www.nice.org.uk/guidance/ng123.

Prehabilitation in Head and Neck Cancer Surgery

15

Gouthaman Shanmugasundaram
and Ramkumar Dhanasekaran

Abbreviation

6MWT	6 Minute Walk Test
ACE 27	Adult Comorbidity Evaluation 27
ARISCAT	Assess Respiratory Risk in Surgical Patients in Catalonia
BMI	Body Mass Index
BPI	Brief Pain Inventory
CBC	Complete Blood Count
CPAP	Continuous Positive Airway Pressure
CPET	Cardiopulmonary Exercise Testing
CT	Computed Tomography
CVD	Cardiovascular Disease
FEES	Fiberoptic Endoscopic Evaluation of Swallowing Studies
FEV1	Forced Expiratory Volume
FRS	Framingham Risk Score
HADS	Hospital Anxiety and Depression Scale
HbA1c	Glycosylated Haemoglobin
HIIT	High-Intensity Interval Training
HNC	Head and Neck Cancer
HNSCC	Head and Neck Squamous Cell Carcinoma
IMT	Inspiratory Muscle Training

G. Shanmugasundaram (✉)
Department of Surgical Oncology, Sri Ramachandra Medical College & Research Institute (SRMC&RI), Sri Ramachandra Institute of Higher Education & Research, Chennai, India

R. Dhanasekaran
Department of Anaesthesiology and Pain Medicine, Sri Ramachandra Medical college & Research Institute (SRMC&RI), Sri Ramachandra Institute of Higher Education & Research, Chennai, India

A. Chakraborty, A. Balakrishnan (eds.), *Prehabilitation for Cancer Surgery*,
https://doi.org/10.1007/978-981-16-6494-6_15

LANSS	Leeds Assessment of Neuropathic Signs And Symptoms
MACE	Major Adverse Cardiac Events
MBSS	Modified Barium Swallow Studies
METS	Metabolic Equivalents
MHR	Maximum Heart Rate
MID	Maximum Inter-Incisor Distance
MRI	Magnetic Resonance Imaging
NCCN	National Comprehensive Cancer Network
NCIN	National Cancer Intelligence Network
NMES	Neuromuscular Electrical Stimulation
NPC	Nasopharyngeal Cancers
OSA	Obstructive Sleep Apnea
POCD	Postoperative Cognitive Dysfunction
POD	Postoperative Delirium
QOL	Quality Of Life
RCRI	Revised (Lee) Cardiac Risk Index
RD	Registered Dietitian
RIT	Radiotherapy-Induced Trismus
RT	Radiotherapy
SLP	Speech and Language Pathologist
SpO_2	Oxygen Saturations
TENS	Transcutaneous Electrical Nerve Stimulation
TEP	Tracheoesophageal Puncture/Prosthesis
TLI	Temporal Lobe Injury
TMJ	Temporomandibular Joint
TNM	Tumour–Node–Metastasis
VTE	Venous Thromboembolism

Patients with head and neck cancer (HNC) majorly benefit from prehabilitation program, as they mostly undergo surgery post 4–6 weeks of chemoradiation. This period is ideal enough to implement general prehabilitation interventions such as optimization of cardiopulmonary function and comorbid conditions, pain management, psychological support along with tobacco cessation and HNC specific interventions such as specific exercise therapy to prevent or manage radiation/cancer induced complications, speech/swallowing therapy, and provision of conditioned diet rich in proteins and nutritional supplements.

Patient comorbid illness which is unrelated to HNC can be a significant risk for perioperative morbidity and mortality and therefore requires risk assessment and optimization before the surgery. Alcohol and tobacco use pose a strong risk factor for HNC and also show a causal relationship with coronary heart disease, stroke, renal dysfunction, lung disease and cardiac failure which are all proven risk factors for adverse perioperative outcomes. Therefore, prehabilitation seems vital to optimize the pre-existing comorbidities and to improve patient's functional capacity to overcome the perioperative stress. A collaborative approach is needed at prehabilitation and pre-anaesthetic clinic to assess the functional capacity and comorbidities and to assess the tumour specific prehabilitation measures to plan an individualized approach to address the medical and physical prehabilitation interventions.

The functional capacity is assessed either through simple subjective estimates of the metabolic equivalents (METs) or by dynamic testing such as 6 minute walk test (6MWT) and cardiopulmonary exercise testing (CPET). Exercise is the single most effective approach to increase the functional reserve irrespective of patient's preoperative status. Exercise therapies include aerobic, resistance, and flexibility training to induce a controlled physical stress which improves the body's adaptive responses and functional reserves to withstand future surgical stress. Patients with severe obstructive pulmonary disorders can undergo deep breathing exercises, chest physiotherapies, and specific prehabilitation therapies like Nordic walking and neuromuscular electrical stimulation (NMES) in severely disabled patients. Nasopharyngeal cancers may present as headache or multiple cranial nerve palsies. These patients require further risk evaluation, timely endovascular stenting of carotid artery in case of carotid artery involvement, and early cancer treatment to prevent tumour progression or metastasis.

Patients with HNC are prone to anaemia preoperatively due to poor nutritional intake following dysphagia/trismus, nausea, vomiting, or bone marrow suppression subsequent to chemoradiotherapy. The correction of anaemia enhances effort tolerance and decreases requirement of perioperative transfusion which increases the risk of tumour recurrence and decreased survival rates.

Patients with head and neck cancer are prone to psychological stress. The stressors associated with HNC are uncertainty associated with prognosis, intrusive treatments, body disfigurement, dependency, disability, threat of recurrence, and mortality. Undetected and untreated psychological needs are associated with poor quality of life and intentions to cooperate with caregivers during prehabilitation. Swelling and scarring, pain or numbness, and functional impairment such as dysphagia or radiation induced fibrosis also have a significant impact on one's psychological well-being, social functioning, and overall QOL. The impact of such disfigurement and dysfunction on personal identity, ability to communicate or relate to others, and ability to feel successful interpersonally are all important considerations for the treatment team. Psychological counselling, behavioural pain therapy, relaxation techniques, and other appropriate psychotherapy interventions form an important part of the prehabilitation program.

Smoking and alcohol abuse are associated with increased risk of primary and secondary cancers, cancer recurrence, and other complications involving cardiopulmonary, neurological and renal systems leading to increased perioperative morbidity and mortality. Most cancer institutions have developed smoking cessation programs that incorporate behavioural therapy and pharmacotherapy in accordance with NCCN guidelines.

HNC specific prehabilitation measures include assessment and optimization of HNC specific modifiable risk factors. Dysphagia and odynophagia are common symptoms of HNC patients. Impaired mastication contributes to dysphagia.

Odynophagia usually results from mucositis during and immediately following chemoradiation treatment. Odynophagia needs appropriate pain medication to improve oral intake. A baseline speech and swallowing function are often assessed using videostroboscopy, Modified Barium Swallow Studies (MBSS) and/or Fiberoptic Endoscopic Evaluation of Swallowing studies (FEES) by specialists. Exercises like Mendelsohn manoeuver followed by effortful swallow, Shaker and Masako manoeuver were recommended to improve or prevent swallowing difficulties. Patients planned for laryngectomy are explained about oesophageal speech and a tracheoesophageal puncture/ prosthesis (TEP) to prepare and educate them to face the future challenges. Perilaryngeal cancers are associated with drooling, choking, or coughing during or following food intake, which can lead to aspiration. Specialists like Speech and Language Pathologist (SLP) should assess the patient's ability to swallow different liquids and food textures to determine the consistency needed to prevent aspiration.

Mucositis, an inflammatory ulcerated lesions in the mouth and throat is a common problem due to chemoradiotoxicity. Glutamine supplementation can be used to reduce the incidence and severity of oral mucositis. Xerostomia or dry mouth is the most common late side effect of radiation treatment to the head and neck. Increased dental caries and infections are sequelae of dry mouth. Dietary management techniques like intake of moist foods, increased consumption of fluids, and frequent mouth rinsing are the solutions to xerostomia.

Trismus is a significant complication that has to be addressed preoperatively. The causes include tumour invasion of the temporomandibular joint (TMJ), fibrosis of masticatory muscles, and buccal tissues following radiation therapy. It is important to delineate radiotherapy-induced trismus (RIT) from other types to start a specific prehabilitation exercise. Pain and inability to open one's mouth may lead to improper nutrition, poor oral hygiene, psychological stress, and decreased social interactions. The physical therapist should perform the assessment of posture and range of joint mobility to decide upon appropriate exercises and use of supportive devices. Exercises, in combination with jaw-mobilizing devices like TheraBite and Dynasplint, have proven to be the most effective strategy in the management of trismus. Studies have shown that any irradiated area could become 5–6 times thicker due to collagen formation. The prehabilitation goal here is to prevent the development of torticollis in patients who are prone for fibrotic neck. Headmaster cervical collar prevents neck extensor weakness and thereby prevents torticollis. Stretching exercises of the anterior neck and chest prevents the development of a flexion contracture. Cervical traction in a horizontal plane seems to be an effective treatment option for both the stiff and the fibrotic neck. The current recommended regime for preoperative head and neck cancer related exercise interventions is to perform ten specific exercise repetitions, three times a day supplemented with health trainer guided individualized physical activity program.

To conclude, the prehabilitation program is proven to be vital in improving the patient's functional reserve and in preventing or treating HNC related complications. Prehabilitation interventions should be implemented as early as possible after the cancer diagnosis using specific exercise therapies, individualized physical activity program combined with simultaneous management of comorbidities, pain, nutrition, and mental health. Thus, a newly diagnosed head and neck cancer patient will enter into the treatment phase having had their physical and mental health optimized with necessary prehabilitation therapies and education to ease their experience during the acute phase of surgical treatment. Future researches are needed to develop cancer specific prehabilitation guidelines that can be incorporated routinely in the head and neck cancer management practice.

15.1 Manuscript

Prehabilitation is defined as 'a process on the cancer continuum of care that occurs between the time of cancer diagnosis and the beginning of acute treatment and includes physical and psychological assessments that establish a baseline functional level, identify impairments, and provide interventions that promote physical and psychological health to reduce the incidence and/or severity of future impairments' [1]. A diagnosis of cancer triggers intense emotions including, but not limited to, fear of the unknown, as well as fear of future disfigurement, loss of function, and pain. Evidence has demonstrated that a multidisciplinary team (Fig. 15.1) approach starting at the time of diagnosis promotes improved outcomes [2].

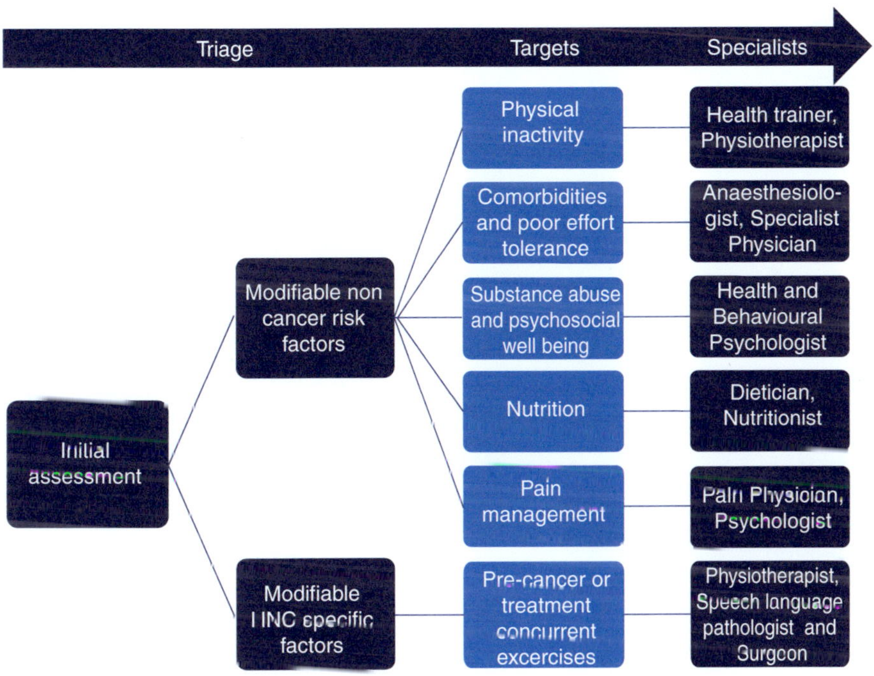

Fig. 15.1 Prehabilitation outline

Patients with head and neck cancer (HNC) undergo surgery either upfront or post chemoradiation as per the stage of the disease at presentation. Prehabilitation starts immediately after diagnosis and chemoradiation as the surgery may be planned 4–6 weeks post chemoradiation. Prehabilitation interventions (Fig. 15.2) include optimization of cardiopulmonary function and comorbid conditions, provision of adequate nutrition, physical therapy, psychological support, pain management, speech and swallowing therapy along with tobacco cessation.

Comorbidities unrelated to head and neck carcinoma (HNC) can be a significant risk for morbidity and mortality than the primary cancer and therefore requires risk assessment and optimization before the surgery. The mortality rate among patients with head and neck squamous cell carcinoma (HNSCC) due to non-cancer ailments is 13% in comparison to 23.8% 5-year incidence of HNSCC-specific mortality and 14.6% second cancer mortality [3]. With the available advanced cancer treatment options, HNSCC-specific mortality has dramatically decreased to 5%, whereas death because of second cancers and non-cancer causes remained 20% to 25% higher in patients with HNSCC compared with matched controls, between 5 and 10 years after treatment [4, 5]. Coronary artery disease (28%), chronic obstructive pulmonary disease (8.5%), and cerebrovascular disease (5.6%) are the common causes for non-cancer mortality [6]. Alcohol and tobacco use not only are strong

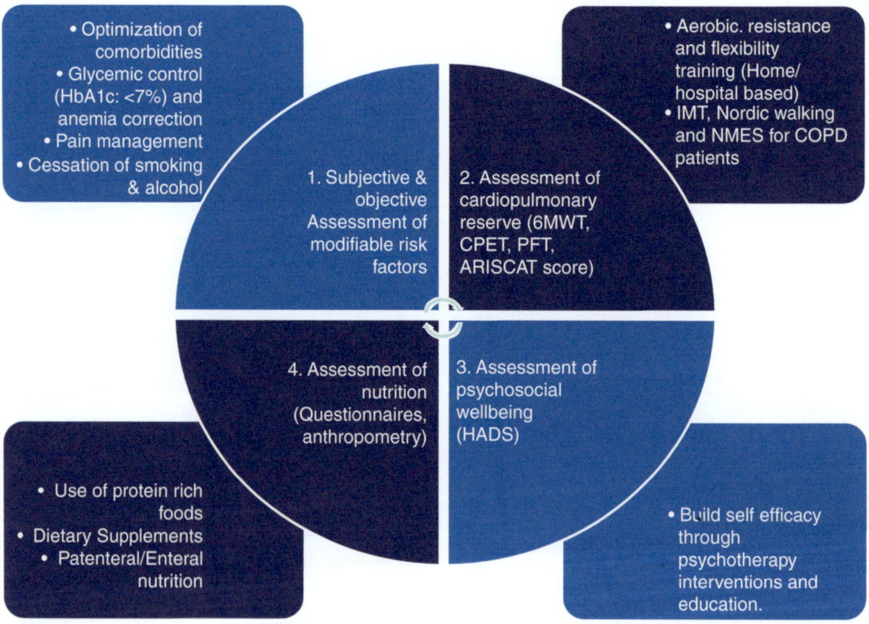

Fig. 15.2 General prehabilitation measures in head and neck cancer (*6MWT* 6 Minute Walk Test, *CPET* Cardio Pulmonary Exercise Testing, *PFT* Pulmonary Function Test, *ARISCAT score* Assess Respiratory Risk in Surgical Patients in Catalonia score, *IMT* Inspiratory Muscle Training, *COPD* Chronic Obstructive Pulmonary Disease, *NMES* Neuro Muscular Electrical Stimulation, *HADS* Hospital Anxiety and Depression Scale

HNC risk factors but also show a causal relationship with coronary heart disease, stroke, renal dysfunction, and cardiac failure which are all proven risk factors for adverse perioperative outcomes. Therefore, prehabilitation is crucial to optimize the pre-existing comorbidities and to improve patient's functional capacity to overcome the perioperative stress.

Prehabilitation process includes identification of modifiable risk factors, optimizing the comorbid ailments and improving one's performance capacity with customized optimization programs. Several instruments like Adult Comorbidity Evaluation 27 (ACE 27) and Revised (Lee) Cardiac Risk Index (RCRI) are available to stratify the perioperative morbidity and mortality risks [7]. ACE 27 is an extensive but thorough instrument to quantify the comorbidity. RCRI is a multivalidated and simple 6-item index which can be easily implemented into preoperative HNC screening protocols. Screening diseases without assessing patient cardiopulmonary performance status is highly incomplete. Performance tests such as cardiopulmonary exercise testing (CPET) or 6 minute walk test (6MWT) are used to assess the effect of illness/age on functional capacity. These assessments are still inadequate to measure the pretreatment comorbid burden and prognosis without assessing the stage of cancer. Hence, National Cancer Intelligence Network (NCIN) recommended the development of 'prognostigrams' relating to tumour–node–metastasis (TNM) stage, comorbidity, and the performance status, which can adversely influence on disease specific survival, prehabilitation approach, and the treatment selection [7].

15.2 Cardiovascular System and HNC

Previous study data demonstrates a high prevalence and risks for cardiovascular disease (CVD) at the time of HNSCC diagnosis. Specifically, 15% of patients with HNSCC had coronary artery disease and 9% had carotid artery disease which is comparatively higher or similar among the men belonging to the general population aged between 40 and 59 years and 60 and 79 years, respectively [6]. HNSCC patients without any previous history of CVD had a 58% 10-year risk estimate for developing a CVD critical event in comparison to 33% among the general population [6, 8]. Data published by Okoye et al. showed that the Framingham Risk Score (FRS) was not only high among laryngeal cancer patients which usually has high mortality rate but also even among patients with HPV-positive oropharyngeal cancer which has a most favourable prognosis [6]. This indicates that there were no major differences in the cardiac risks among subtypes of HNCC. The study also recommends the use of statin therapy to reduce major adverse cardiac events (MACE). Therefore, it is important to consider CVD prevention and prehabilitation measures among all HNSCC cancer subgroups.

As per United Kingdom National multidisciplinary guidelines [7] on preclinical assessment of patients with head and neck cancers, thyroid dysfunction and extraadrenal pheochromocytoma or head and neck paragangliomas can present with hypertension. Severe hypertension should be controlled below 160/100 mm Hg with careful introduction of antihypertensives. There is also possibility of postural hypotension due to baroreceptor failure due to radiation therapy or may be due to cisplatin induced autonomic neuropathy [9]. Aged patients and those with diabetes or with poor effort tolerance or with other cardiac risks should be referred to cardiologist for further evaluation and optimization with early introduction or continuation of anti-ischemic drugs. Dobutamine stress echocardiography can provide a dynamic assessment of cardiac status where CPET is not possible. A patient with severe valvular heart disease especially aortic stenosis, which is not uncommon among aged individuals may need appropriate medical or percutaneous interventions before or during prehabilitation process. Atrial fibrillation and other cardiac arrhythmias are quite common among surgical patients and are found to be cause for poor outcomes including sudden death during the perioperative period. A preoperative Holter monitoring can guide the prehabilitation team in the management of patients focusing mainly on the heart rate control, appropriate anticoagulation therapies, and identifying the right candidate for preoperative pacing. Cardiac pacemakers should have their battery and threshold check as per treating physician's advice or manufacturer's recommendations.

15.3 Vascular Complications

Vascular complications occur in patients with HNSCC, both as a result of either the disease or the treatments which can affect the quality of life and the survival. The causes for the development of vascular complications are invasion or occlusion of major vessels by the primary cancer itself or by the deep cervical lymph nodes which are in close proximity to the carotid sheath. It may lead to 'carotid blowout'—a haemorrhage from extracranial carotid arteries which carries a risk of 40% mortality or carotid stenosis/occlusion, with resultant neurological sequelae. Endovascular stenting, a major advancement in interventional radiology over the last decade has significantly reduced the vascular related complications [10]. Clinicians should always suspect cardiac metastasis in patients with primary tumour from tonsils, larynx, and sinuses. They can present with either cardiac complications or embolisms causing pulmonary embolism related complications, stroke, or acute limb ischemia [11]. These patients need prompt workup with transthoracic echocardiogram, appropriate level computed tomography (CT) angiogram, and positron emission tomography CT scans for early diagnosis and radiological interventions preoperatively, which can aid in implementing prehabilitation programs and improving clinical outcomes.

15.4 Respiratory System and HNSCC

Upper aerodigestive tumours, advanced age, tobacco and alcohol abuse, and other comorbidities share common characteristics with HNSCC patients which predispose to severe adverse pulmonary outcomes [12]. The prevalence of respiratory comorbidities such as respiratory infections, bronchiectasis, and aspiration pneumonitis in HNSCC patients approximates 10–15%, nearly twice as common as healthy controls [13, 14]. Age at diagnosis, sex, body mass index (BMI), tobacco use, treatment modality, primary tumour site and stage, malnutrition, and presence of tracheostomy tube were also identified as significant risk factors for adverse respiratory outcomes. HNSCC patients are also at increased risk for a variety of viral and bacterial pulmonary infections due to immunosuppression following disease complications or chemotherapy. Cytomegalovirus, herpes, influenza, parainfluenza, respiratory syncytial virus, rhinovirus, and adenovirus are identified as common viral pathogens and pseudomonas aeruginosa, staphylococcus aureus predominated among bacterial infections in HNSCC patients [13]. Poor oral hygiene has been identified as an independent risk factor for the development of HNSCC and has been associated with poor survival rates [15].

Patients with HNC are at increased risk for the development of synchronous or metachronous primary lung cancers, which requires to be evaluated and managed simultaneously during prehabilitation process along with evaluation of pre-existing lung disorders [16]. Patients with perilaryngeal and thyroid malignancies may have obstructed larynx or trachea, respectively, by their mass effect or may be due to vocal cord palsy following direct infiltration or by recurrent laryngeal nerve palsy. Airway compromise may be indicated by subtle changes to the voice, dysphagia, orthopnoea, and new onset of snoring. Such patients may develop frequent aspirations, pneumonia, atelectasis, fistula formation, lung collapse, and fatal pulmonary complications. Therefore patients with HNSCC must undergo CT scans and spirometry evaluation for diagnosis of lung disease, grading of disease severity, and for the assessment of bronchodilator therapy response. Assess Respiratory Risk in Surgical Patients in Catalonia (ARISCAT) score is a useful and validated method to assess the perioperative pulmonary risks [17]. Patients with abnormal predicted forced expiratory volume (FEV1) during spirometry evaluation pose a marked risk for postoperative pulmonary complications. Such patients can be optimized preoperatively by using multi-model approach using optimal bronchodilators, trial of steroid therapy in moderate to severe disease, incentive spirometry, deep breathing exercises, inspiratory muscle training (IMT), chest physiotherapy, good nutrition, good oral hygiene, and appropriate antibiotic/antiviral therapy for intercurrent infections [12]. It is also important to identify patients with obstructive sleep apnea (OSA) with or without pulmonary hypertension preoperatively using polysomnography, echocardiogram, and their baseline oxygen saturations (SpO_2). Patients with OSA benefit from exercises and continuous positive airway pressure (CPAP) therapy to improve oxygenation, prevent hypercarbia related complications, enhance the sense of well-being, and more importantly prevent the perioperative pulmonary complications [18].

15.5 Assessment of Cardiopulmonary Reserve

A collaborative approach is needed at prehabilitation and pre-anaesthetic clinic to assess the patient comorbidities, anthropometric data, range of joint motion, and assessment of functional capacity to plan an individualized approach to medical and physical prehabilitation programs. The functional capacity is assessed either through simple subjective estimates of the metabolic equivalents (METs) or by dynamic testing such as 6MWT and CPET. One MET equates to the oxygen consumption of a 70 kg man at rest and climbing up one flight of stairs indicates 4 METS. The patients who fail to achieve 4 METS or anaerobic threshold of 11 ml/kg/minute during CPET are associated with increased perioperative risk and are identified as prime candidates for prehabilitation programs [19].

CPET is currently the most reliable and an objective assessment of the integration of the cardiovascular, respiratory, haematological, and cellular functions. The morbidity and mortality in the perioperative period are well correlated with anaerobic threshold and peak oxygen consumption (VO_2 max) assessed during CPET [17, 19]. Its application in head and neck oncosurgery is still being evaluated. CPET results have been used to guide prehabilitation measures to improve preoperative functional capacity and thereby the postoperative clinical outcomes. 6 minute walk Test (6MWT) is simple and inexpensive test which assesses how far the patient can walk in 6 minute. Repetition of test after appropriate prehabilitation interventions allows the quantification of changes in cardiopulmonary reserve [20].

15.6 Cardiopulmonary Prehabilitation Interventions

The approach to modify the risks assessed during screening is done through endurance and resistance exercise, respiratory muscle training, pharmacological interventions, and cessation of smoking/alcohol in the available time before surgery.

15.7 Exercise

Exercise is the single most effective approach to increase the functional reserve, especially in older adults. The principle behind the exercise therapy is that it induces a physical stress that causes an adaptive response in the body which increases the capacity to withstand future surgical and intraoperative hemodynamic stresses. The type of interventions is based on the CPET/6MWT, disease nature, patient characteristics, and the possible chemoradiotoxicity related sequelae. Whole body exercise programs like outdoor or treadmill walking, stationary cycling at 60–80% of predetermined maximal walking speed/cycling load for 20–30 min are recommended for patients who are mainly restricted during CPET by reaching their maximal heart rate [11]. Exercises can be systemic or tissue-specific. Such specific exercise protocol helps us to assess the improvements in the functional capacity, allows us to identify the site of functional limitations, and finally guides us to set the rehabilitation goals.

The three main types of physical activity are aerobic, resistance, and flexibility training. *Aerobic exercise* aims to increase cardiovascular and respiratory endurance, defined as the ability to take up, deliver, and utilize oxygen. The stationary and recumbent type bikes, stair-climbing machines, and treadmills are the commonly used methods. *Resistance exercise* training is the main intervention for optimizing the impaired muscle function and structure, especially in older individuals. Flexibility and individual/group muscle strengthening exercises are also encouraged as a part of physiotherapy program. The *World Health Organization's* recommendation includes 150 minutes of moderate activity or 75 min of vigorous physical activity per week with 2 or more days of muscle strengthening exercise per week or Borg scale of 12–16 in prehabilitation setting [17, 19, 20]. *Borg scale* may have an advantage over heart rate (HR) monitoring approach in patients taking beta-blockers which can alter HR response to exercise. The target for a heart rate-based approach is 70–80% of maximum heart rate (MHR) which falls in the aerobic training zone. High-intensity interval training (HIIT) programs are also found useful during exercise therapy which mainly concentrates on alternate workout between short work periods at 70–90% of MHR and rest intervals at 60–65% of MHR [20].

Patients with severe obstructive pulmonary disorders with or without heart failure can undergo specific prehabilitation therapies like Nordic walking and neuromuscular electrical stimulation (NMES). Nordic walking [21] that involves the use of whole body muscles in walking is recommended for patients with preserved effort tolerance and NMES for patients who are mostly dyspnoeic and sick, an ideal substitute to resistance training [22]. If there is oxygen desaturation during CPET or exercise therapy, patient should be supplemented with portable oxygen therapy. Patients with poor mobility should perform physical activity three or more days per week in order to enhance body balance skills and prevent falls. Home-based programs are encouraged nowadays, as they are cheaper and more convenient. Other measures to mitigate the adverse functional impacts of surgery and radiation induced fibrosis are early dysphagia intervention programs, optimization of comorbid respiratory diseases, specialist referral, multidisciplinary care and frequent disease surveillance should be implemented during prehabilitation among higher risk HNSCC patients.

15.8 Glycaemic Control [7, 23]

Patients with diabetes or on chronic steroid therapy with poor glycaemic control are associated with increased wound infections, postoperative morbidity, and prolonged hospital stay. Glycemic control over the last 3 months can be assessed by the glycosylated haemoglobin (HbA1c) level. A level below 7% is vital to avoid microvascular complications and bad perioperative outcomes. The ideal perioperative glycaemic target of 6–10 mmol/L should be achieved by strict glycaemic surveillance, optimal insulin/drug therapy, modified diet plan, and timely referral to a diabetologist.

15.9 Neurological Concerns

Nasopharyngeal cancers (NPC) may present as headache or multiple cranial nerve palsies, which may occur in 15–30% of cases [24]. It usually involves the cranial nerves III, V, VI, and VII, due to invasion of para-cavernous sinus of tumour. Further dorsolateral spread can produce vagus nerve paralysis resulting in aspiration, dysphagia, and palatal paralysis. Distant metastatic bone involvement may produce epidural spinal cord compression. Previous studies show that radiotherapy (RT) increases the risk for carotid artery stenosis which can lead to a cerebrovascular event in 12–34% of patients with HNSCC [6, 25, 26]. Patients with recent stroke are not ideal candidates for early surgery. Hence, they can be prehabilitated both medically and physically during the neurological recovery periods. Temporal lobe injury (TLI) ipsilateral to the NPC is well known complication and often discovered by CT or magnetic resonance imaging (MRI). Patients with TLI may manifest from asymptomatic to marked dementia like cognitive impairment, deficits in memory, dysphasia, and executive function [24]. Every effort should be made to look for patients with age >70 years, previous history of cognitive impairment, delirium, alcohol abuse, renal dysfunction, visual impairment, and depression. These patients are prone to postoperative cognitive dysfunction (POCD) and postoperative delirium (POD) which is permanent and debilitative. Echocardiogram, carotid angiogram, and MRI brain will help us to identify the cause and severity of neurological conditions. These patients require further risk evaluation, optimization of cardiovascular status, timely endovascular stenting of carotid artery, and early cancer treatment to prevent tumour progression or metastasis.

15.10 Cancer Anaemia

Patients with HNSCC are prone to anaemia preoperatively due to malignant process itself, poor nutritional intake following dysphagia/trismus, nausea, vomiting or bone marrow suppression subsequent to chemoradiotherapy [27]. There is significant correlation between anaemia and poor prognosis in patients with HNSCC due to the fact that anaemia leads to tumour hypoxia which leads to poor patient's response rates to chemoradiotherapy [28].

A thorough screening for causes and types of anaemia followed by haematinics and B12/folic acid supplementations or intravenous iron therapy should be done to improve patient's oxygen delivering capacity. Anaemia is one of the important predictors of poor clinical outcomes that can be identified and optimized before planning the cancer treatment.

The objectives of anaemia correction are as follows [27, 29]:

- Prevention of local tumour relapse or metastasis
- Enhance their perioperative effort tolerance and overall quality of life
- Alleviation of symptoms and related end organ dysfunction
- Decrease in requirement of perioperative transfusion which increases the risk of tumour recurrence and decreased survival rates

A meta-analysis report suggested that erythropoietin reduces cancer associated anaemia [30]. The recommended dose is 150 U/ kg body weight given subcutaneously thrice weekly and it can be used to prevent or correction of anaemia and prior to chemo- or radiotherapy when routine treatment measures fail [28]. Patients treated with erythropoietin can develop hypertension, hence haemoglobin value and blood pressure must be regularly monitored. If indicated, it is advisable to initiate or intensify anti-hypertension medications.

15.11 Venous Thromboembolism (VTE)

The overall incidence of VTE in head and neck surgery patients is 0.4% as against the incidence of 0.1% in general population [31]. Patients with one or more risk factors for VTE should receive either mechanical or pharmacological prophylaxis preoperatively balancing the risk of bleeding. The knee or thigh high stockings, regular physical exercises, and adequate hydration are the ways to address the concerns during prehabilitation phase [7].

15.12 Cancer Pain

Pain is one of the most feared consequences of cancer and is identified in 80% of patients with HNC. Chronic pain is most common type of HNC pain and it is associated with disturbed sleep, impaired appetite, depression, and altered psychosocial behaviours. Brief pain inventory (BPI) and hospital anxiety and depression scale (HADS), Leeds assessment of neuropathic signs and symptoms (LANSS) questionnaire are useful assessment tools for an objective analysis of the pain [32]. Addressing pain concerns encourage patients to get actively involved in prehabilitation program. Pain management options include early antineoplastic therapies, multi-model approach using NSAIDS, opioids, head and neck nerve blocks including neurolytic (alcohol/phenol) blocks of trigeminal nerve divisions, behaviour pain therapies and other physical therapies such as muscle stretching and strengthening exercises, transcutaneous electrical nerve stimulation (TENS), relaxation techniques, hypnosis, and acupuncture [20, 32].

15.13 Nutrition

Early detection of malnutrition in HNC patients is important to prevent or minimize weight loss during and after treatment. A Registered Dietitian (RD) consult for nutrition assessment should be sought before treatment to establish a patient's baseline nutrition status on an outpatient basis. With focus on symptom management and weight maintenance, HNC patients should be reassessed on a weekly basis [33].

15.14 Components of Nutrition Assessments

Medical history: Location of head and neck tumour, planned treatment regimen and anticipated side effects, comorbidities (e.g., diabetes, hypertension, cardiovascular disease), and dental history (full, partial, or absent dentition).

Social history: Focus on personal resources and social support to aid in food preparation, food access, and nutrition supplementation.

Physical exam: Look for signs of muscle wasting, ascites/oedema, pressure ulcer/wound, mucositis, stomatitis, and glossitis.

Anthropometric assessment: Height, usual weight, current weight, weight change over time, BMI, fluid status.

Relevant laboratory Data: Albumin, pre-albumin, glucose, electrolytes, CBC (complete blood count) panel, lipid panel, liver function, renal function.

15.15 Nutrition Intake

History: Detailed usual oral intake versus current oral intake, use of food records if appropriate, personal or prescribed diet restrictions (e.g., diabetic diet), food allergies and intolerances, nutrition impact symptoms (e.g., swallowing/chewing difficulty), use of dietary supplements (e.g., vitamins, herbs, probiotics), use of high calorie high protein oral supplements (e.g., Ensure, Boost), use of appetite stimulants (medicinal marijuana), use of enteral nutrition or parenteral nutrition prior to treatment. The goal of nutrition intervention is to continue a safe oral diet, manage symptoms, and supplement as necessary during treatment.

The following are the common symptoms that have to be addressed during HNC specific prehabilitation (Fig. 15.3).

15.16 Dysphagia and Odynophagia

Dysphagia is a common symptom of HNC patients. Impaired mastication contributes to dysphagia. Masticatory difficulty is the most significant predictor of reduced food intake following anorexia. Poor baseline oral health also may result in masticatory difficulty [34]. Odynophagia usually results from mucositis during and immediately following radiation and/or chemotherapy treatment [35]. Odynophagia may need pain medication prior to oral intake. Patients are provided dietary guidelines for mucositis to minimize pain from food choices. Observational symptoms such as drooling, choking, or coughing during or following food and beverage intake are present in patients experiencing dysphagia. Signs include the inability to suck from a straw or hold food in the buccal recesses, gurgled voice quality, and an absent gag reflex. Dysphagia can lead to aspiration. This may result in pneumonia from the bacteria in the oral cavity or the food or beverage entering the lungs referred to as aspiration pneumonia [36]. Swallowing assessment should be a part of the routine care for the HNC patient. Patient's ability to masticate and swallow different liquids and food textures is assessed by the Speech and Language Pathologist (SLP) to determine the consistency needed to prevent aspiration. The SLP works in association with the RD to ensure safe and adequate nutrition for the patients. RDs provide modified consistency diet education and dietary recommendations to promote optimal oral intake.

Problem	Prehabilitation measures
Dysphagia and Odynophagia	Modified consistency diet (Thickend liquids and Pureed diets) Diet modification strategies, monitoring and education
Speech and swallowing problems	Mendelsohn manoeuver with effortful swallow, Shanker or Masako manoeuvers (10 repetitions x 3 times a day) Electrolarynx, Tracheoesophageal puncture/prosthesis (TEP)
Mucositis	Glutamine supplementation Pain management before food intake
Xerostomia	Use salive substitutes and intake of moist foods Xerodent™ tablets can be tried
Trismus	Mouth opening with jaw-mobilizing devices Manual therapies such as masticatory muscle stretching and massage
The stiff or fibrotic neck	Anterior neck and chest stretching exercises Cervical traction in a horizontal plane Headmaster cervical collar to prevent torticollis

Fig. 15.3 Head and neck cancer specific problems and its prehabilitation measures

Liquids need to be thickened for many patients with dysphagia. Patients may have difficulty controlling the fast flow of thin liquids. Thickened liquids move slower and allow the patient to coordinate a bolus for safe swallowing. Modified liquid consistencies range from thin to thick and in order of increasing viscosity include thin, nectar, honey, and pudding thick liquids. Commercial thickeners or modified starches such as tapioca or cornstarch are used to thicken liquids to the desired consistency. Thickeners may be added to beverages such as water, tea, coffee, juice, broth, milk, and liquid consistency foods such as soups. Food is preconditioned to the following consistencies for dietary management of dysphagia and masticatory difficulty namely, pureed, mechanically altered, and advanced. The pureed diet is the most restrictive and recommended for patients with minimal or no dentition. Mechanically altered, advanced, and regular diets require mastication. The advanced diet is used as a transition to a regular diet for patients with mild dysphagia [37].

15.17 Mucositis

Mucositis is a common side effect associated with chemotherapy and radiation therapy for HNC. It is manifested by inflammatory ulcerated lesions in the mouth and throat [38, 39]. L-glutamine (glutamine) is an amino acid derived from foods rich in protein such as fish, red meat, beans, and dairy products. During times of serious illness and stress, decreased protein consumption and diminished ability to extract glutamine from consumed foods place the body in a significant glutamine deficit and supplementation is recommended [40, 41]. Glutamine supplementation can mitigate the incidence and severity of oral mucositis as shown in multiple studies [42–44] recommending supplemental glutamine to HNC patients.10 g of glutamine mixed into a liquid suspension and administered orally 3 times per day has been analysed in majority of clinical trials [41, 45]. Patients are cautioned against mixing glutamine into acidic or hot liquids as these can denature the glutamine.

15.18 Xerostomia

Xerostomia or dry mouth is the most common late side effect of radiation treatment to the head and neck. Dry mouth can impact eating by affecting chewing, forming a bolus, swallowing, taste sensitivity, and speech. Increased dental caries and infections are sequelae of dry mouth [46]. Dietary management guidelines of food preparation techniques include intake of moist foods, increasing fluid consumption, frequent rinsing of the mouth during the day, and good dental hygiene [36]. Xerodent™ tablets containing malic acid with and without fluoride have been investigated for their impact on dry mouth. Increase in saliva flow rate by 15-fold compared to unstimulated levels has been observed and is well tolerated by most patients. These sugar-free tablets also increased the saliva bicarbonate secretion along with pH [47]. Diet modification strategies for xerostomia help the patient to eat more comfortably while staying well-nourished to foster healing. Patients are encouraged to use saliva substitutes, alcohol-free rinses, to gargle with dilute peroxide solution, consume a low-sucrose diet, and eat moist foods at room temperature. Patients should avoid caffeine, spicy and highly acidic foods, tobacco, and dehydration by drinking fluoridated tap water [48].

15.19 Physical Therapy

To date, it remains controversial as to whether a head and neck cancer patient should be seen by physical therapist before their cancer treatment has begun. The ideal pre-evaluation in this patient population includes a baseline functional assessment of the neck and shoulder, overall strength, mouth opening including any deviation, and/or TMJ involvement. The issues arising with prehabilitation include whether it would unnecessarily increase the already considerable high anxiety level of the patient in addition to visits to other providers. However, other patients may benefit from an informed visit that adjusts their expectations, should physical therapy be needed after treatments. To date, there is no data to support this approach for physical therapy in the head and neck cancer population. A selective approach may be more effective and could affect the outcome and the post-functional quality of life of the patient.

15.20 Trismus

Trismus is defined as a decrease in the maximum inter-incisor distance (MID) to <35 mm [49]. Causes of trismus include tumour invasion in the temporomandibular joint (TMJ) and neighbouring muscles, fibrosis of masticatory muscles, and buccal tissues from radiation therapy. It is important to delineate radiotherapy-induced trismus (RIT) from other types, as its management is significantly more intensive and the impact on the patient's quality of life can also be very severe [50]. Pain and inability to open one's mouth preclude proper nutrition, oral hygiene, breathing, tumour surveillance, communication, and social interactions [51, 52]. Lack of physical therapy in many head and neck patients would be deleterious to the return of functional abilities and quality of life for patients as well as their families [53].

Exercise therapy is the centrepiece of RIT management and must begin early after radiation is complete [54–58]. The physical therapist commonly performs an assessment of posture, neck mobility, and the TMJ including intra-oral joint testing and palpation of muscles of mastication. In most cases of RIT, muscles of mastication become stiff and rigid, limiting muscle extensibility. Exercises, in combination with jaw-mobilizing devices, have proven to be the most effective strategy in increasing MID [59]. The first 4 weeks is also when patients can regain the largest increase in mouth opening with jaw-mobilizing device [60]. Manual therapies such as masticatory muscle stretching and massage, temporomandibular/cervical joint mobilization, and myofascial release to neck musculature also augment the effectiveness of treatment [61]. Two of the most commonly utilized and studied jaw-mobilizing devices include TheraBite and Dynasplint. With TheraBite, patients manually squeeze the handle to apply torque, while with Dynasplint, patients incrementally increase torque and jaw opening by turning a handle. Such differences become important when chemotherapy-induced neuropathy impairs grip strength for TheraBite usage [62].

15.21 The Stiff or Fibrotic Neck

The fibrotic neck after head and neck radiation remains poorly understood and often wrongly diagnosed as lymphedema in the presence of neck swelling. Studies have shown that any irradiated area could become 5–6 times thicker in collagen formation due to the hyperactivity of the fibroblast cell in the connective tissue, especially of collagen type I and III [63]. The prehabilitation goal is to prevent the development of torticollis in patients who are prone for fibrotic neck. Stretching the anterior neck and chest prevents the development of a flexion contracture. Anterior neck and chest stretching exercises such as done for thoracic outlet syndrome are also helpful. Cervical traction in a horizontal plane seems to be an effective treatment option for both the stiff and the fibrotic neck. Strengthening of the interscapular muscles and neck extensors are meaningful, since the interscapular muscles are phasic muscles and will weaken over time when sedentary. One effective neck brace to prevent neck extensor weakness, but also to prevent a torticollis from occurring is the Headmaster Cervical Collar [64].

15.22 Psychological Distress

Psychological distress encompasses a wide spectrum of symptoms ranging from transient feelings of fear or sadness to the more disabling symptoms of anxiety or depression. Patients with head and neck cancer face the gamut of stressors and challenges inherent to cancer in general (e.g., uncertainty, intrusive treatments, dependency, disability, threat of recurrence, and mortality). In addition, their distress can be magnified by unique issues stemming from specific functional difficulties (e.g., speaking, eating, and breathing) and the stigma of disfigurement [65]. Studies have shown that patients with HNC have experienced increased distress at the time of diagnosis, as well as during and following treatment. Undetected and untreated psychological needs are associated with reduction in patient quality of life (QOL), extended hospital stays, malnutrition, complications with treatment, and treatment non-compliance [66].

The Distress Management Panel of the National Comprehensive Cancer Network (NCCN) has established guidelines for the recognition, monitoring, documentation, and treatment of distress [67]. According to these guidelines, all patients should be screened for distress during their initial visit and at appropriate intervals thereafter, particularly during changes in disease status and treatment. A number of cancer centres have implemented distress screening tools in order to identify and flag distress in head and neck cancer patients at risk for illness-related biopsychosocial complications [68].

Body image is the subjective picture of one's own physical appearance established both by self-observation and by noting the reactions of others [69]. According to Rhoten et al. [70] conceptual model, the two primary causes of body image disturbance are disfigurement and dysfunction. Patients with HNC often not only experience changes to their physical appearance but also to function. Swelling and scarring, sensory changes such as pain or numbness, and functional impairment such as dysarthria or dysphagia may be temporary or long term and have a significant impact on one's psychological well-being, social functioning, and overall QOL. Numerous studies have shown that body image concerns in patients with HNC have been associated with higher levels of anxiety and depression, poorer quality of life, and difficulties with sexual functioning [71–78]. The impact of such disfigurement and dysfunction on personal identity, ability to communicate or relate to others, and ability to feel successful interpersonally are all important considerations for the treatment team [79].

15.23 Depression and Anxiety

When patients are first confronted with the diagnosis of HNC, anticipatory anxiety is commonly seen, along with symptoms of distractibility and poor sleep. However once the patients are more adapted to the disease and treatment, the rate of anxiety significantly declines [80]. Conversely, fear of recurrence and the unknowns related to mortality are common concerns for patients with cancer. Changes in appearance often create a visible reminder that one has, or has had, cancer and so does the ability to swallow or salivate. These reminders can contribute to anxiety, whether conscious or unconscious. Simply looking in the mirror can often trigger an anxiety response. Depression is seen in HNC patients with a frequency ranging from 11 to 52% [79]. The potential triggering factors for depression include difficulties with eating and communicating, body disfigurement, changes in sexuality, presence of comorbidities, a history of substance abuse, impaired ability to work, dissatisfaction with care, and poor delivery of information by the medical team. Psychological counselling and appropriate psychotherapy interventions form part of the prehabilitation program.

15.24 Speech and Swallowing

Patients benefit from a team to navigate their journey through cancer to recovery. Speech pathologists are an integral part of that team. A baseline of voice, speech, and swallowing function is often achieved by a myriad of studies including videostroboscopy, Modified Barium Swallow Studies (MBSS), and/or Fiberoptic Endoscopic Evaluation of Swallowing studies (FEES).Beyond the baseline data, prehabilitation sessions provide the patient and family with much-needed education regarding strategies to compensate for any current deficits (i.e., communication strategies, diet modifications, or aspiration precautions), as well as what to expect for recovery given their diagnosis.

Exercises like Mendelsohn manoeuver followed by effortful swallow, Shaker and Masako manoeuver were recommended to improve or prevent swallowing difficulties (Fig. 15.4).

During the Mendelsohn manoeuver, patients were asked to hold the larynx for 3–5 s after swallowing. Effortful swallowing involves pushing the tongue firmly against the hard palate while squeezing the neck muscles and were allowed to swallow as forcefully as possible [81]. Shaker exercise is an isometric or isokinetic exercise to improve the strength of the suprahyoid musculature resulting in both improved hypolaryngeal movement and upper oesophageal sphincter opening. This exercise involves the sustained lifting of neck for one-minute repeated three times in a supine position with a one-minute rest period between each lift, followed by the patient is advised to lift the neck 30 times in the same position without any rest period between the lifts and without sustaining each lift [82]. The Masako or tongue-hold manoeuver is shown to improve swallowing by helping the coordination of the larynx and improving the constriction of the pharynx. It is done by protruding the tongue and holding the anterior tongue between the central incisor teeth while swallowing [83]. As per current literature evidence, these exercises are recommended at the rate of ten repetitions done three times a day [84].

During these prehabilitation evaluation and counselling sessions, post-treatment potential to regain speech, voice, and swallow function are reviewed as well as the importance of the patient's active participation in the treatment planning and

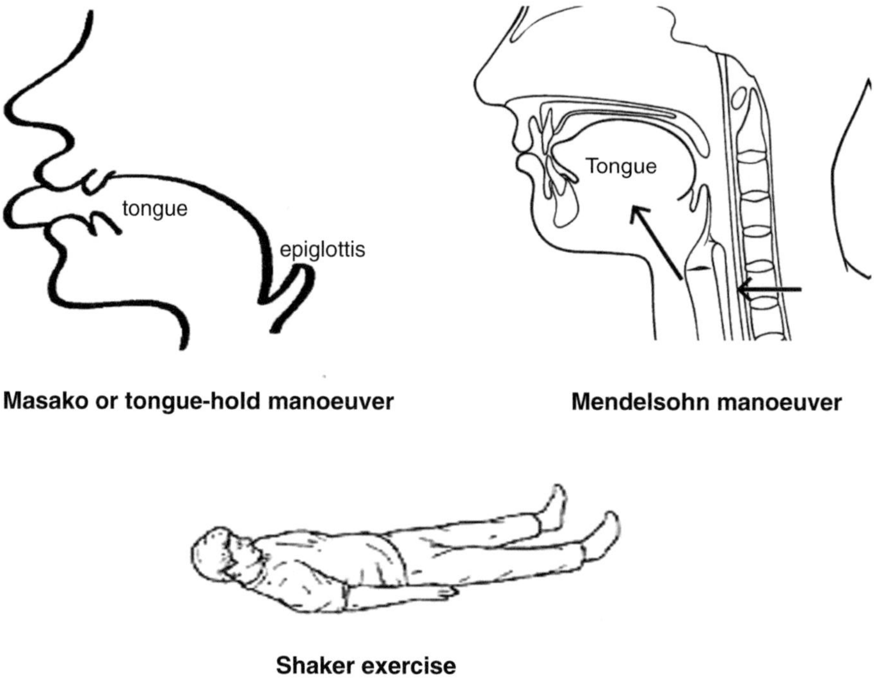

Fig. 15.4 Swallowing exercises

program. The severity of baseline impairments may not always be self-perceived, as the frequency of subjective dysphagia before treatment has been reported as high as 59%. Severity of baseline speech and swallow dysfunction is highly predictive of post-treatment functioning [85]. It is very important to consider the patient's specific condition, coping style, access to therapy, and rehabilitative preferences when developing the treatment plan.

Pre-laryngectomy patients, for example, are shown an electrolarynx (their own device is ordered so it is ready for them during their acute hospitalization phase) and offered the opportunity whenever logistically possible to meet with another laryngectomy patient in order to get a more vivid understanding of what to expect following treatment. If pertinent for the pre-laryngectomy patient, oesophageal speech and a tracheoesophageal puncture/ prosthesis (TEP) are explained to the patient and family. All of these discussions may help to ease anxiety and fear of the unknown and lead to improved outcomes [86]. The newly diagnosed head and neck cancer patient thus enters into the treatment phase of their care having had the necessary guidance and education to ease their experience during the acute phase of treatment. The use of prehabilitation in cancer treatment results in the highest quality care for this population, as the newly diagnosed patient feels well supported in their treatment plan.

15.25 Tobacco Cessation

Tobacco and alcohol use accounts for an estimated 75% of HNC cases [87–89]. Although many HNC patients will quit smoking before or during treatment, 14–60% will relapse [90–94]. Continued smoking is associated with several negative outcomes including increased risk of other smoking-related illnesses (e.g., coronary artery disease), secondary cancers, and primary cancer recurrence [95–97]. In addition, smoking reduces treatment efficacy [98, 99] and worsens treatment side effects [100–103]. One study found that depression was a significant predictor of continued smoking among HNC survivors, surpassing poor QOL and social support [104]. Most cancer institutions have developed smoking cessation programs that incorporate behavioural therapy and pharmacotherapy in accordance with NCCN guidelines.

15.26 Conclusion

Prehabilitation is a continuous process of identifying and improving the baseline functional capacity of the patients, preventing the anticipated impairments and optimizing the existing functional loss. The program is started as early as possible after the cancer diagnosis with specific exercise interventions and it is followed by early rehabilitation as well. Though there are limited consensus on the optimal design and duration of preoperative head and neck cancer related exercise interventions, the current recommended regime is to perform ten specific exercise repetitions, three times a day supplemented with specialist guided individualized physical activity program along with management of comorbidities, pain, nutrition, and mental health. Thus, a newly diagnosed head and neck cancer patient will enter into the treatment phase having had their physical and mental health optimized with necessary guidance and education to ease their experience during the acute phase of surgical treatment. Future researches are needed to develop cancer specific prehabilitation guidelines that can be incorporated routinely in the head and neck cancer management practice.

References

1. Silver JK, Baima J, Mayer RS. Impairment-driven cancer rehabilitation: an essential component of quality care and survivorship. CA Cancer J Clin. 2013;63(5):295–317. https://doi.org/10.3322/caac.21186.
2. Silver JK, Baima J. Cancer prehabilitation: an opportunity to decrease treatment-related morbidity, increase cancer treatment options, and improve physical and psychological health outcomes. Am J Phys Med Rehabil. 2013;92(8):715–27. https://doi.org/10.1097/PHM.0b013e31829b4afe.
3. Rose BS, Jeong JH, Nath SK, Lu SM, Mell LK. Population-based study of competing mortality in head and neck cancer. J Clin Oncol. 2011;29(26):3503–9. https://doi.org/10.1200/JCO.2011.35.7301.

4. Argiris A, Brockstein BE, Haraf DJ, Stenson KM, Mittal BB, Kies MS, Rosen FR, Jovanovic B, Vokes EE. Competing causes of death and second primary tumors in patients with locoregionally advanced head and neck cancer treated with chemoradiotherapy. Clin Cancer Res. 2004;10(6):1956–62. https://doi.org/10.1158/1078-0432.ccr-03-1077.
5. van der Schroeff MP, van de Schans SA, Piccirillo JF, Langeveld TP. Baatenburg de Jong RJ, Janssen-Heijnen ML. Conditional relative survival in head and neck squamous cell carcinoma: permanent excess mortality risk for long-term survivors. Head Neck. 2010;32(12):1613–8. https://doi.org/10.1002/hed.21369.
6. Okoye CC, Bucher J, Tatsuoka C, Parikh SA, Oliveira GH, Gibson MK, et al. Cardiovascular risk and prevention in patients with head and neck cancer treated with radiotherapy. Head Neck. 2017;39(3):527–32. https://doi.org/10.1002/hed.24646.
7. Robson A, Sturman J, Williamson P, Conboy P, Penney S, Wood H. Pre-treatment clinical assessment in head and neck cancer: United Kingdom National Multidisciplinary Guidelines. J Laryngol Otol. 2016;130(S2):S13–22. https://doi.org/10.1017/S0022215116000372.
8. Goff David C, Lloyd-Jones Donald M, Glen B, Sean C, D'Agostino Ralph B, Raymond G, et al. ACC/AHA guideline on the assessment of cardiovascular risk. Circulation. 2014;129(25_suppl_2):S49–73.
9. Goyal M, Shukla P, Gupta D, Bisht S, Verma NS, Tiwari S, et al. Cardiovascular sequel of neck irradiation in head and neck cancer patients. Int J Radiat Biol. 2017;93(7):711–6.
10. Rimmer J, Giddings CEB, Vaz F, Brooks J, Hopper C. Management of vascular complications of head and neck cancer. J Laryngol Otol. 2012;126(2):111–5.
11. Wouters EF, Posthuma R, Koopman M, Liu W-Y, Sillen MJ, Hajian B, et al. An update on pulmonary rehabilitation techniques for patients with chronic obstructive pulmonary disease. Expert Rev Respir Med. 2020;14(2):149–61.
12. Silverman DA, Lin C, Tamaki A, Puram SV, Carrau RL, Seim NB, et al. Respiratory and pulmonary complications in head and neck cancer patients: evidence-based review for the COVID-19 era. Head Neck. 2020;42(6):1218–26.
13. Landis SH, El-Hariry IA, van Herk-Sukel MPP, van den Haak P, Janssen-Heijnen MLG, Penning-van Beest FJA, et al. Prevalence and incidence of acute and chronic comorbidity in patients with squamous cell carcinoma of the head and neck. Head Neck. 2012;34(2):238–44.
14. Kawakita D, Abdelaziz S, Chen Y, Rowe K, Snyder J, Fraser A, et al. Adverse respiratory outcomes among head and neck cancer survivors in the Utah cancer survivors study. Cancer. 2020;126(4):879–85.
15. Chang C-C, Lee W-T, Hsiao J-R, Ou C-Y, Huang C-C, Tsai S-T, et al. Oral hygiene and the overall survival of head and neck cancer patients. Cancer Med. 2019;8(4):1854–64.
16. Bentz BG, Snyderman CH. Pulmonary complications in patients with head and neck and lung neoplasms. Arch Otolaryngol Head Neck Surg. 2000;126(3):429–32.
17. Durrand J, Singh SJ, Danjoux G. Prehabilitation. Clin Med. 2019;19(6):458.
18. Marin JM, Soriano JB, Carrizo SJ, Boldova A, Celli BR. Outcomes in patients with chronic obstructive pulmonary disease and obstructive sleep apnea: the overlap syndrome. Am J Respir Crit Care Med. 2010;182(3):325–31.
19. Gonçalves CG, Groth AK. Pré-habilitação: como preparar nossos pacientes para cirurgias abdominais eletivas de maior porte? Rev Colégio Bras Cir. 2019;46:e20192267.
20. Banugo P, Amoako D. Prehabilitation. BJA Educ. 2017;17(12):401–5.
21. Breyer M-K, Breyer-Kohansal R, Funk G-C, Dornhofer N, Spruit MA, Wouters EFM, et al. Nordic walking improves daily physical activities in COPD: a randomised controlled trial. Respir Res. 2010;11(1):112.
22. Sillen MJH, Speksnijder CM, Eterman R-MA, Janssen PP, Wagers SS, Wouters EFM, et al. Effects of neuromuscular electrical stimulation of muscles of ambulation in patients with chronic heart failure or COPD: a systematic review of the English-language literature. Chest. 2009;136(1):44–61.
23. Myatra S, Divatia JV, Jibhkate B, Barreto GS, Shrikhande SV. Preoperative assessment and optimization in periampullary and pancreatic cancer. Indian J Cancer. 2011;48(1):86–93.

24. Aiken RD. Neurologic complications of head and neck cancers. Semin Oncol. 2006;33(3):348–51.
25. Dorth JA, Patel PR, Broadwater G, Brizel DM. Incidence and risk factors of significant carotid artery stenosis in asymptomatic survivors of head and neck cancer after radiotherapy. Head Neck. 2014;36(2):215–9.
26. Smith GL, Smith BD, Buchholz TA, Giordano SH, Garden AS, Woodward WA, et al. Cerebrovascular disease risk in older head and neck cancer patients after radiotherapy. J Clin Oncol Off J Am Soc Clin Oncol. 2008;26(31):5119–25.
27. Munting KE, Klein AA. Optimisation of pre-operative anaemia in patients before elective major surgery - why, who, when and how? Anaesthesia. 2019;74(Suppl 1):49–57.
28. Becker A, Hänsgen G, Bloching M, Weigel C, Lautenschläger C, Dunst J. Oxygenation of squamous cell carcinoma of the head and neck: comparison of primary tumors, neck node metastases, and normal tissue. Int J Radiat Oncol Biol Phys. 1998;42(1):35–41.
29. Oettle H, Riess H, Raguse JD, Bier J, Gath HJ. Recombinant human erythropoietin in the treatment of head and neck tumour anaemia. Int J Oral Maxillofac Surg. 2001;30(2):148–55.
30. Zhao F, Wang Y, Liu L, Bian M. Erythropoietin for cancer-associated malignant anemia: a meta-analysis. Mol Clin Oncol. 2017;6(6):925–30.
31. Moubayed SP, Eskander A, Mourad MW, Most SP. Systematic review and meta-analysis of venous thromboembolism in otolaryngology–head and neck surgery. Head Neck. 2017;39(6):1249–58.
32. Ghei A, Khot S. Pain Management in Patients with head and neck carcinoma. Otorhinolaryngol Clin Int J. 2010;2:69–75.
33. Grant B. Pocket guide to the nutrition care process and cancer. Chicago: Academy of Nutrition and Dietetics; 2015.
34. Farhangfar A, Makarewicz M, Ghosh S, Jha N, Scrimger R, Gramlich L, Baracos V. Nutrition impact symptoms in a population cohort of head and neck cancer patients: multivariate regression analysis of symptoms on oral intake, weight loss and survival. Oral Oncol. 2014;50:877–83.
35. Hayward MC, Shea AM. Nutritional needs of patients with malignancies of the head and neck. Semin Oncol Nurs. 2009;25:203–11.
36. Mahan L, Escott-Stump S, Raymond J, Krause M. Krause's food & the nutrition care process. Amman: Elsevier; 2017.
37. American Academy of Nutrition and Dietetics. Nutrition care manual. Chicago: Academy of Nutrition and Dietetics; 2017.
38. Kumar NB. Nutritional management of cancer treatment effects, vol. 206. Berlin: Springer Science & Business Media; 2012.
39. Sideras K, Hallemeier CL, Loprinzi CL. Oral complications. Abeloff's Clin Oncol. 2014;43:635–647.e4.
40. Noé JE. L-glutamine use in the treatment and prevention of mucositis and cachexia: a naturopathic perspective. Integr Cancer Ther. 2009;8:409–15.
41. Tsujimoto T, Yamamoto Y, Wasa M, Takenaka Y, Nakahara S, Takagi T, Tsugane M, Hayashi N, Maeda K, Inohara H, Uejima E, Ito T. L-glutamine decreases the severity of mucositis induced by chemoradiotherapy in patients with locally advanced head and neck cancer: a double-blind, randomized, placebo-controlled trial. Oncol Rep. 2015;33:33–9.
42. Silverman S. Diagnosis and management of oral mucositis. J Support Oncol. 2007;5:13–21.
43. Chang PH, Wang CH, Huang JS, Lai CH, Wu TH, Lan YJ, Tsai JCS, Chen EYC, Yang SW, Yeh KY. Low body mass index at 3 months following adjuvant chemoradiation affects survival of postoperative locally advanced oral cavity cancer patients. Laryngoscope. 2012;122:2193–8.
44. Anderson PM, Schroeder G, Skubitz KM. Oral glutamine reduces the duration and severity of stomatitis after cytotoxic cancer chemotherapy. Cancer. 1998;83:1429–33.
45. Leung HWC, Chan ALF. Glutamine in alleviation of radiation-induced severe oral mucositis: a meta-analysis. Nutr Cancer. 2016;68:734–42.
46. Paterson C, Caldwell B, Porteous S, McLean A, Messow CM, Thomson M radiotherapy-induced xerostomia, pre-clinical promise of LMS-611. Support Care Cancer. 2016;24:629–36.

47. Lajer C, Buchwald C, Nauntofte B, Specht L, Bardow A. Jensdottir T erosive potential of saliva stimulating tablets with and without fluoride in irradiated head and neck cancer patients. Radiother Oncol. 2009;93:534–8.
48. Zheng WK, Inokuchi A, Yamamoto T, Komiyama S. Taste dysfunction in irradiated patients with head and neck cancer. Fukuoka Igaku Zasshi. 2002;93(4):64–76.
49. Dijkstra PU, Huisman PM, Roodenburg JL. Criteria for trismus in head and neck oncology. Int J Oral Maxillofac Surg. 2006;35(4):337–42.
50. Pauli N, et al. The incidence of trismus and long-term impact on health-related quality of life in patients with head and neck cancer. Acta Oncol. 2013;52(6):1137–45.
51. Epstein JB, et al. Neuropathic and nociceptive pain in head and neck cancer patients receiving radiation therapy. Head Neck Oncol. 2009;1:26.
52. Weber C, et al. Limited mouth opening after primary therapy of head and neck cancer. Oral Maxillofac Surg. 2010;14(3):169–73.
53. Guru K, Manoor UK, Supe SS. A comprehensive review of head and neck cancer rehabilitation: physical therapy perspectives. Indian J Palliat Care. 2012;18(2):87–97.
54. Rapidis AD, et al. Trismus in patients with head and neck cancer: etiopathogenesis, diagnosis and management. Clin Otolaryngol. 2015;40(6):516–26.
55. Kamstra JI, et al. Dynasplint trismus system exercises for trismus secondary to head and neck cancer: a prospective explorative study. Support Care Cancer. 2016;24(8):3315–23.
56. Kamstra JI, et al. TheraBite exercises to treat trismus secondary to head and neck cancer. Support Care Cancer. 2013;21(4):951–7.
57. Nagaraja S, et al. Trismus in head and neck cancer patients treated by telecobalt and effect of early rehabilitation measures. J Cancer Res Ther. 2016;12(2):685–8.
58. Pauli N, et al. Exercise intervention for the treatment of trismus in head and neck cancer —a prospective two-year follow-up study. Acta Oncol. 2016;55(6):686–92.
59. Scherpenhuizen A, et al. The effect of exercise therapy in head and neck cancer patients in the treatment of radiotherapy-induced trismus: a systematic review. Oral Oncol. 2015;51(8):745–50.
60. Pauli N, et al. Treating trismus: a prospective study on effect and compliance to jaw exercise therapy in head and neck cancer. Head Neck. 2015;37(12):1738–44.
61. Calixtre LB, et al. Manual therapy for the management of pain and limited range of motion in subjects with signs and symptoms of temporomandibular disorder: a systematic review of randomised controlled trials. J Oral Rehabil. 2015;42(11):847–61.
62. Addington J, Freimer M. Chemotherapy-induced peripheral neuropathy: an update on the current understanding. F1000Res. 2015;5:F1000.
63. Riekki R, et al. Increased expression of collagen types I and III in human skin as a consequence of radiotherapy. Arch Dermatol Res. 2002;294(4):178–84.
64. Stubblefield MD. Radiation fibrosis syndrome: neuromuscular and musculoskeletal complications in cancer survivors. PM&R. 2011;3(11):1041–54.
65. Devins GM. Head and neck cancer. In: Holland JC, Breitbart WS, Jacobsen PB, Loscalzo MJ, McCorkle R, Butow PN, editors. Psycho-oncology (3rd edn). Oxford: Oxford University Press; 2015. p. 92–7.
66. Neilson K, Pollard A, Boonzaier A, et al. A longitudinal study of distress (depression and anxiety) up to 18 months after radiotherapy for head and neck cancer. Psycho-Oncology. 2013;22(8):1843–8.
67. Holland JC, Andersen B, Breitbart WS, et al. Distress management. J Natl Compr Cancer Netw. 2010;8(4):448–85.
68. Loscalzo M, Clark K, Dillehunt J, Rinehart R, Strowbridge R, Smith D. SupportScreen: a model for improving patient outcomes. J Natl Compr Cancer Netw. 2010;8(4):496–504.
69. Merriam-Webster.com. Body image. https://www.merriamwebster.com/medical/body%20image. Accessed 13 Sept 2016.
70. Rhoten BA, Murphy B, Ridner SH. Body image in patients with head and neck cancer: a review of the literature. Oral Oncol. 2013;49(8):753–60.

71. Gamba A, Romano M, Grosso IM, et al. Psychosocial adjustment of patients surgically treated for head and neck cancer. Head Neck. 1992,14(3):218–23.
72. Newell R. Psychological difficulties amongst plastic surgery ex-patients following surgery to the face: a survey. Br J Plast Surg. 2000;53(5):386–92.
73. Rumsey N, Clarke A, White P, Wyn-Williams M, Garlick W. Altered body image: appearance-related concerns of people with visible disfigurement. J Adv Nurs. 2004;48(5):443–53.
74. Low C, Fullarton M, Parkinson E, et al. Issues of intimacy and sexual dysfunction following major head and neck cancer treatment. Oral Oncol. 2009;45(10):898–903.
75. Fingeret MC, Vidrine DJ, Reece GP, Gillenwater AM, Gritz ER. Multidimensional analysis of body image concerns among newly diagnosed patients with oral cavity cancer. Head Neck. 2010;32(3):301–9.
76. Fingeret MC, Yuan Y, Urbauer D, Weston J, Nipomnick S, Weber R. The nature and extent of body image concerns among surgically treated patients with head and neck cancer. Psycho-Oncology. 2012;21(8):836–44.
77. Fingeret MC, Teo I, Goettsch K. Body image: a critical psychosocial issue for patients with head and neck cancer. Current Oncol Rep. 2015;17(1):422.
78. Rhoten BA, Deng J, Dietrich MS, Murphy B, Ridner SH. Body image and depressive symptoms in patients with head and neck cancer: an important relationship. Support Care Cancer. 2014;22(11):3053–60.
79. Katz MR, Irish JC, Devins GM, Rodin GM, Gullane PJ. Reliability and validity of an observer-rated disfigurement scale for head and neck cancer patients. Head Neck. 2000;22(2):132–41.
80. Wu YS, Lin PY, Chien CY, et al. Anxiety and depression in patients with head and neck cancer: 6-month follow-up study. Neuropsychiatr Dis Treat. 2016;12:1029–36.
81. Kim J-H, Kim Y-A, Lee H-J, Kim K-S, Kim S-T, Kim T-S, et al. Effect of the combination of Mendelsohn maneuver and effortful swallowing on aspiration in patients with dysphagia after stroke. J Phys Ther Sci. 2017;29(11):1967–9.
82. Shaker R, Easterling C, Kern M, Nitschke T, Massey B, Daniels S, et al. Rehabilitation of swallowing by exercise in tube-fed patients with pharyngeal dysphagia secondary to abnormal UES opening. Gastroenterology. 2002 May;122(5):1314–21.
83. Byeon H. Effect of the Masako maneuver and neuromuscular electrical stimulation on the improvement of swallowing function in patients with dysphagia caused by stroke. J Phys Ther Sci. 2016 Jul;28(7):2069–71.
84. Loewen I, Jeffery CC, Rieger J, Constantinescu G. Prehabilitation in head and neck cancer patients: a literature review. J Otolaryngol - Head Neck Surg. 2021 Jan 6;50(1):2.
85. Carnaby-Mann G, Crary MA, Schmalfuss I, Amdur R. "Pharyngocise": randomized controlled trial of preventative exercises to maintain muscle structure and swallowing function during head-and-neck chemoradiotherapy. Int J Radiat Oncol Biol Phys. 2012;83(1):210–9.
86. Silver JK. Cancer prehabilitation and its role in improving health outcomes and reducing healthcare costs. Semin Ocol Nurs. 2015;31(1):13–30.
87. IARC Working Group on the Evaluation of Carcinogenic Risks to Humans. Personal habits and indoor combustions. Volume 100 E. A review of human carcinogens. IARC Monogr Eval Carcinog Risks Hum. 2012;100(Pt E):1–538.
88. Chaturvedi AK, Engels EA, Pfeiffer RM, et al. Human papillomavirus and rising oropharyngeal cancer incidence in the United States. J Clinic Oncol. 2011;29(32):4294–301.
89. Blot WJ, McLaughlin JK, Winn DM, et al. Smoking and drinking in relation to oral and pharyngeal cancer. Can Res. 1988;48(11):3282–7.
90. Ostroff JS, Jacobsen PB, Moadel AB, et al. Prevalence and predictors of continued tobacco use after treatment of patients with head and neck cancer. Cancer. 1995;75(2):569–76.
91. Gritz ER, Nisenbaum R, Elashoff RE, Holmes EC. Smoking behavior following diagnosis in patients with stage I non-small cell lung cancer. Cancer Causes Control: CCC. 1991;2(2):105–12.
92. Dresler CM, Bailey M, Roper CR, Patterson GA, Cooper JD. Smoking cessation and lung cancer resection. Chest. 1996;110(5):1199–202.

93. Davison AG, Duffy M. Smoking habits of long-term survivors of surgery for lung cancer. Thorax. 1982;37(5):331–3.
94. Walker MS, Larsen RJ, Zona DM, Govindan R, Fisher EB. Smoking urges and relapse among lung cancer patients: findings from a preliminary retrospective study. Prev Med. 2004;39(3):449–57.
95. Parsons A, Daley A, Begh R, Aveyard P. Influence of smoking cessation after diagnosis of early stage lung cancer on prognosis: systematic review of observational studies with meta-analysis. BMJ. 2010;340:b5569.
96. Kawahara M, Ushijima S, Kamimori T, et al. Second primary tumours in more than 2-year disease-free survivors of small-cell lung cancer in Japan: the role of smoking cessation. Br J Cancer. 1998;78(3):409–12.
97. Do KA, Johnson MM, Doherty DA, et al. Second primary tumors in patients with upper aerodigestive tract cancers: joint effects of smoking and alcohol (United States). Cancer Causes Control CCC. 2003;14(2):131–8.
98. Browman GP, Wong G, Hodson I, et al. Influence of cigarette smoking on the efficacy of radiation therapy in head and neck cancer. N Engl J Med. 1993;328(3):159–63.
99. Zhang J, Kamdar O, Le W, Rosen GD, Upadhyay D. Nicotine induces resistance to chemotherapy by modulating mitochondrial signaling in lung cancer. Am J Respir Cell Mol Biol. 2009;40(2):135–46.
100. Zevallos JP, Mallen MJ, Lam CY, et al. Complications of radiotherapy in laryngopharyngeal cancer: effects of a prospective smoking cessation program. Cancer. 2009;115(19):4636–44.
101. Arcavi L, Benowitz NL. Cigarette smoking and infection. Arch Intern Med. 2004;164(20):2206–16.
102. Moller AM, Pedersen T, Villebro N, Schnaberich A, Haas M, Tonnesen R. A study of the impact of long-term tobacco smoking on postoperative intensive care admission. Anaesthesia. 2003;58(1):55–9.
103. Smith JB, Fenske NA. Cutaneous manifestations and consequences of smoking. J Am Acad Dermatol. 1996;34(5 Pt 1):717–32. quiz 733–714
104. Berg CJ, Thomas AN, Mertens AC, et al. Correlates of continued smoking versus cessation among survivors of smoking-related cancers. Psycho-Oncology. 2013;22(4):799–806.

Prehabilitation for Musculoskeletal Cancer Surgery

16

Naresh Kumar, Sirisha Madhu, and Gurpal Singh

16.1 Introduction

Musculoskeletal tumors are a group of rare benign or malignant growths that develop within the bone or soft tissues and severely affect the functioning and quality of life (QoL) of patients. Management of these tumors is challenging and requires a multidisciplinary approach ranging from chemotherapy, surgery, radiation therapy, palliative care, or their combination [1–3].

Surgical resection of bone and soft tissue tumors is often preceded by chemotherapy which may be associated with significant side-effects that may in turn affect post-surgical clinical and functional outcomes [4, 5]. Therefore, optimization of patients through appropriate and timely prehabilitation is an emerging concept for achieving better outcomes in patients undergoing musculoskeletal cancer surgery.

Prehabilitation or preventative therapy is a process in the continuum of cancer care that is provided between cancer diagnosis and the initiation of acute cancer treatment [6–8]. It incorporates physical and psychological interventions that help: (1) improve baseline functional level and physical/cardiopulmonary/psychological health; (2) address modifiable risk factors; (3) accelerate recovery and decrease hospital length of stays; and (4) reduce the incidence and severity of future complications/unplanned hospital readmissions [6, 8, 9]. The concept of "prehabilitation" has been explored with successful outcomes in various cancer settings, including lung, oesophageal, colorectal, gastrointestinal, hepatobiliary, pancreatic, breast, and

N. Kumar (✉) · S. Madhu
Department of Orthopaedic Surgery, National University Health System, Singapore, Singapore
e-mail: dosksn@nus.edu.sg

G. Singh
Centre for Orthopaedic Oncology and Reconstructive Surgery, Connexion Farrer Park Medical Centre, Singapore, Singapore

A. Chakraborty, A. Balakrishnan (eds.), *Prehabilitation for Cancer Surgery*,
https://doi.org/10.1007/978-981-16-6494-6_16

bladder cancer [10–18]. However, literature on the use and outcomes of preventative therapy for musculoskeletal cancer surgery is sparse.

The objectives of this chapter are to discuss: (1) the goals and benefits of prehabilitation; (2) preoperative evaluation; (3) prehabilitation interventions; (4) the role of a multidisciplinary team; (5) examples of multimodal prehabilitation programs; and (6) current barriers and future prospects of prehabilitation in patients undergoing musculoskeletal cancer surgery.

16.2 Prehabilitation for Musculoskeletal Cancer Surgery

16.2.1 Goals

The goals of a prehabilitation plan prior to musculoskeletal cancer surgery are to:

- Establish baseline functional level through appropriate physical/psychological assessments
- Identify impairments that may affect post-surgical morbidity
- Provide optimal interventions to rectify the impairments and improve patient functioning prior to surgery
- Provide patient counselling, including setting appropriate expectations/goals of functional recovery
- Individualize and optimize the surgical plan
- Facilitate early hospital discharge and prevent/reduce the severity of anticipated musculoskeletal cancer surgery-related adverse effects/disability.

16.2.2 Benefits

The benefits of prehabilitation in patients undergoing musculoskeletal tumor surgery are multifarious, as shown in Box 16.1 [3, 9, 19–22]. The physical function gains with prehabilitation are further enhanced when combined with appropriate and timely rehabilitation measures [9].

Box 16.1 Benefits of Prehabilitation Interventions in Patients Undergoing Musculoskeletal Tumor Surgery

Improvement in adherence to chemotherapy prior to surgery
Improvement in response to chemotherapy
Reduction in anxiety and improvement in overall health status/QoL
Improvement in muscle strength and endurance, physical fitness, and functional mobility
Optimization of the surgical plan to reduce post-surgical morbidity
Improvement in postoperative outcomes and facilitation of early recovery

16.2.3 Preoperative Evaluation

Preoperative evaluation of functional and psychological condition of the patient alongside risk assessment is a crucial step in optimizing the prehabilitation and surgical plan for the treatment of musculoskeletal tumors. A comprehensive list of preoperative evaluations and corresponding prehabilitation considerations in patients undergoing musculoskeletal cancer surgery is shown in Table 16.1 [5, 21, 23].

16.2.4 Prehabilitation Interventions

The common multimodal approaches for prehabilitation in cancer care include supervised exercise (resistance, aerobic, and range of motion); nutritional assessment and intervention; psychoeducation; psychosocial support; smoking cessation; and stress/anxiety reduction techniques [6, 9, 11, 13, 16]. Studies specific for prehabilitation modalities in patients undergoing musculoskeletal cancer surgery are limited. An overview of plausible prehabilitation approaches in this patient cohort is outlined below.

16.2.4.1 Patient Counselling and Setting Expectations

Functional recovery after musculoskeletal tumor surgery is often unpredictable due to the difficulty in elucidating the involved neurovascular structures until the time of surgery. Furthermore, the extent and duration of recovery is dependent on various tumor and patient related factors. For example, distal femoral, tibial, and pelvic tumor resections and reconstructions may be technically challenging with unpredictable outcomes and prolonged/aggressive rehabilitation. Similarly, significant loss of function may be noted in most patients after resection of upper extremity sarcomas. Surgical resection of spine tumors may also be associated with sensory and neurological changes and significant loss of physical functioning and bladder functions. Hence, preoperative counselling and setting up expectations on the plausible extent and duration of post-surgical rehabilitation and functional recovery are an important aspect of an optimal prehabilitation plan. Additionally, optimizing the surgical plan based on the patients' expectations and desired level of activity after surgery is also vital for better long-term QoL in patients with bone and soft tissue tumors [2].

16.2.4.2 Appropriate Management of Comorbid Risk Factors

Advanced age and high comorbidity burden [Charlson Comorbidity Index (CCI) ≥4] have been reported to be associated with a significantly high risk of morbidity and mortality in patients undergoing musculoskeletal tumor surgery [24]. Additionally, being underweight has been linked with a significantly high risk of severe adverse events post musculoskeletal tumor surgery even after adjusting for confounding risk factors such as age, gender, CCI, and type of surgery [25]. Hence, an ideal prehabilitation plan should include comprehensive screening and

Table 16.1 Preoperative assessment and prehabilitation considerations in patients undergoing musculoskeletal tumor surgery

Preoperative assessment *(purpose)*	Assessment tools/risk factors	Prognostic significance	Prehabilitation considerations
Functional and psychological assessments *(for preoperative detection of potential/actual disability)*	Karnofsky performance status	General Well-being and functional impairment	• Appropriate prehabilitation intervention tailored to patients' functional needs • Psychological counselling • Setting expectations on postoperative functional recovery and outcomes
	ECOG scores	Functional impairment and patients' ability to tolerate treatment	
	Pulmonary function test	Lung function	
	Tokuhashi or Tomita scoring system	Survival prognosis	
	SMII	Surgical invasiveness prognosis	
	Brief pain inventory	Severity of pain and its impact on functioning	
	Numeric pain rating scale	Severity of pain	
	Musculoskeletal tumor society score	Physical function	
	6/9-min walk test	Exercise tolerance and endurance	
	Manual muscle testing	Muscle strength and function	
	Kinematic gait analysis	Gait dysfunction	
	SF-36/SF-12	Quality of life	
	SOSG outcome scores	Quality of life	

Risk assessment *(to identify high-risk patients with poor prognosis, or risk of greater postoperative morbidity)*	Comorbid risk factors • Older age • High CCI • Malnutrition	Poor postoperative outcomes	• Appropriate management of risk factor • Setting nutritional care goals • Individualizing the surgical plan • Patient counselling • Setting appropriate expectations on functional recovery and outcomes
	Preoperative chemotherapy and/or radiotherapy	Poor response and/or side-effects to preoperative cancer therapy	• Taking specific precautions/actions based on side-effects to preoperative chemotherapy and/or radiotherapy • Patient counselling
	Risk factors for bleeding and perioperative anaemia • Large and hypervascular tumors • Presence of risk factors for blood transfusion • Low preoperative haemoglobin	• Delayed wound healing • Delayed postoperative recovery • Postoperative morbidity (e.g., infections)	• Individualizing the surgical plan based on associated risk of bleeding • Blood management *Preoperatively* – Administration of targeted ESAs – Autologous predonation – Preoperative embolization *Intraoperatively* – Acute normovolemic hemodilution – IOCS – Allogeneic blood transfusion • Taking appropriate precautions/action to prevent infections while using blood products
	Medical history or risk factors for DVT	Postoperative DVT	• Antithrombotic prophylaxis
	Presence of risk factors for wound complications • Preoperative radiotherapy • Smoking • Diabetes mellitus • Vascular disease	Postoperative infections	• Appropriate management of risk factor • Appropriate postoperative wound management
	Personal/family history of depression or any psychological conditions	Post-surgical depression	• Psychological counselling and appropriate management

CCI Charlson comorbidity index, *DVT* Deep vein thrombosis, *ECOG* Eastern Cooperative Oncology Group, *ESA* Erythropoiesis stimulating agents, *IOCS* Intraoperative cell salvage, *SMII* Spinal metastasis invasiveness index, *SOSG* Spine Oncology Study Group identification of risk factors, such as older age, primary tumors with worse prognosis, malnutrition, high CCI, blood coagulation disorders, or high probability of blood transfusion requirement during surgery. It is important that all the modifiable risk factors be addressed adequately during prehabilitation to optimize the intra- and post-surgical outcomes in patients undergoing musculoskeletal cancer surgery [5, 9].

16.2.4.3 Preoperative Chemotherapy and/or Radiotherapy Planning

Musculoskeletal tumors are often treated with chemotherapy and/or radiotherapy to shrink the tumor prior to surgical resection. Both these interventions significantly affect the patient's clinical condition due to associated adverse effects, which may in turn influence the post-surgical outcomes. Therefore, a thorough patient' history and all possible adverse effects of chemotherapy given prior to surgery should be taken into consideration. Appropriate precautions/steps may be considered to mitigate the effects of prior chemotherapy as shown in Table 16.2 [4, 5].

16.2.4.4 Blood Management

Patients with soft tissue sarcoma are more likely to present with anaemia after tumor diagnosis when compared to cancer-free controls [26]. Chemotherapy and/or

Table 16.2 Adverse effects of chemotherapy and recommendations to mitigate the adverse effects

Chemotherapeutic class/agent	Common adverse effects	Precautions/actions
Anthracycline antibiotics (doxorubicin, daunorubicin)	Cardiac toxicity	• Specific care in elderly patients or patients with prior cardiac disease, or MI • Presurgical cardiac evaluation • Care with anaesthetics inducing myocardial depression (isoflurane) • Care wit QT-prolonging drugs
Taxanes (paclitaxel, docetaxel)	Neuropathy	• Careful neurological examination preoperatively (neuropathy should be considered when regional anaesthesia is planned)
Platinum analogues (cisplatin, carboplatin)	Nephrotoxicity, cardiotoxicity, hepatotoxicity, peripheral neuropathy	• Adequate hydration and diuresis • Monitoring of electrolyte levels • Evaluation of hepatic function • Care with QT-prolonging drugs • Consider neuropathy while planning regional anaesthesia
Antimetabolites (methotrexate)	Hepatic fibrosis, cirrhosis, non-cardiogenic pulmonary oedema	• Dose reduction of drugs metabolized in the liver • Caution during intubation
Trabectedin	Hepatotoxicity, rhabdomyolysis, arthralgias	• Evaluate hepatic function • Consider dose reduction of drugs metabolized in liver • Check electrolyte levels

radiotherapy prior to surgery in musculoskeletal tumor patients may also result in significant anaemia and thrombocytopenia. Additionally, patients undergoing musculoskeletal tumor surgery often experience high rates of blood loss, both intraoperatively and postoperatively, leading to anaemia and necessitating blood transfusion. Kawai et al. [27] retrospectively reviewed 1047 consecutive operations for musculoskeletal tumors. Blood transfusions were required in 20.1% (210/1047) of the musculoskeletal operations with total blood loss ranging from 0 to 26,050 ml. Of the musculoskeletal tumor surgeries, the requirement of transfusion occurred in 0.4% of biopsies, 20.8% of curettages, 34.1% of amputations and disarticulations, 5.0% of marginal resections, and 37.9% of wide resections. Wide resections of bone tumors experienced significantly more median blood loss than soft tissue tumors (2155 ml vs. 180 ml). Similarly, Pennington et al. [28] highlighted the requirement for blood transfusions in spine surgery for vertebral metastases. They found that open metastatic spine surgery resulted in an average of 1418 ml (713.3–3120 ml) of intraoperative blood loss and minimally invasive metastatic spine surgery resulted in an average of 745 ml (184–1320 ml) of intraoperative blood loss.

Preoperative anaemia has been noted to be a significant and independent risk factor for poor survival in soft tissue sarcoma patients [29, 30]. Hence, appropriate blood management strategies such as preoperative administration of erythropoiesis stimulating agents (ESAs), preoperative embolization, autologous predonation, and intraoperative salvage should be considered.

Several recent studies suggest that arterial embolization prior to musculoskeletal tumor surgery is feasible, safe, and beneficial in reducing intra- and postoperative blood loss and transfusion requirements in patients with highly vascular musculoskeletal tumors [23, 31]. In a retrospective study by Wong et al. [23] 13 patients underwent preoperative embolization followed by surgery of musculoskeletal tumors with 100% technical success and no major complications. The authors suggested that transarterial embolization prior to musculoskeletal tumor surgery is feasible and safe and may help in reducing intraoperative blood loss and intra/postoperative blood product usage. Kumar et al. [32] conducted a retrospective study in 218 patients undergoing open surgery for metastatic spine tumors and suggested that the success of preoperative embolization is dependent on the extent of embolization and the time duration between embolization and index surgery. The authors reported that total embolization and index surgery within 24 h of embolization may be associated with reduced blood loss when compared to partial/subtotal embolization or increased embolization–surgery interval. Another retrospective review of patients undergoing spinal oncologic surgery revealed primary tumors to also be an influencing factor for success of preoperative embolization with metastases from hepatocellular carcinoma, thyroid, and primary spine tumors experiencing favourable outcomes with the procedure [33]. Additionally, the use of magnetic resonance imaging over angiography to evaluate hypervascularity prior to transarterial embolization has been found to be associated with significantly reduced blood loss during surgical treatment of vertebral tumors [34].

Literature is sparse on the role of autologous predonation for blood management in patients undergoing musculoskeletal tumor surgery. Nakai et al. [35] conducted sacral tumor resection in six patients using preoperatively collected autologous blood and suggested this strategy to be useful in reducing blood transfusion requirements. In another study by Lichtiger et al. [36] in 23 patients undergoing bone and soft tissue tumor surgery, the use of pre-deposited autologous blood was found to be a viable option with reduced need for additional blood transfusions.

Allogenic blood transfusion is one of the blood management strategies to replenish the blood lost during or after musculoskeletal tumor surgery. However, allogenic blood transfusion may not be ideal as it has been associated with adverse effects such as immune-system compromise, transfusion-related acute lung injury, and longer intensive care unit and hospital stays [37]. Intraoperative cell salvage (IOCS) is a process whereby the blood lost during surgery is salvaged (centrifuged and washed), and the salvaged blood is transfused back into the patient, thereby decreasing the dependency on allogenic blood transfusion. However, IOCS was previously contraindicated in tumor surgeries due to the fear of metastasis through the reinfusion of autologous salvaged blood containing tumor cells [37, 38]. Several studies have since evaluated the use of IOCS in musculoskeletal tumor surgeries. In a prospective observational study, Kumar et al. [37] collected blood samples from 50 patients undergoing metastatic spine tumor surgery. These blood samples were subjected to IOCS processing with a leukocyte depletion filter (LDF). In their study, it was found that blood subjected to IOCS-LDF processing contained no viable malignant tumor cells. Conversely, they found that 8% (4/50) of blood samples subjected to IOCS alone contained malignant tumor cells. However, in an advanced cellular evidence study by Kumar et al. [39], it was proven that such malignant tumor cells present in blood after IOCS alone represented a significantly decreased cell count when compared to the patients' own circulating tumor cell count. Furthermore, such malignant tumor cells were damaged by the IOCS process, rendering them unable to replicate and unlikely to metastasize [40]. Similar results were reported by Muller et al. [41], whereby osteosarcoma cells from an established cell line were added to red cell concentrates and Ringer solution. These were then subjected to the IOCS-LDF process. It was found that osteosarcoma cells were still present after the IOCS process alone. However, with the combined IOCS-LDF process, no osteosarcoma cells were evident. With the safety of the IOCS process with and without LDF supported for musculoskeletal tumor surgeries, prehabilitation efforts are eased as the burden attributed to blood loss of musculoskeletal tumor surgeries is reduced.

A holistic approach to optimal blood management in patients undergoing musculoskeletal tumor surgery using the various interventions described above is shown in Fig. 16.1.

16.2.4.5 Anti-Thromboembolic Prophylaxis

Patients undergoing musculoskeletal tumor surgery are at a high risk of deep vein thrombosis (DVT) and pulmonary embolism (PE) when compared to patients undergoing standard orthopaedic surgical procedures [42, 43]. The risk of DVT is high even after mechanical antithrombotic prophylaxis [44]. While the risk of PE is higher after resection of bone tumors versus soft tissue resections [43]. A

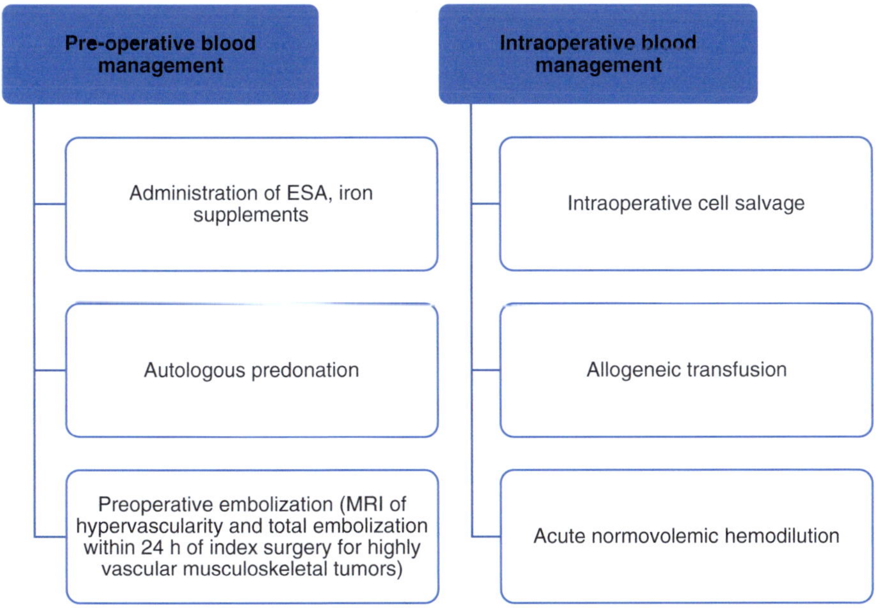

Fig. 16.1 Prehabilitative blood management strategies in patients undergoing musculoskeletal tumor surgery. *MRI*: Magnetic resonance imaging

recent systematic review of the literature on prophylactic management of venous thromboembolism (VTE) in orthopaedic oncology patients revealed that the incidence of VTE in these patients is 10.7% (VTE with and without pharmacologic prophylaxis: 7.9% and 8.7%, respectively) and DVT 8.8% (asymptomatic DVT: 10.9%; symptomatic DVT: 2.9%). Furthermore, the review concluded that all musculoskeletal tumor patients undergoing surgery should be assessed for VTE risk factors and considered for both mechanical and pharmacological VTE prophylaxis [45]. Some of the VTE risk factors highlighted in this review and other relevant studies in the literature include pelvic or hip resections, duration of surgery >3 h, prosthetic reconstruction, malignancy diagnosis, elevated D-dimer (DD) levels, elevated preoperative platelet count, tumor diameter exceeding 8 cm, age $\geq$ 30 years, and presence of comorbidities such as ischemic heart disease, pulmonary disease, paralysis, neurological disorders, or coagulopathy [45–48].

Surgeons and clinicians should evaluate all musculoskeletal tumor surgical patients for VTE risk factors as a part of the prehabilitation plan. Weighing the risk of VTE versus the risk of haemorrhage is also crucial during the decision-making process for initiating anti-thromboembolic prophylaxis [45, 49]. Both mechanical and pharmacological prophylaxis are needed and have been found to be feasible, safe, and effective in preventing VTE in patients undergoing musculoskeletal tumor surgery [44, 45, 50, 51].

16.2.4.6 Individualized Exercise Therapy

Patients with bone and soft tissue tumors are at an increased risk of physical activity limitations and poor functional quality of life. Prehabilitation prior to surgery of musculoskeletal tumors, especially in patients undergoing preoperative chemotherapy increases muscle strength and endurance, reduces activity limitations, and improves postoperative outcomes [3]. In a study by Corr et al. [19] prehabilitation exercise sessions were found to be feasible in patients with osteosarcoma and included endurance, strengthening, and stretching exercises such as ambulation (with or without support), video simulation of sport, bicep/tricep curls, calf raises, squats or press-ups from a mat or wheel-chair. Patients who took part in exercise sessions had a significant improvement in functional mobility than the control group in this study. In another study, high compliance and increase in muscle strength were noted to aerobic and strengthening exercises in patients with bone tumors [20].

In addition to increase in muscle strength and endurance, exercise during chemotherapy has been noted to have positive effects on QoL and physical functioning [52]. Experimental studies have suggested the beneficial effect of exercise in increasing chemotherapy efficacy by improving vascular structure and function and enhancing drug delivery to the tumor, thereby promoting inhibition of tumor growth [22, 53]. Improvement in blood vessel function after exercise may also reduce tumor hypoxia, potentially increasing efficacy of radiation therapy [3]. These plausible favourable effects of exercise in improving chemotherapy and radiation therapy efficacy are however noted in experimental settings and need to be proven in clinical studies.

Exercise sessions need not be restricted to traditional aerobic exercises, upper extremity ergometry, or muscle strengthening exercises. Supervised alternative physical activity sessions such as yoga, qigong, and tai chi also provide therapeutic benefits in terms of reduction of fatigue, anxiety, depression, and improvement in appetite, sleep, immunity, general well-being, and QoL both for cancer patients and caregivers [54, 55].

Several clinical oncologic and sports societies and cochrane systematic reviews recommend that healthcare professionals should discuss the role of exercise with cancer patients and encourage them to participate in supervised and targeted multimodal moderate-intensity exercise programs tailored to individual needs in order to improve the health-related QoL of cancer patients [56–58].

16.2.4.7 Setting Nutrition Care Goals

Severe thinness and being underweight have been proven to be significant risk factors for adverse postoperative events in patients undergoing musculoskeletal tumor surgery [25, 59]. Regional clinical oncology societies recommend screening of all cancer patients for malnutrition and sarcopenia at the time of diagnosis, to identify high-risk patients. Treatment of cancer-related malnutrition and sarcopenia should be individualized under the supervision of a multidisciplinary team with the help of targeted medical nutrition therapy, exercise prescription, and behavioural and psychological therapy [60].

16.2.5 Multidisciplinary Team for Musculoskeletal Tumor Surgical Prehabilitation

The successful implementation of an optimal prehabilitation plan prior to musculoskeletal tumor surgery and complementary rehabilitation plan requires the combined effort of a multidisciplinary team comprising of surgeon, oncologist, neurologist, nurse, physical and occupational therapist, orthotist, prosthetist, psychologist, nutritionist, social worker, and family and friends. The roles played by each member of this team have been described in Table 16.3 [2, 3].

16.3 Examples of Multimodal Prehabilitation for Musculoskeletal Tumor Surgery

A timeline diagram for implementation of plausible prehabilitation approaches prior to and during index musculoskeletal tumor surgery is shown in Fig. 16.2, supported later with two real-life case examples.

Table 16.3 Roles of members of a multidisciplinary prehabilitation team for patients undergoing musculoskeletal tumor surgery

Team member	Roles and responsibilities
Surgeon	Presurgical planning, surgery, post-surgical management, optimizing motion restrictions based on healing, patient counselling
Oncologist	Tumor treatment planning while considering individual physiologic and functional thresholds for nausea, fatigue, and pain, patient counselling
Neurologist	Treatment planning to mitigate neuropathy, balance, and pain
Nurse	Provide adequate guidance to patients to improve their compliance to the treatment plan
Physical and occupational therapist	Optimization of physical function and fitness, enhancing patient's independence and ability to perform activities of daily living, and prevention or reduction of functional disability with appropriate and targeted exercise prescriptions
Orthotist	Design and application of individualized orthoses
Prosthetist	Design and application of individualized prostheses
Psychologist	Emotional and psychosocial health and support, patient counselling
Nutritionist	Medical nutrition treatment to prevent or treat malnutrition/sarcopenia
Social worker	Psychosocial support
Family and friends	Behaviour modelling and emotional support

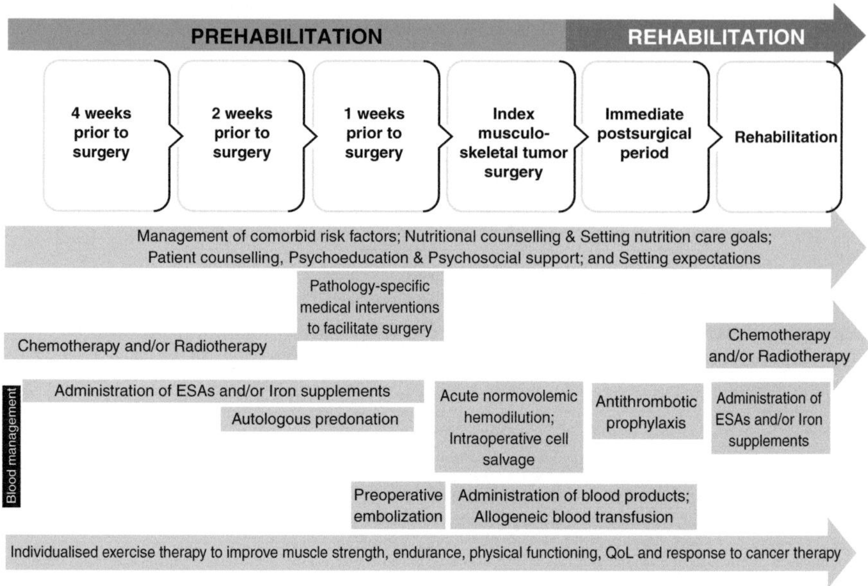

Fig. 16.2 Timeline diagram of prehabilitation approaches prior to and during index musculoskeletal tumor surgery. *ESA* Erythropoiesis stimulating agents, *QoL* Quality of life

Case Example 1

A 16-year-old male presented with progressive swelling and fixed flexion attitude of the right knee for the past 2 months. The patient complained of severe pain in the right lower limb at night from the past 2 weeks (numerical pain rating scale score: 8). He, however, did not divulge his condition to his family due to social stigma and inhibition, until visible swelling was noted. A weight loss of 5 kg was noted over the past 2 months, and the patient was anaemic (haemoglobin levels: 10.2 g/dL). A diagnosis of osteosarcoma was made based on clinical presentation and plain radiographs. The patient was scheduled for distal femur resection and prosthetic replacement.

Prehabilitation plan:

The patients' anaemia was addressed by starting him on oral hematinics.

High protein diet was supplemented to improve albumin level and facilitate better wound healing.

Skin injuries were avoided to improve local skin care, facilitate better skin closure during surgery and improve wound healing after surgery.

Exercise prescription:

Open-chain exercises were prescribed to develop and build the gastrocnemius muscle, and make the flap more viable and be able to rotate

Chest physiotherapy was provided for improving lung function to be able to tolerate the effects of chemotherapy.

The patient was provided psychological counselling to overcome his social inhibitions.

Case Example 2

A 57-year-old female presented with severe back pain for 3–4 weeks, reduced mobility, subtle weakness in the left lower limb and recent loss of appetite. She was treated 4 years ago for carcinoma breast and was in remission. Magnetic resonance imaging and computed tomography of the thorax, abdomen, and pelvis revealed metastasis to L4. She was scheduled for metastatic spine tumor surgery.

Prehabilitation plan:

High protein diet was supplemented to improve albumin level and facilitate better wound healing.

Iron supplementation was started to improve the haemoglobin levels.

Pre-operative bracing: Improved mobility and reduced back pain with bracing helped ascertain the diagnosis of pathological fracture secondary to metastatic spine tumor cord compression.

Preoperative physiotherapy was provided to improve mobility, facilitate better adaptation to physical exercises, and complement exercise therapy during rehabilitation.

The patient was counselled on the need for post-operative rehabilitation

The postoperative stereotactic body radiation therapy plan (dose, surgery-radiation therapy interval) was finalized with the radiotherapist.

Prior to index surgery, angio-embolization was done to reduce intraoperative blood loss and subsequent risk of anaemia.

16.4 Current Barriers to Prehabilitation

The existing barriers to prehabilitation in patients undergoing musculoskeletal tumor surgery include: [6, 9]

- Lack of skilled clinicians trained in prehabilitation care delivery
- Lack of insurance benefits covering prehabilitation therapy/exercise services
- Difficulty in tailoring prehabilitation approaches to individual patient' needs
- High probability of co-existing comorbid conditions that may reduce physical functioning of the patient and complicate treatment

- Lack of clinical studies on effectiveness of prehabilitation in patients undergoing surgery for musculoskeletal tumors
- Difficulty in achieving right balance between time duration of prehabilitation interventions and need for acute cancer treatment

16.5 Future Directives

Prehabilitation prior to musculoskeletal tumor surgery helps in optimizing the surgical plan and postoperative recovery as well as outcomes. It acts as a useful complement to rehabilitation after surgery. The existing lacuna on the effectiveness of preventative therapy in these patients should be addressed in future by conducting well-designed, short-term studies and publishing expert group consensus opinions. Multidisciplinary teams involved in treatment of musculoskeletal tumors should be encouraged to embrace this concept and participate in conferences and focus group meetings on prehabilitation in cancer care.

Acknowledgements We would like to acknowledge Keith Gerard Lopez, Sridharan Alathur Ramakrishnan, and Laranya Kumar for their contributions to the chapter.

References

1. Binitie O, Alvero C, Letson GD. Chapter 34 - Musculoskeletal bone and soft tissue tumors. In: Magee DJ, Zachazewski JE, Quillen WS, Manske RC, editors. Pathology and intervention in musculoskeletal rehabilitation. 2nd ed. Philadelphia: W.B. Saunders; 2016. p. 1175–94.
2. Andrews CC, Siegel G, Smith S. Rehabilitation to improve the function and quality of life of soft tissue and bony sarcoma patients. Patient Relat Outcome Meas. 2019;10:417–25. https://doi.org/10.2147/prom.S130183.
3. Garcia MB, Ness KK, Schadler KL. Exercise and physical activity in patients with osteosarcoma and survivors. In: Kleinerman ES, Gorlick R, editors. Current advances in osteosarcoma clinical perspectives: past, present and future, Chap 16. *Advances in experimental medicine and biology*, vol. 1257. 2nd ed. Cham: Springer International Publishing; 2020. p. 193–207.
4. Anderson MR, Jeng CL, Wittig JC, Rosenblatt MA. Anesthesia for patients undergoing orthopedic oncologic surgeries. J Clin Anesth. 2010;22(7):565–72. https://doi.org/10.1016/j.jclinane.2010.02.011.
5. Karmaniolou I, Makris A, Lamprou K, Staikou C. Perioperative management of patients with bone and soft tissue tumors: a narrative review. Acta Anaesthesiol Belg. 2017;68:1–12.
6. Silver JKRV, Wisotzky EM. Oncology rehabilitation. In: MM HP, editor. Quality cancer care. 1st ed. Cham: Springer International Publishing; 2018. p. 119–47. chap 9.
7. Nagpal A FJ, Bickelhaupt B, Eckmann MS, Boies B, Benfield J. Cancer rehabilitation. In: Gulati A, Puttanniah, V., Bruel BM, Rosenberg W, Hung JC, ed. Essentials of interventional cancer pain management. 1st ed. Springer International Publishing: Cham; 2019:363–373.:chap 40.
8. Carli F, Silver JK, Feldman LS, et al. Surgical prehabilitation in patients with cancer: state-of-the-science and recommendations for future research from a panel of subject matter experts. Phys Med Rehabil Clin N Am. 2017;28(1):49–64. https://doi.org/10.1016/j.pmr.2016.09.002.
9. Faithfull S, Turner L, Poole K, et al. Prehabilitation for adults diagnosed with cancer: a systematic review of long-term physical function, nutrition and patient-reported outcomes. Eur J Cancer Care (Engl). 2019;28(4):e13023. https://doi.org/10.1111/ecc.13023.

10. Driessen EJ, Peeters ME, Bongers BC, et al. Effects of prehabilitation and rehabilitation including a home-based component on physical fitness, adherence, treatment tolerance, and recovery in patients with non-small cell lung cancer: a systematic review. Crit Rev Oncol Hematol. 2017;114:63–76. https://doi.org/10.1016/j.critrevonc.2017.03.031.
11. Ferreira V, Minnella EM, Awasthi R, et al. Multimodal prehabilitation for lung cancer surgery: a randomized controlled trial. Ann Thorac Surg. 2020; https://doi.org/10.1016/j.athoracsur.2020.11.022.
12. Halliday LJ, Doganay E, Wynter-Blyth VA, et al. The impact of prehabilitation on post-operative outcomes in oesophageal cancer surgery: a propensity score matched comparison. J Gastrointest Surg. 2020; https://doi.org/10.1007/s11605-020-04881-3.
13. Minnella EM, Bousquet-Dion G, Awasthi R, et al. Multimodal prehabilitation improves functional capacity before and after colorectal surgery for cancer: a five-year research experience. Acta Oncol. 2017;56(2):295–300. https://doi.org/10.1080/0284186x.2016.1268268.
14. Steffens D, Young J, Beckenkamp PR, et al. Feasibility and acceptability of a preoperative exercise program for patients undergoing major cancer surgery: results from a pilot randomized controlled trial. Pilot Feasibility Stud. 2021;7(1):27. https://doi.org/10.1186/s40814-021-00765-8.
15. Bundred JR, Kamarajah SK, Hammond JS, et al. Prehabilitation prior to surgery for pancreatic cancer: a systematic review. Pancreatology. 2020;20(6):1243–50. https://doi.org/10.1016/j.pan.2020.07.411.
16. Wu F, Laza-Cagigas R, Pagarkar A, et al. The feasibility of prehabilitation as part of the breast cancer treatment pathway. PM R. 2020; https://doi.org/10.1002/pmrj.12543.
17. Lambert J, Hayes L, Keegan T, et al. The impact of prehabilitation on patient outcomes in hepatobiliary, colorectal, and upper gastrointestinal cancer surgery: a PRISMA-accordant meta-analysis. Ann Surg. 2020; https://doi.org/10.1097/sla.0000000000004527.
18. Nahon I, Paterson C, Sayner A. The impact of exercise and nutrition as part of a person-centered approach to prehabilitation in patients with bladder cancer. Semin Oncol Nurs. 2020;36(5):151072. https://doi.org/10.1016/j.soncn.2020.151072.
19. Corr AM, Liu W, Bishop M, et al. Feasibility and functional outcomes of children and adolescents undergoing preoperative chemotherapy prior to a limb-sparing procedure or amputation. Rehabil Oncol. 2017;35(1):38–45.
20. Fiuza-Luces C, Padilla JR, Soares-Miranda L, et al. Exercise intervention in pediatric patients with solid tumors: the physical activity in pediatric cancer trial. Med Sci Sports Exerc. 2017;49(2):223–30. https://doi.org/10.1249/mss.0000000000001094.
21. Morii T, Kishino T, Shimamori N, et al. Preoperative evaluation of intraoperative blood loss during malignant soft tissue tumor resection by ultrasonography. J Orthop Sci. 2018;23(2):403–7. https://doi.org/10.1016/j.jos.2017.12.011.
22. Morrell MBG, Alvarez-Florez C, Zhang A, et al. Vascular modulation through exercise improves chemotherapy efficacy in Ewing sarcoma. Pediatr Blood Cancer. 2019;66(9):e27835. https://doi.org/10.1002/pbc.27835.
23. Wong SJ, Urlings T, Seng C, et al. Pre-operative embolisation of musculoskeletal tumours - a single centre experience. Malays Orthop J. 2020;14(1):42–8. https://doi.org/10.5704/moj.2003.007.
24. Ogura K, Yasunaga H, Horiguchi H, et al. What is the effect of advanced age and comorbidity on postoperative morbidity and mortality after musculoskeletal tumor surgery? Clin Orthop Relat Res. 2014;472(12):3971–8. https://doi.org/10.1007/s11999-014-3889-y.
25. Ogura K, Yasunaga H, Horiguchi H, et al. Nomogram predicting severe adverse events after musculoskeletal tumor surgery: analysis of a national administrative database. Ann Surg Oncol. 2014;21(11):3564–71. https://doi.org/10.1245/s10434-014-3760-0.
26. Herk-Sukel MPPV, Shantakumar S, Overbeek LIH, et al. Occurrence of comorbidities before and after soft tissue sarcoma diagnosis. Sarcoma. 2012;2012:402109. https://doi.org/10.1155/2012/402109.
27. Kawai A, Kadota H, Yamaguchi U, et al. Blood loss and transfusion associated with musculoskeletal tumor surgery. J Surg Oncol. 2005;92(1):52–8. https://doi.org/10.1002/jso.20375.

28. Pennington Z, Ahmed AK, Molina CA, et al. Minimally invasive versus conventional spine surgery for vertebral metastases: a systematic review of the evidence. Ann Transl Med. 2018;6(6):103. https://doi.org/10.21037/atm.2018.01.28.
29. Szkandera J, Gerger A, Liegl-Atzwanger B, et al. Pre-treatment anemia is a poor prognostic factor in soft tissue sarcoma patients. PLoS One. 2014;9(9):e107297. https://doi.org/10.1371/journal.pone.0107297.
30. Nakamura T, Grimer R, Gaston C, et al. The relationship between pretreatment anaemia and survival in patients with adult soft tissue sarcoma. J Orthop Sci. 2013;18(6):987–93. https://doi.org/10.1007/s00776-013-0454-6.
31. Sare A, Jain N, Chandra V, et al. Perioperative blood loss after embolization of hypervascular musculoskeletal tumors outside of the spine: a single-center ten year experience and systematic review of the literature. Clin Imaging. 2021;79:24–9. https://doi.org/10.1016/j.clinimag.2021.04.001.
32. Kumar N, Tan B, Zaw AS, et al. The role of preoperative vascular embolization in surgery for metastatic spinal tumours. Eur Spine J. 2016;25(12):3962–70. https://doi.org/10.1007/s00586-016-4494-4.
33. Tan BWL, Zaw AS, Rajendran PC, et al. Preoperative embolization in spinal tumour surgery: enhancing its effectiveness. J Clin Neurosci. 2017;43:108–14. https://doi.org/10.1016/j.jocn.2017.05.021.
34. Zhang J, Kumar NS, Tan BWL, et al. Pre-operative embolisation of spinal tumours: neither neglect the neighbour nor blindly follow the gold standard. Neurosurg Rev. 2019;42(4):951–9. https://doi.org/10.1007/s10143-018-1003-8.
35. Nakai S, Yoshizawa H, Kobayashi S, et al. Role of autologous blood transfusion in sacral tumor resection: patient selection and recovery after surgery and blood donation. J Orthop Sci. 2000;5(4):321–7. https://doi.org/10.1007/s007760070037.
36. Lichtiger B, Huh YO, Armintor M, Fischer HE. Autologous transfusions for cancer patients undergoing elective ablative surgery. J Surg Oncol. 1990;43(1):19–23. https://doi.org/10.1002/jso.2930430106.
37. Kumar N, Ahmed Q, Lee VK, et al. Are we ready for the use of intraoperative salvaged blood in metastatic spine tumour surgery? Eur Spine J. 2016;25(12):3997–4007. https://doi.org/10.1007/s00586-015-4112-x.
38. Waters JH, Donnenberg AD. Blood salvage and cancer surgery: should we do it? Transfusion. 2009;49(10):2016–8. https://doi.org/10.1111/j.1537-2995.2009.02379.x.
39. Kumar N, Lam R, Zaw AS, et al. Flow cytometric evaluation of the safety of intraoperative salvaged blood filtered with leucocyte depletion filter in spine tumour surgery. Ann Surg Oncol. 2014;21(13):4330–5. https://doi.org/10.1245/s10434-014-3950-9.
40. Kumar N, Zaw AS, Khoo BL, et al. Intraoperative cell salvage in metastatic spine tumour surgery reduces potential for reinfusion of viable cancer cells. Eur Spine J. 2016;25(12):4008–15. https://doi.org/10.1007/s00586-016-4478-4.
41. Müller M, Kuhn DF, Hinrichs B, et al. Is the elimination of osteosarcoma cells with intraoperative "mesh autotransfusion" and leukocyte depletion filters possible? Anaesthesist. 1996;45(9):834–8. Ist die Elimination von Osteosarkomzellen durch "maschinelle Autotransfusion" und Leukozyten-Depletionsfilter möglich? https://doi.org/10.1007/s001010050318.
42. Fu D, Zhao Y, Shen J, et al. Comparison of venous thromboembolism after Total artificial joint replacement between musculoskeletal tumors and osteoarthritis of the knee by a single surgeon. PLoS One. 2016;11(6):e0158215. https://doi.org/10.1371/journal.pone.0158215.
43. Ogura K, Yasunaga H, Horiguchi H, et al. Incidence and risk factors for pulmonary embolism after primary musculoskeletal tumor surgery. Clin Orthop Relat Res. 2013;471(10):3310–6. https://doi.org/10.1007/s11999-013-3073-9.

44. Yamaguchi T, Matsumine A, Niimi R, et al. Deep-vein thrombosis after resection of musculoskeletal tumours of the lower limb. Bone Joint J. 2013;95-b(9):1280–4. https://doi.org/10.1302/0301-620x.95b9.30905.
45. Lex JR, Evans S, Cool P, et al. Venous thromboembolism in orthopaedic oncology. Bone Joint J. 2020;102-b(12):1743–51. https://doi.org/10.1302/0301-620x.102b12.Bjj-2019-1136.R3.
46. Morii T, Mochizuki K, Tajima T, et al. Venous thromboembolism in the management of patients with musculoskeletal tumor. J Orthop Sci. 2010;15(6):810–5. https://doi.org/10.1007/s00776-010-1539-0.
47. Iwata S, Kawai A, Ueda T, Ishii T. Symptomatic Venous Thromboembolism in Patients with Malignant Bone and Soft Tissue Tumors: A Prospective Multicenter Cohort Study. Ann Surg Oncol. 2020; https://doi.org/10.1245/s10434-020-09308-6.
48. Congiusta DV, Amer KM, Thomson J, et al. Risk factors of venous thromboembolism in patients with benign and malignant musculoskeletal tumors: a dual database analysis. Int Orthop. 2020;44(10):2147–53. https://doi.org/10.1007/s00264-020-04707-6.
49. Patel AR, Crist MK, Nemitz J, Mayerson JL. Aspirin and compression devices versus low-molecular-weight heparin and PCD for VTE prophylaxis in orthopedic oncology patients. J Surg Oncol. 2010;102(3):276–81. https://doi.org/10.1002/jso.21603.
50. Tuy B, Bhate C, Beebe K, et al. IVC filters may prevent fatal pulmonary embolism in musculoskeletal tumor surgery. Clin Orthop Relat Res. 2009;467(1):239–45. https://doi.org/10.1007/s11999-008-0607-7.
51. Tang BQ, Guo W, Yang RL, et al. Evaluation of efficacy and safety of rivaroxaban in the prevention of postoperative venous thromboembolism in adult patients with primary bone tumor undergoing knee operation. Zhonghua Yi Xue Za Zhi. 2012;92(39):2768 71.
52. Cave J, Paschalis A, Huang CY, et al. A systematic review of the safety and efficacy of aerobic exercise during cytotoxic chemotherapy treatment. Support Care Cancer. 2018;26(10):3337–51. https://doi.org/10.1007/s00520-018-4295-x.
53. Schadler KL, Thomas NJ, Galie PA, et al. Tumor vessel normalization after aerobic exercise enhances chemotherapeutic efficacy. Oncotarget. 2016;7(40):65429–40. https://doi.org/10.18632/oncotarget.11748.
54. Lopez G, Chaoul A, Powers-James C, et al. Group yoga effects on cancer patient and caregiver symptom distress: assessment of self-reported symptoms at a Comprehensive Cancer Center. Integr Cancer Ther. 2018;17(4):1087–94. https://doi.org/10.1177/1534735418795301.
55. Zeng Y, Luo T, Xie H, et al. Health benefits of qigong or tai chi for cancer patients: a systematic review and meta-analyses. Complement Ther Med. 2014;22(1):173–86. https://doi.org/10.1016/j.ctim.2013.11.010.
56. Cormie P, Atkinson M, Bucci L, et al. Clinical oncology Society of Australia position statement on exercise in cancer care. Med J Aust. 2018;209(4):184–7. https://doi.org/10.5694/mja18.00199.
57. Hayes SC, Newton RU, Spence RR, Galvão DA. The exercise and sports science Australia position statement: exercise medicine in cancer management. J Sci Med Sport. 2019;22(11):1175–99. https://doi.org/10.1016/j.jsams.2019.05.003.
58. Mishra SI, Scherer RW, Snyder C, et al. Exercise interventions on health-related quality of life for people with cancer during active treatment. Cochrane Database Syst Rev. 2012;2012(8):Cd008465. https://doi.org/10.1002/14651858.CD008465.pub2.
59. Tsuda Y, Ogura K, Kobayashi E, et al. Impact of geriatric factors on surgical and prognostic outcomes in elderly patients with soft-tissue sarcoma. Jpn J Clin Oncol. 2017;47(5):422–9. https://doi.org/10.1093/jjco/hyx016.
60. Kiss N, Loeliger J, Findlay M, et al. Clinical oncology Society of Australia: position statement on cancer-related malnutrition and sarcopenia. Nutr Diet. 2020;77(4):416–25. https://doi.org/10.1111/1747-0080.12631.

MIX
Papier aus verantwortungsvollen Quellen
Paper from responsible sources
FSC® C105338

If you have any concerns about our products,
you can contact us on
ProductSafety@springernature.com

In case Publisher is established outside the EU,
the EU authorized representative is:
Springer Nature Customer Service Center GmbH
Europaplatz 3, 69115 Heidelberg, Germany

Printed by Libri Plureos GmbH
in Hamburg, Germany